# Child survival in developi

## Can demographic and health

## to understand the determinants?

Academisch proefschrift
ter verkrijging van de graad van doctor
aan de Universiteit van Amsterdam,
op gezag van de Rector Magnificus Prof. dr P.W.M. de Meijer,
ten overstaan van een door het college van dekanen ingestelde
commissie in het openbaar te verdedigen in de Aula der Universiteit
op maandag 6 mei 1996 te 15.00 uur

door
Jan Ties Boerma
geboren te Zaandam

## Promotiecommissie

| | |
|---|---|
| *Promotor* | Prof. dr A S Muller |
| *Co-promotor* | Dr J K S van Ginneken |
| | |
| *Leden* | Prof. dr G A M van den Bos, Prof. dr C Varkevisser, Prof. dr P J Willekens, Prof. dr J A Kusin, Dr G T Bicego, Prof. dr D J van de Kaa |
| | |
| *Faculteit* | Faculteit der Geneeskunde |

## Credits

Chapter 3 and 7 are reprinted from *DHS Methodological Reports*, no 2, 1994, pages 1-20 and pages 145-157, by permission of Demographic and Health Surveys, Macro International Inc., Calverton, MD, U.S.A.

Chapter 4 is reprinted by permission of Oxford University Press, from *International Journal of Epidemiology*, vol 20, no 4, pages 1073-1080

Chapter 5 is reprinted by permission of Union Internationale pour l'Etude Scientifique de la Population (UIESP), from the book *Measurement of Maternal and Child Mortality, Morbidity and Health Care*, Liège, 1993.

Chapter 8 is reprinted by permission of Population Association of America Inc., from *Demography*, vol 30, no 3, pages 459-475

Chapter 9 is reprinted with permission of the World Health Organization, from Bulletin of the World Health Organization, vol. 74, no. 2 in press.

Chapter 10 is reprinted with permission by The John Hopkins University School of Hygiene and Public Health, from *American Journal of Epidemiology*, Vol 135, No 4, pages 438-449.

Chapter 11 is reprinted with the permission of the Population Council, from *Studies in Family Planning*, vol. 23, no.4 (Jul/Aug 1992): 243-256.

Chapter 12 was reprinted from *Social Science and Medicine*, Vol 36, No 9, George T. Bicego and J. Ties Boerma, 'Maternal education and child survival: a comparative study of survey data from 17 countries', pages 1207-1227, 1993, with kind permission from Elsevier Science Ltd, The Boulevard, Langford Lane, Kidlington OX5 1GB, UK.

*Cover*: A sandstone statue of *Men Brayut*. *Men Brayut* is the heroine of a wellknown folktale from Bali, Indonesia. She is poor in money but rich in children; her statue is always accompanied one of *Pan Brayut*, her husband, who also carries nine children on his head, back and shoulders. Together they symbolize the happiness of family. Carved in Ubud, Bali, about 1935, by an unknown artist. (Collection Tropenmuseum -Amsterdam)

# Table of contents

# Acknowledgement

If a PhD is obtained 15 years after completing one's medical studies and 13 years after being awarded a Master's Degree in demography, the chances are that this acknowledgement will turn into a kind of *memoires*. I do feel, however, that the foundation for my PhD was laid in 1981 when I struggled towards the end of my medical studies. Clinical work was not as exciting as I had expected and I was searching for ways to satisfy my numerical and research interests. A small advertisement in the weekly newspaper of the University of Groningen drew my attention to a course in demography by Harrie van Vianen. The course fascinated me, but what was more important, Harrie turned out to be an inspiring lecturer who patiently broadened my medical perspective to include quantitative and social science perspectives during the following four years. Teachings by the late Bert van Norren also made a long-lasting impact on my scientific thinking. I was also fortunate to be able to carry out field work in Machakos, Kenya, during 1982, which became the basis for my first scientific publication and reinforced my desire to work in Africa.

With the biomedical and demographic training in my baggage I got a job as associate expert in a joint UNICEF/WHO assignment in 1984: first in the regional office for Eastern and Southern Africa, later in Coastal Kenya under the UNICEF Kenya programme. Again, I was fortunate to meet and work with very inspiring people. John Bennett and Mburu taught me how to conduct evaluations, conduct workshops and how to link research and interventions. Moreover, they gradually made me understand more about Africa and its peoples during the five years that we worked together in eight countries, from Somalia to Lesotho.

For the following four years I worked for the Demographic and Health Surveys programme (DHS). This PhD is mostly based on work done during those years. DHS is a well-oiled survey machine operated by mainly demographers and data processing experts with an amazingly high output level. Martin Vaessen recruited me to take part in this, but his flexible management style gave me the freedom to utilize my strengths and dual background as much as possible. I enjoyed being part of DHS and working with the staff. In particular, I benefited from my interactions with George Bicego – who never got tired of questioning what we were doing – and Elisabeth Sommerfelt – always working hard behind the scenes.

When I left DHS to join the TANESA project of the Royal Tropical Institute, Amsterdam, and moved to Mwanza, Tanzania, I did not have a clear plan of the thesis I was going to write on child survival and surveys. In fact, the initial plan was different, based on data from a longitudinal study of maternal and child health in coastal Kenya and I enjoyed the technical support of Stan Becker and Ron Gray. The plan, however, was not feasible, given the workload of the TANESA assignment. I therefore had to change the original plan, which has led to a less original but probably more interesting thesis. It was only through the flexibility and enduring support of Lex Muller and Jeroen van Ginneken that I finally managed to complete my thesis. They went through multiple drafts of the introduction and conclusions never losing sight of the overall context.

I am grateful to all the aforementioned individuals (and many others whom I did not mention) who made a major contribution to my scientific development, which has culminated in this thesis.

Financial aid is indispensable and I thank my parents for their patience during my prolonged studies, USAID for funding DHS, and the Royal Tropical Institute for funding this publication.

Psycho-social support came from my wife Francien and our three children, Marije, Pieter and Inge, to whom I am much indebted for keeping me away from work when necessary.

I

# Introduction

During the past four decades we have witnessed a substantial decline of infant and child mortality in developing countries (Hill and Pebley, 1989, Sullivan et al., 1994). This has been documented by data from censuses, demographic surveys and, to a much lesser extent, small-scale multi-round surveys or longitudinal studies. Surveys conducted in the context of large-scale programmes, such as the World Fertility Survey (WFS) and the Demographic and Health Surveys programme (DHS), have been the principal sources of data on child survival levels and trends during the past three decades.

Demographers have used the same survey data sources to increase our knowledge of child mortality differentials (Hobcraft et al., 1984, 1985, Cleland et al., 1992, Sullivan et al., 1994). Presently, a rich body of evidence is available on the existence of childhood mortality differentials by socioeconomic characteristics of the household or parents (e.g. mother's education) and biodemographic characteristics of the mother and child (e.g. birth intervals, birth order, sex of the child). The description of such mortality differentials is useful for the identification of special target groups for interventions and may enhance our understanding of the reasons for the infant and child mortality decline in developing countries.

Initially, the collection and analysis of child health data were not in the domain of demography. Most information on child health status, health practices and health services utilization originated from health interview surveys, health facility statistics, hospital-based studies and a few longitudinal epidemiological studies (e.g. on the interaction of malnutrition and infection). The WFS focused on the collection of data on fertility, family planning and child mortality during the 1970s, and only incidentally included health-related topics. Its successor, DHS, which fielded its first survey in 1985, expanded the goal of demographic surveys to include maternal and child health information. The main areas are antenatal and maternity care, child morbidity and treatment, immunization, breastfeeding, child anthropometry, and causes of death. This information was collected for all live births in the five years preceding the survey. In 10 years more than 50 nationally representative DHS surveys have been completed. Thus, currently, DHS is the leading source of maternal and child data in the world.

This thesis is an attempt to assess the contribution of cross-sectional surveys, notably DHS, to our understanding of the determinants of child survival in developing countries. Two basic issues will be addressed. The first relates to data quality and concerns the measurement of health variables in demographic surveys. To what extent can cross-sectional demographic surveys, primarily aimed at the collection of mortality and fertility data, become useful instruments for the collection of data on causes of death, morbidity, anthropometry, health services utilization, and feeding practices? The second is whether these data can actually enhance our understanding of the determinants of child survival in developing countries. For instance, can we, by including anthropometric and health services utilization data, understand why there is such a strong association between preceding birth intervals and infant mortality? Does the association between maternal education and the indicators of health services utilization help us explain why maternal education exerts such a clear effect on child survival?

To understand the determinants of child survival, we need to have a framework conceptualizing how we think they affect child survival. The Mosley-Chen framework for the study of child survival in developing countries was published in 1984 and has dominated child survival research during the last decade (Mosley and Chen, 1984). The framework is particularly suitable for cross-sectional surveys and has had a major influence on DHS. In Chapter 2 the Mosley-Chen framework is presented, and its advantages and limitations discussed.

The following ten chapters involve analyses of DHS data on various aspects related to the determinants of child survival in developing countries. The quality of health data in DHS surveys is considered in Chapters 3, 4 and 5. Chapter 3 synthesizes the results of a large evaluation of health data quality in the first 27 DHS surveys. Data quality is assessed for demographic aspects related to birth data, antenatal and maternity care, child vaccinations, child morbidity and treatment, breastfeeding and supplementary feeding patterns, child anthropometry and causes of death in childhood.

Morbidity reporting is one of the most problematic areas of health interview surveys. Chapter 4 analyzes the specific problems associated with the collection of data on childhood diarrhoea in DHS surveys.

An external validation of survey data on child health is done through a substantive comparison between the results of demographic surveys and longitudinal epidemiological studies (Chapter 5). Results are compared for child morbidity (diarrhoea, respiratory infections), vaccination, and neonatal tetanus mortality.

Chapters 6, 7 and 8 are concerned with collection of data on causes of death in surveys. A validation study of the verbal autopsy method to ascertain the probable cause of death in childhood was carried out in Namibia prior to the DHS survey (Chapter 6). The aims were to improve the questions in the subsequent DHS survey and to facilitate the interpretation of child mortality data generated by the main survey. Chapter 7 analyzes the results on causes of death obtained in seven DHS surveys through a verbal autopsy module. Tetanus is one of the leading causes of neonatal death in many developing countries. Chapter 8 shows how age-specific mortality data from DHS surveys can be used to assess the magnitude of this mortality.

Birthweight is also an important determinant of child survival. National data on the incidence of low birthweight are often limited to health facilities. Birthweight data from household surveys are also restricted to those who were weighed at birth, but there is even a greater disadvantage, because of an additional recall bias. Chapter 9 examines the usefulness of recalled data on the size of the child at birth for better estimates of the incidence of low birthweight.

Child anthropometric data have been collected from surviving children in most DHS surveys. Chapter 10 utilizes the availability of both mortality and anthropometric data in the same anthropometric survey to assess the potential impact of a survivor bias on estimates of undernutrition.

Child spacing and maternal education are two of the most important determinants of child survival in developing countries. Chapter 11 presents a comparative analysis of 17 DHS countries using the Mosley-Chen conceptual framework in an attempt to assess why the preceding birth interval has such a strong effect on child survival. The same approach is employed to study the link between mother's education and child survival (Chapter 12).

Finally, the contribution of DHS and other surveys to our understanding of the determinants of child survival in developing countries is reviewed (Chapter 13). Specific suggestions are made to accommodate more qualitative approaches in the context of cross-sectional surveys.

## References

Cleland J, Bicego G, Fegan G (1992). Socioeconomic inequalities in childhood mortality: the 1970s to the 1980s. *Health Transition Review* 2: 1-18.

Hill KH and Pebley AR (1989). Child mortality in the developing world. *Population and Development Review* 15: 657-687.

Hobcraft J, McDonald JW and Rutstein SO (1985). Demographic determinants of infant and early child mortality: a comparative analysis. *Population Studies* 39: 363-385.

Hobcraft J, McDonald JW and Rutstein SO (1984). Socioeconomic factors in infant and child mortality: a cross-national comparison. *Population Studies* 38: 193-223.

Mosley WH and Chen LC (1984). An analytical framework for the study of child survival in developing countries. In Mosley WH and Chen LC (eds.). Child survival; strategies for research. *Population and Development Review* 10 (suppl): 25-45.

Sullivan JM, Rutstein SO and Bicego GT (1994). Infant and child mortality. *DHS Comparative Studies* No. 15. Calverton, Maryland: Macro International Inc.

**2**

# Understanding the determinants of child survival in developing countries:

# the Mosley-Chen conceptual framework

## Introduction

To study the determinants of child survival, a conceptualization is required which links them through behavioural and eventually biological mechanisms to survival. About ten years ago, Mosley and Chen (1984) proposed a conceptual framework for the study of the determinants of child survival in developing countries, incorporating both social and biological variables and aiming to integrate research methods from demography and epidemiology. During the decade following its publication, attempts have been made to improve and operationalize the framework. It has been used in a range of longitudinal and cross-sectional studies of child survival in developing countries. In particular, demographers have made efforts to collect more information on the processes linking underlying determinants and child survival. The Mosley-Chen framework has greatly influenced the formulation of the health questions in the core questionnaires of the largest global survey programme, the Demographic and Health Survey (DHS).

This chapter describes the basic features of the Mosley-Chen framework and its relevance to the study of child survival in developing countries.

## Conceptual framework

The two main disciplines concerned with the population-based study of child survival are demography and epidemiology. Demographers and epidemiologists have different approaches with regard to study methodology, interpretation of mortality data, and design of health interventions (Mosley and Chen, 1984, Gray, 1989). Epidemiological research primarily focuses on specific diseases and often pays limited attention to underlying socioeconomic and other characteristics. Demographic research is predominantly concerned with the association between socioeconomic and biodemographic background characteristics and child survival, and pays less attention to the behavioural

**Figure 1** Operation of the five groups of proximate determinants on the health dynamics of a population

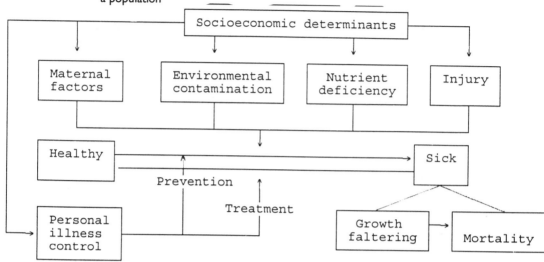

and biological processes leading to death. The purpose of developing a conceptual framework for the study of child survival was primarily to facilitate and promote inter-disciplinary communication and to lay the theoretical groundwork for further investigation.' (Mosley, 1984). The basic feature of the Mosley-Chen framework is the specification of a set of proximate or intermediate determinants which directly link the influence to the risk of morbidity and mortality in children[2] (see Figure 1). All social and economic determinants must operate through the proximate determinants to affect child survival. The framework redefines causes of death to emphasize the social dimension. Diseases and malnutrition are no longer causes of death, but are considered a consequence of interaction between the social and biological systems. As such, a specific disease state of an individual is a marker of the operation of the proximate determinants.

The proximate variables are specified as maternal factors (age of childbearing, parity, birth interval, which are affected by reproductive practices); environmental contamination with infectious agents (contamination of air, water and food, skin and soil, and insect vectors, which is influenced by hygienic practices); availability of nutrients to the fetus and infant (calories, protein, micro-nutrients, affected by feeding practices); injuries (accidents and intentional injury, which are affected by care); and personal disease control factors (personal preventive measures, medical treatment). Socio-economic determinants, such as mother's education and household income, operate through the proximate determinants to influence child growth and mortality.

During the past decade the Mosley-Chen conceptual framework has been shown to be very useful in the study of the determinants of child survival in developing countries. Demographers have made extensive use of the conceptual framework and health data collection has become part and parcel of many demographic studies. In epidemiology, much less use has been made of the framework, as, for instance, evidenced by the limited number of publications referring to the framework in epidemiological journals. However, like any attempt to conceptualize real life, the Mosley- Chen framework has its limitations, which are discussed below.

## Oversimplification

Most criticisms on the proximate determinant framework originate from demographers with an anthropological orientation. Caldwell and Hill (1988) have argued that proximate determinant frameworks, while advancing our knowledge on a small set of factors affecting fertility or mortality, lead to pre-occupation with the effects of single determinants of the demographic outcome at the cost of the search for the more complex, influence of 'remote determinants'. Also, they are uni-directional, deterministic frameworks, which favour the use of cross-sectional surveys as the main instrument of data collection. Such a simplification facilitates the interpretation and use of the framework by researchers from different disciplines and by policy makers, but is not conducive to considering complicated effects involving feedback. Proximate determinant frameworks are more likely to lead to research focusing on individual level decision-making rather than broader society processes with its complex web of factors influencing behaviour (Ewbank, 1994) or analyses at other levels such as family, community, etc. Caldwell and Hill argued that more can be gained using micro-level approaches research in demography, with a strong qualitative component.

These concerns present important caveats for users of the proximate determinant framework for child survival. The basic structure of Mosley and Chen should, however, continue to guide the study of the determinants of child survival, because it can be used by different disciplines and helps to integrate information from the biomedical and social sciences. An example of a such a study focusing on the 'remote' or underlying determinants of child survival using a micro-approach and the proximate determinant framework was conducted in India by Das Gupta (1990). The basic abilities and personality characteristics of the mother were considered an important individual level determinant, independently of education and economic indicators. Although the analysis shows that education increases maternal skills, the main conclusion of this study is that the two should not be equated. Das Gupta suggested that the personal ability of the caretaker be added to the Mosley-Chen framework as an underlying determinant.

## Specification of proximate determinants

Bert van Norren, an anthropologist, improved the conceptual clarity of the Mosley-Chen framework by a better specification of the proximate determinants (Van Norren and Van Vianen, 1986). He argued that, in analogy with work by Davis and Blake (1956) on fertility determinants, the proximate determinants (or 'truly intermediate' variables) have to be both biological and behavioural. In the original Mosley-Chen framework the proximate determinants are either biological or behavioural or both. In Van Norren's framework, all of them are both behavioural and biological and directly affect a set of four biological risk factors: physical constitution at birth, nutritional intake, exposure to infectious agents and susceptibility to infections (Figure 2). These risk factors have biological effects on the probability of occurrence of malnutrition-infections. The set of proximate determinants, which focused on priority child survival interventions, included 13 variables, mostly health-related practices of the child's caretaker. Van Norren's framework can thus be used for the evaluation of contemporary primary health care programmes (Van Norren et al., 1989).

To be able to assist in the analysis of empirical data, the concepts have to be translated into measurable indicators. One problem involves the measurement of the extent of the effects of the biological risk factors, as specified by Van Norren. Existing data are only partially adequate to quantify these effects on child health and nutritional status (frailty) and on mortality in different settings. Thus, while Van Norren's specification of the proximate determinants was a theoretical improvement, it does not appear to further our attempts to understand the determinants of child survival in developing countries, or to bring us closer to being able to quantify the effects of health interventions on child survival.

## Quality of care and proximate determinants

Most of the proximate determinants have a quality dimension which is not well expressed in the Mosley-Chen conceptual framework. Variation in the quality of care weakens the relationships between the proximate determinants and child health/survival, and thus undermines the ability to disentangle causal pathways through which underlying socioeconomic determinants affect child mortality. Some aspects of quality of care are under the control of the caretakers, others are clearly outside their control. For instance, in Bangladesh the risk of neonatal tetanus was not reduced by a maternal history of two doses of tetanus toxoid (Hlady et al., 1992). Low vaccine potency was found to be the cause for the lack of an effect, a factor clearly outside the control of the caretakers. Evaluations of diarrhoea treatment practices in health facilities in eight African countries showed suboptimal compliance with diagnostic and treatment standards established by the WHO (Foster, 1993). Generally, too little attention has been paid to the quality of care as opposed to the coverage of care. Methods have been designed to measure the quality of primary health care and to assist managers to institute and moni-

**Figure 2** A model of the malnutrition-infections syndrome and its demographic outcome in terms of the categories: risk factors, intermediate variables and household characteristics

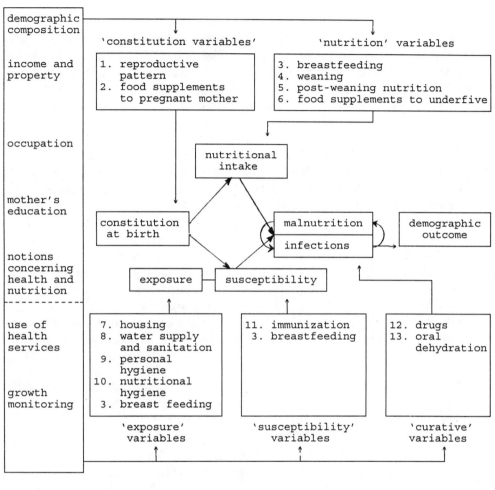

Legenda: ——→ effect
——— connection

tor a quality improvement process (Newman et al., 1992). These include exit surveys at health facilities, use of observational techniques and simulated cases. Cross-sectional surveys are less useful instruments to measure the quality of health care, and linking survey results with health facility or other data for the purpose of explanatory analysis is very difficult. Similarly, the quality of care given by the caretakers at home is difficult to evaluate and not clearly specified in the framework.

## Road-to-death concept

An important feature of the conceptual framework is that '.. Growth faltering and ulti-mately mortality in children (the dependent variable) are the cumulative consequences of multiple disease processes (including their biosocial interactions). Only infrequently is a child's death the result of a single isolated disease episode' (Mosley and Chen, p.27). In other words, it assumes the existence of a 'road-to-death' for the majority of deaths, which was later elaborated in statistical terms (labelled frailty) by Mosley and Becker (1991). The child's anthropometric status is considered a useful indicator of the 'road to death', is relatively easy to measure, and is probably the best single indicator of individual mortality risk. Indeed, mortality risks are greatly increased for children with severe protein energy malnutrition (PEM), but also, to a lesser extent, for children with mild to moderate PEM (Pelletier, 1991). The latter group of children is much larger than those with severe malnutrition, so that the contribution of mild/moderate PEM to the overall mortality is greater. In addition, the majority of children who die do not have anthropometric deficits. Pelletier concluded from 15 studies that an estimated 25-50% of child deaths are statistically attributable to anthropometric deficits. This sug-gests that the majority of children die without growth faltering (PEM) and that only a minority of children follow the anthropometric 'road-to-death'. The innovative work on measles mortality by Peter Aaby (1989) also presents a challenge to the anthro-pometric dimension of 'road-to-death' concept. Case fatality was greatly increased among children secondarily infected with measles virus in the household compared with children who brought the infection into the household, presumably due to the in-fectious dose. This elevated mortality risk was independent of nutritional status prior to the measles episode.

A second argument weakening the 'road-to-death' assumption follows from an analysis of age-specific mortality data. The assumption is probably least correct for children 1-5 months of age. During this period mortality is high (often 20-25% of all under five deaths), nutritional status is better than later in infancy and early childhood, and condi-tions with established effects on children's nutritional and health status (measles, vita-min A deficiency, diarrhoea) are much less common than at later ages. Some of these children may be more frail because of prenatal influences, but the most severely af-fected cases will already have died during the critical perinatal and neonatal periods. It is, therefore, likely that the high case fatality due to single disease episodes is even more important during this age interval. At other ages, this may also be the case, but less prominently so.

## Age specificity

The age factor is not explicit in the conceptual framework, yet it is one of the most im-portant variables affecting the level of mortality (rapid decrease with age). All biomedi-cal causes of death have explicit age patterns of mortality, which can partly be explained by immunology (e.g. maternal antibodies, building of child's own immunity) and exposure to infectious agents. The incidence and case fatality of diseases such as neonatal tetanus, rotavirus diarrhoea, whooping cough, measles, etc. vary with age. Accordingly, the relative importance of proximate determinants will vary considerably with age. As examples, maternal factors and maternity care have their largest effect during the first month of life, water quality becomes more important as exclusive breast-feeding ends, and measles immunization can only improve survival chances from the age of vaccination. Finally, the underlying determinants may also have age-specific influences on mortality, which may help us understand causal mechanisms. Examples of analyses using age in its conceptual framework are presented by Barnum and Barlow (1984) and Bicego and Boerma (1993). Different proximate determinant frameworks can be used for neonatal, postneonatal and child mortality.

## Endogeneity

From conceptual and statistical perspectives, proximate determinant conceptual frameworks may be misleading because of endogeneity (Cebu Study Team, 1991, Trussell and Menken, 1984). Exogenous variables are those determined by forces outside the model, and endogenous variables are those specified within the model as the effects of variables included in the model. Endogenous variables are thus affected by choice. A problem occurs when choice variables appear as explanatory variables in the analysis. For instance, an analysis of the effects of delivery care on infant mortality may show a higher neonatal mortality for hospital births. It should, however, be taken into account that mothers may be more likely to use health services if they consider their child at risk or if they have been advised to do so by the health worker because of possible complications. To solve this problem, information on these choices (was advice given to deliver in a hospital? were there complications during the pregnancy?) needs to be available. Statistical solutions to this problem have also been proposed (Cebu Study Team, 1991, Trussell and Menken, 1984).

## Quantification: towards a statistical model

The proximate determinant framework of fertility was successfully translated into a statistical model by Bongaarts (Bongaarts and Potter, 1983). A quantification of the effects of the proximate determinants on child health (malnutrition and infections) and its demographic outcome may be crucial to further our understanding of the determinants of child survival and to design more effective health programmes. Mosley and Becker (1991) developed an analytical model based on the Mosley-Chen framework to demonstrate how multiple disease conditions interact through the mechanisms of competing risks and acquired frailty, resulting in high childhood mortality. Children in high-risk settings experience multiple bouts of infections in short periods of time, and survival following a disease-specific intervention can be smaller than expected because of competing risks. Furthermore, morbidity associated with most childhood diseases may increase the child's frailty, i.e. greater susceptibility to die from the next illness episode. The model focuses on the interaction between disease states and malnutrition and its demographic outcome. The Mosley-Becker model requires measurable indicators at the population level of the operation of acquired frailty to produce mortality differentials. Birthweight, anthropometric status and vitamin A levels were proposed as useful indicators of frailty. The results of their analysis clearly challenged the current emphasis in child survival programmes on single-disease life-saving interventions. Modest simultaneous reductions in multiple risk factors (e.g. low birth weight, parasitic infections) were shown to have had a more beneficial effect on frailty and child survival.

Attempts to explain the substantial and prolonged infant and child mortality decline in developing countries have had only limited success, particularly regarding the role of health programmes (Ewbank and Gribble, 1993, Chen et al., 1993, Hill and Pebley, 1989). The Mosley-Becker model suggests that relatively small improvements in nutrition and hygiene can result in substantial mortality reductions, if they occur simultaneously. If such minor improvements can be brought about by modest social and economic development or by health programmes, this could be an explanation for the decline.

Mosley and Becker acknowledge the importance of heterogeneity in exposure to risk (e.g. male versus female children, children of uneducated mothers versus children of educated mothers). Their statistical model, however, does not fully take into account the social dimension of child survival and how the social system interacts with the biological system through the proximate determinants. It focuses on the biological aspects, and neglects the underlying and proximate determinants of child survival. The latter may not only affect the number of health 'insults', but also the consequences of an insult for frailty. For instance, the child of an educated mother may recover completely from an episode of diarrhoea because of appropriate feeding during the convalescence period, while it takes a child of an uneducated mother much longer to recover because no special efforts were made (if recovery is ever achieved).

The parameters in the model are highly dependent upon the inputs and assumptions. For a number of key parameters, notably the proportion of children becoming more frail with a given disease, no data are available (Black and Becker, 1994). Thus, while UNICEF's estimates of numbers of children's lives saved by immunization or diarrhoeal disease control may be biased by accepting a single cause of death concept or ignoring frailty, the Mosley-Becker analysis may suffer from overemphasizing the importance of frailty for child survival. It appears the strongest support for the validity of the model is derived from studies describing the mortality impact of measles immunization (Koenig et al., 1990) and vitamin A (Beaton et al., 1992). Interventions had a much larger mortality-reducing effect than expected on the basis of simply counting directly attributed death. The enhanced mortality impact could be explained by the presumably large effect of measles and vitamin A deficiency on frailty among survivors.

The development of a model including all possible interventions to assess health impact or to study the determinants of child survival is not considered feasible (Mosley and Becker, 1991). Perhaps the best example of a comprehensive study using a longitudinal data set to assess the underlying and proximate determinants of child health is the Cebu longitudinal health and nutrition study (Cebu Study Team, 1991). This study includes indicators of all levels of the Mosley-Chen framework, and illustrates this with an analysis of the effects of maternal education on child diarrhoea incidence. They show how a one-year increase in education reduces the probability of exclusive breastfeeding (reduction 36%) or of any breastfeeding (-5%), but improves caloric intake (+7%), use of preventive health services (+4%), and excreta disposal (+9%), and increases soap use (+2%). The net effect of a one-year increase in maternal education would be to reduce the incidence of diarrhoea by 5% due to better feeding practices (more calories), improved use of preventive health services, and better excreta disposal, in part offset by a reduction in the number of mothers who breastfed. Clearly, such detailed studies require high quality data on a large number of variables, which can only be collected in prospective studies.

## Conclusion

The Mosley-Chen conceptual framework has been shown to be very useful in the study of the determinants of child survival in developing countries. It has facilitated interdisciplinary communication between the two main disciplines involved (demography and epidemiology), but could also be used to integrate information collected by social scientists using qualitative methods. The framework has greatly influenced the development of health data collection and analysis in demographic surveys, such as DHS.

A number of limitations of the conceptual framework have been pointed out, and should be taken into account when using it. At present, there is no good alternative to the Mosley-Chen proximate determinant framework, which could be used by different disciplines studying the determinants of child survival. Perhaps the greatest challenge is to incorporate the complex social dimension of health further into the framework.

Using this framework, the contribution of cross-sectional demographic surveys in enhancing our knowledge of the determinants of child survival is assessed in the following chapters.

## Notes

1 A conceptual or analytical framework can be defined as a systematic construction of a set of statements about determinants and causal mechanisms affecting the phenomenon of interest (Palloni, 1987, Duchene and Wunsch, 1989). A conceptual framework is the product of accumulated knowledge in one or more areas of study. It is a way of structuring reality according to assumptions

and depends on theory or at least hypotheses about relations between phenomena. Frameworks may lead to the formulation of statistical models for the testing of hypotheses.

2   Such a proximate determinant framework has been successful in clarifying the determinants of fertility in developing countries (Bongaarts and Potter, 1983). This framework assumes a biological maximum fecundity level, which is reduced through the fertility-inhibiting effects of proximate determinants (not-marrying, contraceptive use, pregnancy loss, lactational infecundity, and pathological sterility). The effect of each proximate determinant on the demographic outcome has been quantified in a statistical model to successfully explain variation in fertility between populations and population sub-groups.

## References

Aaby P (1989). Malnourished or overinfected. An analysis of the determinants of acute measles mortality. *Danish Medical Bulletin* 36: 93-113

Barnum HN and Barlow R (1984). Modelling resource allocation for child survival. In: Mosley WH and Chen LC (eds.). Child survival; strategies for research. *Population and Development Review* suppl to vol 10: 367-387.

Beaton GH, Martorell R, L'Abbe KA et al. (1992). Effectiveness of Vitamin A supplementation in the control of young child morbidity and mortality in developing countries. International Nutrition Program. University of Toronto.

Bicego GT and Boerma JT (1993). Maternal education and child survival: a comparative study of survey dat from 17 countries. Social Science and Medicine 36: 1207-1277.

Black RE and Becker S (1994). Potential effect on child mortality of interventions for control of diarrheal diseases. In: Rashad H, Gray RH and Boerma JT (eds.). *Evaluation of the health impact of interventions.* Liege: Ordina Editions for IUSSP.

Bongaarts J and Potter JE (1983). *Fertility, biology and behavior.* New York: Academic Press.

Caldwell JC and Hill AG (1988). Recent developments using micro-approaches to demographic research: introduction. In: Caldwell JC, Hill AG, Hull VJ (eds.). *Micro-approaches to demographic research.* London: Kegan Paul International, pp. 1-9.

Cebu Study Team (1991). Underlying and proximate determinants of child health: the Cebu longitudinal health and nutrition study. *American Journal of Epidemiology* 133: 185-201.

Chen LC, Hill AG, Murray CJL et al. (1993). A critical analysis of the design, results and implications of the mortality and use of health services surveys. *International Journal of Epidemiology* 22 Suppl 1: S73-S80.

Das Gupta M (1990). Death clustering, mother's education and the determinants of child mortality in rural Punjab. *Population Studies* 44: 489-505.

Davis K and Blake J (1956). Social structure and fertility: an analytic framework. *Economic Development & Cultural Change* 4: 211-235.

Duchene J and Wunsch G (1989). Conceptual frameworks and causal modelling. In: Ruzicka L, Wunsch G and Kane P (eds.). *Differential mortality: methodological issues and biosocial factors.* Oxford: Clarendon Press, pp. 21-35.

Ewbank DC (1994). Maternal education and theories of health behaviour: a cautionary note. *Health Transition Review* 4: 214-223.

Ewbank DC and Gribble JN (1993). Effects of health programs on child mortality in sub-Saharan Africa. National Academy Press. 1993.

Foster SO (1993). Monitoring child survival programmes in Africa: the Child Survival Initiative -Background. *International Journal of Epidemiology* 22 Supplement 1: S2-S7.

Gray RH (1989). The integration of demographic and epidemiologic approaches to studies of health in developing countries. In: Ruzicka L, Wunsch G and Kane P (eds.). *Differential mortality: methodological issues and biosocial factors.* Oxford: Clarendon Press, pp. 36-63.

Hill KH and Pebley AR (1989). Child mortality in the developing world. *Population and Development Review* 15: 657-687.

Hlady WG, Bennett JV, Samadi AR et al. (1992). Neonatal tetanus in rural Bangladesh: risk factors and toxoid efficacy. *American Journal of Public Health* 82: 1365-1369.

Koenig MA, Khan MA, Wojtyniak B et al. (1990). Impact of measles vaccination on childhood mortality n rural Bangladesh. *Bulletin of the WHO* 68: 441-447.

Mosley WH (1984). Child survival: research and policy. In Mosley WH and Chen LC (eds.). Child survival; strategies for research. *Population and Development Review* 10 (suppl): 3-23.

Mosley WH and Becker S (1991). Demographic models for child survival and implications for health intervention programmes. *Health Policy and Planning* 6: 218-233.

Mosley WH and Chen LC (1984). An analytical framework for the study of child survival in developing countries. In Mosley WH and Chen LC (eds.). Child survival; strategies for research. *Population and Development Review* 10 (suppl): 25-45.

Newman JS, Hatzell TA, Blumenfeld SN et al. (1992). Assessing the quality of health services. In: Boerma JT (editor): *Measurement issues in maternal and child mortality, morbidity and health care: interdisciplinary approaches.* IUSSP, Derouaux-Ordina Editions, Liege: pp. 387-407.

Palloni (1997). Theory, analytical frameworks and causal approach in the study of mortality at younger ages in developing countries. *Annales de la Société belge de Médecins tropicale* 67 (suppl): 31-45.

Pelletier DL (1991). Relationships between child anthropometry and mortality in developing countries. Cornell Food and Nutrition Policy Program, Monograph 12.

Trussell J and Menken J (1984). Estimating levels, trends and determinants of child mortality in countries with poor statistics. In Mosley WH and Chen LC (eds.). Child survival; strategies for research. *Population and Development Review* 10 (suppl): 325-346.

Van Norren B and Van Vianen HAW (1986). The malnutrition-infections syndrome and its demographic outcome in developing countries. PCDO/Programming Committee for Demographic Research publication no.4, the Hague.

Van Norren B, Boerma JT and Sempebwa EKN (1989). Simplifying the evaluation of primary health care programmes. *Social Science & Medicine* 28: 1091-1097.

3

# Assessment of the quality of health data in DHS-I surveys: an overview

*J. Ties Boerma, A. Elisabeth Sommerfelt, Jeroen K. van Ginneken, George T. Bicego, M. Kathryn Stewart, Shea O. Rutstein*

**DHS Methodological Reports** *no. 2, Macro International Inc., Calverton, Maryland, USA, 1994, pp. 1—20.*

## Introduction

Collection of health data through large-scale cross-national survey programs is a relatively new area. During the 1970s, the World Fertility Survey (WFS) was the main instrument through which extensive experience was gained in the collection of data on fertility, family planning, and mortality. Its successor, the Demographic and Health Surveys (DHS), built upon that experience, and also expanded the goals of the surveys to include health data.

Until the beginning of the 1980s the experience with health interview surveys in developing countries was relatively limited. Except for the United Nations-supported Household Survey Capability Programme, which included information on health-related issues, most of the data on health status and health care utilization was collected through the health services or in small-scale epidemiological studies. An important development was initiated by the Expanded Programme on Immunization (EPI) division of the World Health Organization (WHO). EPI developed a simple and reliable sampling technique for the collection of child immunization coverage data, which made immunization coverage surveys the most popular type of survey during the 1980s. The sampling technique was also used to collect other data, such as neonatal tetanus mortality (Galazka and Stroh, 1986) and diarrhoea case management (WHO, 1986), and further applications are being investigated (Anker, 1991).

Several authors (Kroeger, 1983, Ross and Vaughan, 1986) have pointed to the weaknesses of health interview surveys. The most difficult area is the collection of data on morbidity, which is subject to a reporting bias. Because health and illness are subjective matters, the magnitude of the reporting bias often is very difficult to evaluate. The measurement of health services utilization is also affected by various reporting biases. For example, the use of health services for diarrhoea depends on the reporting of diarrhoea; some respondents only report severe cases, whereas others include even the mildest cases. Reporting may also differ for deceased and living children or for births longer ago and more recent.

During Phase I of DHS (DHS-I 1984–1989), questions to measure health and health care utilization, based on the existing knowledge, were developed. There were four main areas: antenatal and maternity care, immunization, child morbidity and treatment, and breastfeeding. Child anthropometry was included in most surveys and the causes of death in early childhood were optional.

This overview briefly deals with the quality of the health data in the DHS-I surveys; a more detailed assessment can be found in the specific papers cited. Subsequent sections include an outline of the materials and methods used in assessing the quality of the health data and some of the most important findings for each of the health-related topics. Where applicable, the sections end with a summary of the changes made in the DHS-II core questionnaire.

## Data and methods

The DHS project assists developing countries in the organization of nationally representative surveys, which provide information for policy and program decisionmaking and for scientific research. Survey data include information on fertility and childhood mortality levels, use of family planning, and various maternal and child health indicators. Table 1 provides a summary of the DHS-I surveys, including date of fieldwork, sample size (number of women and number of children under five), and health modules used.

The quality of the health data is assessed for the following areas:

- Demographic aspects related to birth data
- Antenatal and maternity care
- Child vaccinations
- Child morbidity and treatment (diarrhoea, respiratory infections)
- Breastfeeding and supplementary feeding patterns
- Child anthropometry
- Causes of death in childhood.

The methods to evaluate the quality of data vary by topic, but generally include the following:

- Frequencies of missing values and 'don't know' responses, and the proportion of responses in 'other' categories;
- Occurrence of digit preference for duration questions, dating of events, and anthropometry;

- Prevalence of inconsistencies between different parts of the health section or between the health section and birth history;
- Quality of data for deceased children compared to data on living children;
- Quality of data if the mother has to report on more than one child in the last five years; and
- Comparison of DHS results with external sources.

## Demographic aspects of the quality of birth data in the last five years

In the DHS surveys, the questions related to health are embedded in a relatively long questionnaire that also includes fertility, family planning, and background characteristics of the respondent. Health data are collected for all children born in the five-year period preceding the survey. The basis for the selection of these births is the birth history, whereby information on birth dates, age, and survival status is collected. All age-specific analysis of health data uses the information from the birth history. The quality of the birth history data, therefore, affects the quality of the health data. Bicego and Boerma (1994) assessed the quality of various aspects of the birth history; their main findings are summarized below.

### Response rates
Response rates, which can be dissected into the levels of household, individual (woman), and health section, were evaluated first. Once a household has been identified in the field, and the household members have been listed, the interviewer ascertains those women who will be eligible for the individual interview (i.e., those women 15–49 years who slept in the household the night before the survey). The individual questionnaire includes a complete birth history, which is administered to each eligible woman. Based on dates of birth, the interviewer identifies those children born since a specific cutoff date, usually 1 January of the fifth year preceding the year of the survey. These children represent the target population for which maternity care data and part of the feeding pattern data are collected (the remaining health information collected is limited to the subsample of living children). Response rates were on average above 95 percent for each of the three sections. Eight surveys had an overall response rate, defined as the product of the three response rates, below 90 percent. This value represents the theoretical percentage of children in the target sample of households for whom health data were collected.

### Completeness and quality of data on birth date and age
The completeness and quality of data on birth date and age are important for two reasons: age data are used in the analysis of health data, and the age of the child is a criterion of inclusion in the health section. Arnold (1990) presented evidence of a bias in age reporting related to the latter: some birth dates were pushed back a year or two so that the health section could be skipped for these children. Indeed, several DHS surveys

Table I    Summary of DHS-I surveys: date of fieldwork, sample sizes (women and children under five), and health modules, demographic and health surveys, 1985–1990

| Country | Date of fieldwork | | Number of women | Children born in last 5 years | | Health modules | |
| --- | --- | --- | --- | --- | --- | --- | --- |
| | | | | Living | Dead | Child anthropometry | Causes of death |
| **Sub-Saharan Africa** | | | | | | | |
| Botswana | Aug–Dec | 1988 | 4368 | 3068 | 146 | | |
| Burundi | Apr–Jul | 1987 | 3970 | 3502 | 385 | x | |
| Ghana | Feb–May | 1988 | 4488 | 3690 | 446 | x | |
| Kenya | Dec–May | 1988/89 | 7150 | 6593 | 539 | | |
| Liberia[1] | Feb–Jul | 1986 | 5239 | 4307 | 873 | | |
| Mali | Mar–Aug | 1987 | 3200 | 2904 | 537 | x | |
| Ondo State, Nigeria | Sep–Jan | 1986/87 | 4213 | 3018 | 264 | x | |
| Senegal | Apr–Jul | 1986 | 4415 | 3708 | 579 | x | x |
| Togo | Jun–Nov | 1988 | 3360 | 2803 | 331 | x | |
| Uganda | Sep–Feb | 1988/89 | 4730 | 4373 | 676 | x | |
| Zimbabwe | Sep–Jan | 1988/89 | 4201 | 3164 | 194 | x | |
| **North Africa** | | | | | | | |
| Egypt | Oct–Jan | 1988/89 | 8911 | 8009 | 723 | x | x |
| Morocco | May–Jul | 1987 | 5982 | 5602 | 500 | x | x |
| Sudan | Nov–May | 1989/90 | 5960 | 6062 | 582 | | |
| Tunisia | Jun–Oct | 1988 | 4184 | 4250 | 227 | x | x |
| **Asia** | | | | | | | |
| Indonesia | Sep–Dec | 1987 | 11884 | 7592 | 650 | | |
| Sri Lanka | Jan–Mar | 1987 | 5864 | 3877 | 104 | x | |
| Thailand | Mar–Jun | 1987 | 6775 | 3519 | 132 | x | |
| **Latin America/Caribbean** | | | | | | | |
| Bolivia | Mar–Jun | 1989 | 7923 | 5208 | 585 | x | x |
| Brazil | May–Aug | 1986 | 5892 | 3224 | 257 | x | |
| Colombia | Oct–Dec | 1986 | 5329 | 2615 | 87 | x | |
| Dominican Republic | Sep–Dec | 1986 | 7649 | 4106 | 337 | x | |
| Ecuador | Jan–Mar | 1987 | 4713 | 2849 | 202 | | x |
| El Salvador | May–Jun | 1985 | 5207 | 3234 | 256 | | |
| Guatemala | Oct–Dec | 1987 | 5160 | 4230 | 397 | x | |
| Mexico | Feb–May | 1987 | 9310 | 5368 | 312 | | |
| Peru | Sep–Dec | 1986 | 4999 | 2836 | 295 | | |
| Trinidad & Tobago | May–Aug | 1987 | 3806 | 1889 | 59 | x | |

1. Last births only in five years preceding the survey.

have a deficit of births five years before the survey, but an excess six years before. There is little or no evidence of displacement in the surveys in Asia, Latin America, and the Caribbean, with the exception of Guatemala and, to a lesser extent, Bolivia and Trinidad and Tobago. In Guatemala, the number of births five years before the survey is 16 percent less than expected compared to years four and six before the survey. The North African surveys also show some indication of displacement and in several countries of Sub-Saharan Africa the problem of displacement is most severe. Three surveys, Kenya, Liberia, and Ondo State (Nigeria), are especially problematic; the expected number of births at five years before the survey falls short by at least 20 percent compared to the numbers of births in the surrounding years. Ghana is the only African country without evidence of displacement, and Uganda and Zimbabwe have very little displacement.

Virtually all analyses of child health data are undertaken using age groupings. It has been noted that birth dates can be intentionally manipulated, but it is also the case in developing countries that the reporting of birth dates and ages is inherently fraught with uncertainty and imprecision. The current age of a child is most precisely defined when a complete birth date (both month and year) is provided by the mother in the birth history. It becomes less well defined when only the year of birth is reported or when a year of birth and a current age (in years) is given. Several points emerge from an analysis of the incompleteness of birth date information:

- The overall level of incompleteness of birth date information varies widely (see Figure 1). Generally, incompleteness is highest in Sub-Saharan Africa and North Africa and lowest in Latin America. Incompleteness in Mali is especially problematic, with nearly half the children lacking complete birthdate information. Three countries (Morocco, Sudan, and Togo) have 20- to 30 percent incompleteness and three others (Egypt, Ghana, and Liberia) have 10- to 20 percent incompleteness for all births in the last five years. Nevertheless, the average for all 27 countries is a surprisingly low 3.5 percent.
- Children no longer alive are, on average, more than four times more likely than surviving children to lack a completely reported birth date. This pattern is particularly pronounced where overall incompleteness is low (i.e., Latin America), but is exhibited in nearly all countries.
- There exists a tendency for the precision of birth date reporting to diminish with increasing age of the child. For example, the birth dates of children born four completed years before the survey are six times more likely to be imprecisely reported than those of children born in the year of the survey.

Becker (1984) has suggested that there is a tendency to misplace the month of birth of young children in birth histories. Using data from four WFS surveys he found overreporting of the month of birth for the survey month and the months immediately preceding it and underreporting of births following the survey month. For example, if the interview was held in August 1992 and the child was born in September 1990, but the respondent cannot recall the month exactly, then the child is likely to be reported as born in July 1990, which implies that the child's age is overreported by two months. Becker suggested it might be easier for the respondent (or interviewer) to recall the names of the months that have just passed than those still to come. Data from 28 DHS-I surveys showed a birth peak in the first month before the interview and in the second and third month before the survey the numbers of births are also higher than expected. There is a shortage of births in the months following the survey months and, contrary to Becker's observations, in the month of interview.

Figure I Incomplete birth date information among births in the last 5 years, Demographic and Health Surveys, 1985–1990

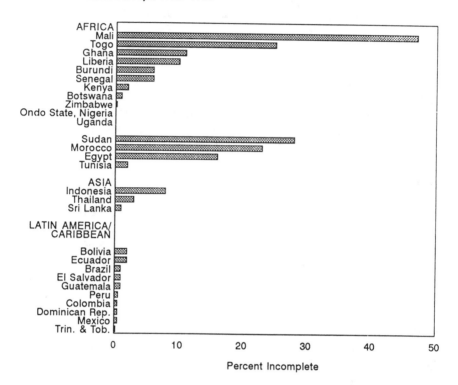

Percent Incomplete

Evidence from both WFS and DHS surveys shows that births have been displaced to the last year before the survey and that births in the last year have been displaced to the more recent months (Grummer-Strawn and Trussell, 1990). A higher number of births were reported for the most recent months than for any other period and for the year preceding the survey than for all other years. Surveys in both Sub-Saharan Africa and Latin America show displacement of births into the first year of life, although the level appears to be much stronger in Sub-Saharan Africa than in Latin America.

It is difficult to find a satisfactory explanation for the observed pattern. Possibly there is a tendency to move birth dates closer to the interview date for births in the two to three years prior to the survey. In this case children's ages would be underreported. This displacement pattern occurs in addition to the displacement of births caused by the preference to report months that have just passed as opposed to months that are still to come. Generally, the effect of this type of displacement is overreporting the age of young children.

### Age-at-death reporting
Age-at-death reporting is more complete than birth date reporting for births in the past five years. In half of the surveys there were no missing data for age at death, and all sur-

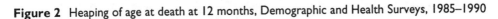

**Figure 2** Heaping of age at death at 12 months, Demographic and Health Surveys, 1985–1990

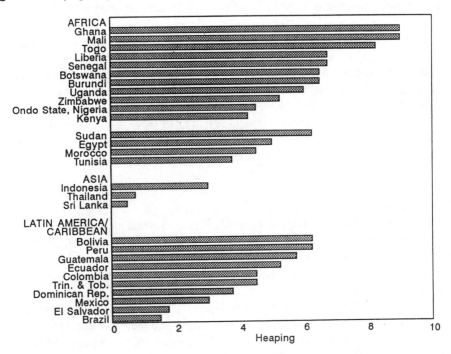

veys had less than 3 percent missing values. The quality of age-at-death data is more difficult to assess. In DHS surveys, deaths under one month had to be recorded in days, deaths under two years in months, and deaths at two years and over in years.

Considerable heaping occurs at 12 months of age in all surveys, except for Sri Lanka and Thailand. There is no precise way to determine the extent of heaping because it assumes knowledge of an 'expected' number of deaths at 12 months of age, which in turn assumes knowledge of the true age pattern to mortality as well as of the age range from which the heaped deaths were drawn. An index of heaping was calculated based on the arbitrary assumptions that heaped deaths were drawn from the 6- to 23–month period, and that the expected number of deaths at 12 months is the average number during months 6 through 23. Figure 2 shows the amount of heaping at 12 months by survey. The level is highest in Sub-Saharan Africa, although Bolivia, Ecuador, Guatemala, Peru, and Sudan also have index values exceeding 5. These figures warn against use of 12 months as a cut-off age for analysis of age-specific determinants of childhood mortality.

## Multiple births

The proportion of live births in the last five years that were part of a multiple birth ranges from 1.0 in Trinidad and Tobago to 5.4 percent in Togo. The mean for 27 countries is 2.3 percent, which corresponds to a twinning rate of approximately 1.1 percent, which is quite plausible. Considerable variation among the countries may be due to poor data quality and to sampling error (small numbers of multiple births), but part of it is probably real, since substantial regional variation has been demonstrated (Pison et al., 1989). The DHS estimate of the frequency of multiple births is a minimum estimate, since there are several reasons to assume that DHS surveys underestimate multiple births. For instance, DHS surveys do not collect data on stillbirths, which are more common for multiple births. Underreporting of deaths may also affect twinning rates, since twins are more likely to die.

## Fostering of children

The proportion of children who were reported by the biological mother not to live with her varied considerably between surveys. The overall level of fostering is highest in Sub-Saharan Africa and lowest in North Africa. In Botswana and Liberia, more than 10 percent of the children under five years were not living with their mothers. In four additional countries, more than 5 percent of the children were 'fostered away' (Dominican Republic, Senegal, Uganda, and Zimbabwe). Fostering is clearly age-dependent: it is rare during infancy (mean for 26 countries 0.3 percent) and increases during the second (mean 1.3 percent), third (2.6 percent), fourth (3.7 percent), and fifth years of life (4.7 percent). Fostering affects the quality of data on feeding, morbidity and treatment patterns, and immunization.

## Density of births in the recent five-year period

DHS surveys collect health data on all live births in the five years preceding the survey. The quality of the data may be affected by the sheer volume of information collected from mothers with more than one birth in the last five years. Indeed, more than half of such mothers had to answer questions about at least two births. On average, 36 percent of these mothers had one birth, 47 percent two births, 15 percent three births, and 2 percent four births or more. In several sections of this volume we will attempt to assess whether either the mother or the respondent is overburdened by being asked questions about all births in the last five years.

Less extensive questionnaires that have been used in other health surveys focus on last births only or on the last two births. From the DHS data it can be shown that last birth samples are only appropriate for studies of infant health, since they capture 98.6 percent of all births (mean for 28 surveys), but they are not suitable for studies that include older children. For example, 10 percent of the children age one year would be missed in a last births sample. Samples that include the last two births could be considered if the focus was on the health of children under three years: 98.1 percent of all births were captured by the last two births (mean for 28 surveys).

## Implications for DHS-II

The efforts to obtain the best possible information on dates of birth and ages of the children in the DHS-II surveys continued along the same lines as in the DHS-I surveys. During the training of the interviewers, field editors, and supervisors, the birth history is the most time-consuming section of the questionnaire. Emphasis is put on consistency of information; use of various methods, such as historical calendars, to obtain a birth date in case the mother does not know the exact month and/or year; and probing of long intervals between births. During fieldwork, data quality tables, including several tables on the accuracy and completeness of children's birth dates, are run repeatedly. The teams in the field receive immediate feedback to improve data collection.

## Maternity care

In DHS-I, pregnant women were asked about tetanus toxoid (TT) immunization and antenatal care received during the current pregnancy. In addition, all women were asked about maternity care received during pregnancies completed in the five years prior to the survey. Specifically, they were asked if they had received tetanus toxoid during pregnancy; who, if anyone, provided antenatal care; and who, if anyone, provided delivery care. Fourteen surveys also included a country-specific question about the place of delivery.

The assessment of the quality of maternity care data focuses on (Stewart et al., 1994):
• The limitations of the questions asked about maternity care;
• The distribution of missing values, 'don't know', and 'other' responses for the maternity care data;
• Internal consistency of responses; and
• Comparison of DHS data with other sources of data on maternity care coverage.

### Current pregnancy

Women were asked if they were currently pregnant and, if so, for how many months. The analysis showed that early pregnancies were underreported in all surveys. This underreporting of early pregnancies may be associated with a lack of awareness or an unwillingness to report early pregnancies. In addition, the data on duration of pregnancy should be interpreted with caution, since the majority of the surveys had markedly higher proportions of women pregnant in the second trimester than in the first or third trimesters.

If the respondent was pregnant, questions were asked about who provided antenatal care and whether or not tetanus toxoid was received. These questions were also asked for births during the five years before the survey (i.e., completed pregnancies). Gross underreporting of these events in previous (completed) pregnancies might be detected by comparing this data with service use reported by women currently in the last trimester of pregnancy. However, the opposite was observed. Coverage of tetanus toxoid and antenatal care among currently pregnant women in their last trimester was in many cases lower than in previous (completed) pregnancies, underscoring the difficulty of obtaining reliable data on service coverage by sampling only currently pregnant women. It is, therefore, likely that there is less underreporting of services received in prior pregnancies than in current pregnancies.

## Data on pregnancies completed in the five years prior to the survey

The data on service coverage for births from pregnancies completed in the five years prior to the survey include information on who provided delivery care in addition to who provided antenatal care and whether a tetanus toxoid injection was received during pregnancy. The questions about maternity care in DHS-I have a number of limitations:

- The data allow a general assessment of tetanus toxoid coverage by the health care system, but do not facilitate examination of individual coverage, because women are not asked the *number* of doses received and because there is no history of vaccinations received prior to the five years before the survey or of doses received outside of pregnancy.
- In asking about antenatal and delivery care, the DHS questions focus only on the 'most qualified' provider of care. Responses to these questions, particularly 'Who provided delivery care?' may be misleading since a woman may delay seeking a trained provider until after developing extremely severe complications which other providers have been unable to manage. This lack of information on both the process involved in seeking care and the actual quality of care received circumscribes the role of the data in studying the specific impact of maternity care *per se.*
- Utilization of health care is determined by a variety of user and service-related factors. Service availability data were collected at the cluster level in more than one-third of the countries surveyed in DHS-I. These data are not assessed in this report. However, the lack of household-level information on available services limits the utility of the DHS-I data in examining individual service-related differences in utilization of care.
- Data on the place of delivery were collected in only half of the DHS-I surveys. Tabulations of type of provider by place of delivery for surveys with both types of information show that it is not always correct to assume that deliveries assisted by medical personnel took place in health facilities. In six of the 13 surveys analyzed, more than 5 percent of all home deliveries were attended by doctors, nurses, or midwives. In two surveys this proportion exceeded 10 percent (Indonesia and Liberia).

In general, the analysis did not reveal striking problems with the recall of antenatal care and delivery care for births in the last five years, but the methods to evaluate the existence of a recall bias are limited. In the majority of surveys the proportion of all births with missing values, 'don't know' responses, or classified as 'other' were within the acceptable range. The length of the recall period did not affect the occurrence of missing values or 'don't know' responses, after controlling for other variables. However, two important problems were identified in bivariate analysis and confirmed by multivariate analysis:

**Figure 3**  Missing values for delivery care by survival status of the child, births in the last 5 years, Demographic and Health Surveys, 1985–1990

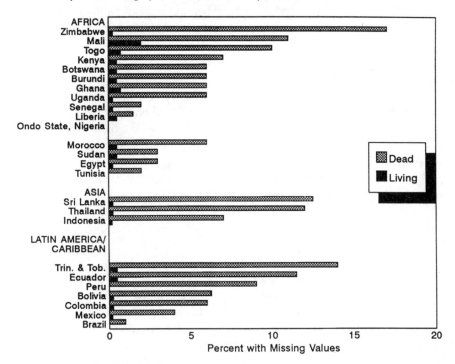

- Missing values are much higher for deceased children (see Figure 3). In seven surveys data on maternity care are missing for more than 10 percent of the deceased children. "Don't know" responses are also more likely to occur for dead children. This indicates that interviewers are more likely to overlook or be reluctant to ask information about events relating to births in these cases.

  Both the respondent and the interviewer may feel uncomfortable discussing events related to a child that has died. In some cultures, this may be a taboo subject, the discussion of which may be perceived as causing further adverse consequences. In addition, a woman may have greater difficulty remembering the details of events surrounding a pregnancy and birth where the child is no longer living, particularly if the death occurred soon after birth. It is also conceivable that the interviewer may lack an understanding of the significance of information about deceased children, resulting in less effort to obtain responses about these births.

- Missing values are more common for the next-to-last births and especially the second-to-last births and before than for last births (most recent births), for which the information is collected first. 'Don't know' responses do not increase by relative birth order (last birth, next-to-last, second-to-last, and before). This suggests that interviewer 'fatigue' is the main reason for the missing values. The magnitude of the problem, however, is within limits. For example, the mean proportion of births with missing values for 26 surveys was 0.4 percent for last births, 1.0 percent for next-to-last births, and 4.2 percent for second-to-last and before births. In multivariate analysis the difference between last and next-to-last births generally was not significant.

## Implications for DHS-II

The maternity section of the DHS-II questionnaire has built upon the experience of DHS-I. First, the questions on use of maternity care for current pregnancies have been omitted. Second, the collection of data on maternity care for all births in the last five years was expanded to accommodate questions on the number of antenatal visits and number of tetanus toxoid injections for each pregnancy, the place of delivery (as a standard question and not an option as in DHS-I) in addition to the provider of delivery care, and, to allow the coding of multiple providers in questions, antenatal and delivery care. There also is a question about whether the mother was given an antenatal card.

# Child vaccination data

Vaccination data differ somewhat from most of the other data in the DHS-I questionnaire, since information is copied from records kept by the respondent. Most DHS-I surveys include questions on the vaccination status of children of the respondents born since January of the fifth year preceding the survey. The standard method of collecting vaccination information was to ask about the presence of a child health card and then request to see it. The interviewer then copied the vaccination dates from the health card (day, month, and year of each vaccination). If no card could be presented, the interviewer then asked whether the child had ever had a vaccination to prevent him/her from getting diseases.

The assessment of the quality of DHS vaccination data, presented in detail in Boerma and Bicego (1994), includes an analysis of the proportion of child health cards seen by the interviewer, the accuracy and completeness of dates of vaccination copied from cards to questionnaires, the reliability of mother's recall of vaccinations to her child(ren), and a comparison of DHS estimates of vaccination coverage with other sources.

## Estimation of coverage

Most DHS-I surveys were limited to the collection of vaccination data from health cards, with only one question for children whose card was not seen (namely whether the child ever received a vaccination). Estimates based only on card information would underestimate coverage if a proportion of cards were not seen or if a substantial proportion of vaccinations could not be confirmed by cards. In nine countries, however, mothers were asked to report information on specific vaccinations, if no card was presented. In Mexico, this was the only source of information, but in the eight other countries it complemented the information collected from the health cards. Vaccination coverage can be estimated from health card and maternal recall information for these eight countries (using the standard procedure for estimation of coverage recommended by WHO). For the other countries, data from the cards and from the proportion ever vaccinated among children without cards can be used to estimate coverage, as has been described elsewhere (Boerma et al., 1990). Due to the different methods of recording vaccinations and the questions used in the survey, coverage estimates for Egypt are less accurate than in most other DHS surveys, and no estimates could be made at all for the Dominican Republic and Togo. These three countries used questions that differed considerably from those included in the DHS core questionnaire.

## Presentation of health cards

Regarding health cards for children under five years of age there were three possibilities in the DHS-I surveys: card reported and seen, card reported but not seen, and no card. Missing values were no problem for this question; almost all countries had less than 0.5 percent missing values. The proportion of children under five with no card at all varies considerably between countries, from 3 percent in Botswana to more than 66 percent in Mali. The large proportion of children for whom the mother said she had a card, but did not show it to the interviewer is striking (see Figure 4). There are various reasons for cards not being seen. These include, the card is kept somewhere else (e.g., a family has more than one residence, health workers keep child health cards), the card could not be found in the house, the mother is reluctant to search for the card, or the interviewer does not insist on seeing the card.

It can generally be assumed that the lower the proportion of cards reported by the respondent and seen by the interviewer, the poorer the quality of the data from this questionnaire section. As Figure 4 shows, more than 70 percent of the cards reported were actually seen by the interviewer in seven countries, which indicates good data quality. In four countries, 60 to 70 percent of the cards were presented, and in six countries the range was 50–60 percent, which may indicate poorer interview quality than the first survey group. In six surveys less than half of the reported cards were presented. The proportion of cards seen among children whose mother said they had a card is particularly low in Bolivia (27 percent), the Dominican Republic (31 percent), Ondo State, Nigeria (35 percent), Mali (39 percent), and Peru (41 percent).

The card problem is age dependent. The older the child, the less likely it is that the interviewer will actually see the card (i.e., the card-present-but-not-seen rate is higher). This situation does not vary much by relative birth order of the child, but there is a slight increase of missing values in the health section: more missing values for the next-to-last and second-to-last children than for the last birth, but the size of the absolute difference is small. This indicates that interviewers become somewhat less attentive for the second, third, and fourth children.

How accurate is the information about the presence of a child health card as reported by the mother? This can be determined somewhat by analyzing data on cards presented

**Figure 4** Proportion of cards seen among children under 5 years with cards, Demographic and Health Surveys, 1986–1989

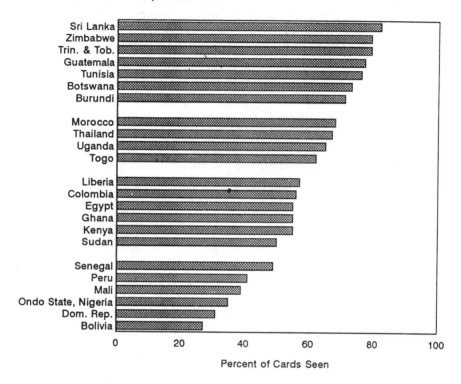

Percent of Cards Seen

and on ever vaccinated status. In seven surveys the proportion ever vaccinated is more than 2 percentage points lower among those with no card presented than for those for whom a card was presented: six surveys in Sub-Saharan Africa (Botswana, Burundi, Ghana, Liberia, Senegal, and Togo) and Morocco. In some cases, it might even be true that the mother had an empty card with no vaccinations on it and did not bother to show this card to the interviewer. In general, however, this can be considered as evidence of a minor inconsistency in mother's reporting of card possession or vaccination status of her children in the seven surveys mentioned above.

## Recall coverage

If no card was presented to the interviewer, mothers in eight surveys were asked to recall specific vaccinations given to their child(ren). Mother's recall of vaccinations is necessary in order to estimate vaccination coverage among all children, with or without cards. In general, coverage is expected to be somewhat lower among children for whom no card was presented to the interviewer, and the discrepancy is expected to be larger for multiple-dose vaccines. Recall coverage is defined as the proportion of children who received a specific vaccination among all children who have no card but had at least one vaccination reported by the respondent.

Recall coverage is indeed lower than card coverage in all eight surveys, with the exception of Sudan. The differences are greatest for the third doses of DPT and polio vaccines. For example, polio3 recall coverage is less than 80 percent of polio3 card coverage in 5 of the 8 surveys. In Sudan, recall coverage is almost as high as card coverage and is even higher for measles vaccination, which suggests some overreporting by mothers.

## Comparison with other data sources

Vaccination coverage rates are usually derived from either special coverage surveys or routine data from health facilities where vaccinations are given. The coverage surveys are conducted using a standard survey methodology recommended by the Expanded Programme on Immunization (EPI) of the World Health Organization (WHO) (Henderson and Sundaresan, 1982). The survey sample consists of 30 clusters selected with probability proportional to population size. In each cluster the first household is randomly chosen and, to reduce survey costs, all subsequent households are selected from neighbouring households until at least seven children in a selected age group are identified. With this method, the level of vaccination coverage can be estimated with a precision of about 10 percent (Lemeshow et al., 1985).

Although the EPI cluster sample coverage surveys are carried out in many countries, two concerns have been raised regarding the reliability of the resulting coverage estimates. First, the sample may be biased by over-representation of households located near health facilities. Second, interviews are often conducted by health workers, which may introduce an additional bias. Further, national coverage estimates can be based on routinely reported data from the vaccination clinics. Data from these health information systems, however, are rarely complete and assumptions have to be made to estimate coverage from such data. In addition, the denominator (number of children eligible for vaccination) often has to be estimated from other sources, such as population projections with census data.

DHS surveys can be compared to official estimates of vaccination coverage based on either of the two methods if the survey period coincides with the reference period for estimates from other sources. Since most EPI cluster coverage surveys focus on children 12–23 months of age, the comparison is limited to this age group. As in EPI cluster sample surveys, information on vaccinations given to the child is copied from the child health card if present. In the EPI surveys, if no health card is presented, the mother is usually asked to recall specific vaccinations.

The comparison shows that DHS estimates of vaccination coverage are generally in the same range as coverage estimates based on the cluster sample coverage surveys, whereas reported data from health facilities often differ considerably from DHS estimates. The latter is most likely due to inaccuracy in the estimates based on routine reports. In most countries, DHS estimates and those from EPI cluster sample surveys were remarkably similar. In some of the more recent DHS-II surveys, however, substantial discrepancies have arisen between results of EPI surveys and DHS surveys in a similar time period. Estimates based on DHS turn out to be considerably lower than the EPI survey results (e.g., Nigeria and Pakistan). The reasons for the discrepancies vary, but mainly appear related to the survey design and execution of the EPI cluster sample surveys. A study is underway to assess the quality of DHS-II vaccination data.

## Implications for DHS-II

In general, DHS data appear to be a useful source of information on childhood vaccinations, but recall of specific vaccinations improves estimates of coverage. For most surveys in the period 1986–90, data on specific vaccinations were not collected from the mother if no card was presented, whereas, in the DHS-II core questionnaire, information was collected from the mother on specific vaccinations if no card was presented. In addition, if the card did not show all vaccinations, the mother was asked whether the child had received any additional vaccinations. Lastly, if the mother had no card for her child, she was asked whether she ever had one.

# Child morbidity and treatment

Data on morbidity and treatment patterns were collected for all living children under five years of age. Most surveys included a question on diarrhoea prevalence, and about half of the surveys collected information on respiratory symptoms (cough and/or difficult breathing) and fever. Although the primary objective of the questionnaire section on morbidity was to assess treatment patterns, the most attention has been paid to the evaluation of the quality of the prevalence data (Boerma and Van Ginneken, 1994). Methods to evaluate the quality of treatment data are not readily available, whereas there are more opportunities to assess the quality of morbidity reporting. In addition, the quality of data on treatment depends to a large extent on the quality of the morbidity data.

## Diarrhoea occurrence

To determine the prevalence of diarrhoea, mothers were first asked whether their children under the age of five years had had diarrhoea in the last 24 hours. If the answer was negative the interviewer asked whether the children had had diarrhoea during the last two weeks. The judgement of what constitutes an episode of diarrhoea was made by the respondent.

Missing values for diarrhoea prevalence are not common; they are observed for less than 1 percent of the children in all but two surveys. However, there is considerable variation in the percentage of 'don't know' responses. Such responses are rare in most surveys, but in seven countries more than 3 percent of the mothers did not know whether diarrhoea had occurred in the last two weeks. This problem is particularly common in Botswana (12 percent), Liberia (9 percent), Uganda (8 percent), Bolivia (8 percent), and Zimbabwe (7 percent). Child fostering is the most important reason for lack of mother's knowledge about the health status of her child(ren): the majority of mothers whose children did not usually live with them did not know whether their child(ren) had had diarrhoea. The percentage of 'don't know' responses is small if the child usually lives with the mother.

The prevalence data can be used to evaluate data quality in DHS surveys where questions were asked about diarrhoea prevalence in the last 24 hours and in the last two weeks. The ratio of the proportion with diarrhoea in the last 24 hours and in the period 2–14 days before the survey is a valuable indicator of data quality (Boerma et al., 1991a). The analysis shows that virtually all DHS surveys suffer from both underreporting of cases that terminated 2–14 days before the interview and overreporting of current cases. Analysis by mother's level of education also suggests some differential reporting by education: either more overreporting of recent diarrhoea or more underreporting of terminated diarrhoea for children of mothers with no education, compared to children of mothers with at least a secondary education.

In eight surveys the duration of diarrhoea episodes was investigated and several irregularities were seen in the distribution of replies, in particular heaping of durations on seven days. This limits the accuracy of this type of information.

## Diarrhoea case management
Except for Ecuador, all the surveys included questions about the use of oral rehydration therapy (ORT) for diarrhoea management. Questions were asked about the use of fluids prepared with ORS packets (oral rehydration salts) and/or home solution (homemade sugar-salt-water solution). Specific questions on both ORS and home solution were asked in five countries, in nine others only ORS packet use was specifically asked, and in another eight surveys both ORS and home solution use were included as response categories in a general question on what was done to treat the diarrhoea. In most surveys, the mother was also asked where she took her child with diarrhoea. In six surveys there was no coding category for traditional medical practitioners. In five surveys, the utilization of health facilities was not asked specifically, and only part of a general question dealt with what was done to treat the diarrhoea. Finally, almost all surveys included a question on what kind of treatment was given, including use of drugs.

The way in which the question was asked strongly affects the results, as was shown in Boerma et al. (1991b). Therefore, comparability of results is limited, particularly comparing the earlier DHS-I surveys and the later ones.

Analysis of the questions on treatment of diarrhoea in 27 DHS surveys shows hardly any missing and 'don't know' replies. No other methods were readily available to assess the quality of the data. There is evidence showing that the relationship of morbidity with treatment is complex, as can be deduced from the finding of a negative association of diarrhoea prevalence with treatment: the higher the diarrhoea prevalence the lower the treatment rate. Therefore the quality of data on type of treatment received could not be evaluated adequately.

The DHS surveys, like most other studies, used a two-week recall period. This time-frame is considered to offer the best balance between the quality of information that can be obtained about treatment (best for current or very recent illness) and the representativeness of that treatment information (possibly best for recent but not current episodes). The selection of a two-week recall period implies that treatment patterns are assessed jointly for a mixed group of sick children: diarrhoea that has terminated, diarrhoea that has just started, and diarrhoea that has been present for a while and still continues. Published DHS data have shown no major differences in treatment patterns for children with terminated diarrhoea and those with current diarrhoea of at least two days duration (Boerma et al., 1991a). Both could be used to evaluate treatment practices. However, the treatment patterns for children with current diarrhoea of less than two days duration differ. These can be analyzed separately to assess home practices in the early stages of diarrhoea.

## Respiratory illness

The questions on respiratory illness are specifically intended to elicit information on the treatment of respiratory infections. There is more variation in the questions on the symptoms of respiratory illness used in the various DHS-I surveys than with the questions on diarrhoea. This variation is partly responsible for the considerable differences in morbidity levels found in these surveys. In the earlier surveys especially, the questions on respiratory illness were rather non-specific and cannot be used to assess treatment patterns of children with symptoms suggestive of acute lower respiratory infections.

There were hardly any missing data and low percentages of 'don't know' responses, which were even lower than for the diarrhoea questions. Comparison of the morbidity levels of respiratory illness as obtained in DHS surveys with epidemiological surveys on acute lower respiratory illnesses showed considerably higher levels in the former than in the latter. This is a strong indication that the DHS questions actually provide data on a wider and more diffuse range of conditions than just pneumonia. It is unknown to what extent these measurement problems influence the quality of the information on treatment patterns for lower respiratory illnesses. In addition, the quality of recalled data on specific treatments received is doubtful. For instance, many respondents may not know whether the syrup their children received was an antibiotic or a cough syrup. An evaluation of the quality of such data is, however, not possible with a DHS survey.

## Implications for DHS-II

These data point to some difficulties associated with morbidity reporting. In DHS-II, the order of the diarrhoea questions was changed because of the suspected overreporting of diarrhoea in the last 24 hours: the general question (diarrhoea in the last two weeks) preceded the specific question. The core questionnaire included one question on diarrhoea with blood and another on duration of current and terminated episodes within the two weeks before the interview. Further improvements in the measurement of diarrhoea morbidity in DHS-type surveys (which were not made in DHS-II) are required. Possibly a question on the severity of diarrhoea might help (Baqui et al., 1991, Peters et al., 1991), e.g., a question on the number of stools on the worst day of the episode or the mother's subjective classification of the severity. In DHS-II, respondents could spontaneously mention ORS packets as a treatment given to children with diarrhoea in the last two weeks. If not mentioned spontaneously, respondents were probed about the use of ORS packets for diarrhoea treatment. The same was done for the recommended home solution.

In DHS-II more standardized questions on respiratory infections were asked and this practice appears to lead to more consistent results, although, as expected, the prevalence of cough with rapid breathing in DHS surveys is considerably higher than the prevalence of pneumonia in epidemiological studies. However, the primary objective of the questions is to identify children who need to be evaluated for pneumonia or other lower respiratory infections. Adding fever (which is a standard question in DHS-II) to the diagnostic algorithm reduces the prevalence and may increase specificity. The treatment-recall questions are similar to the ones in DHS-I.

## Breastfeeding and supplementary feeding

Information was obtained regarding breastfeeding behavior for all children born to respondents in the five years preceding the survey. For each child the respondent was asked if the child was ever breastfed, and if so, for how long. The questionnaire structure assumed that only the last-born child could still be breastfed at the time of the survey. The assessment of the quality of feeding data focuses on the recall data on breastfeeding duration and feeding in the last 24 hours (Boerma and Sommerfelt, 1994).

From earlier work with the World Fertility Survey, it was evident that recall duration data had several problems. Therefore, both the DHS-I and DHS-II reports utilized only current status data for calculating measures of breastfeeding duration.

### Breastfeeding duration recall
How reliable are mothers' reports on the duration of breastfeeding? The marked heaping of breastfeeding duration data on multiples of six months in retrospective surveys (Ferry, 1981, Lesthaeghe and Page, 1980) was noted in several studies. Reinterview surveys in Brazil (Huttly et al., 1990) and Malaysia (Haaga, 1988) have found inconsistencies between the answers in subsequent survey rounds.

Missing values and 'don't know' responses are not common for breastfeeding duration in most surveys. The situation is quite different regarding dead children, where missing values are a problem. Missing values occur for less than 2 percent of the deceased children in only four surveys whereas more than 10 percent of the breastfeeding duration data are missing in seven surveys. In addition, in virtually all countries, there is a strong increase in the proportion of births with missing values for breastfeeding duration with increasing relative birth order (i.e., more serious for births earlier in the five-year period). Multivariate analysis confirmed the importance of survival status of the child and relative birth order for the occurrence of missing values.

Heaping at multiples of six for reported breastfeeding duration is pronounced in most surveys and the amount of heaping varies by background characteristics, such as mother's education. If heaping is a good indicator of the quality of data, then the reported durations of mothers with no education or low levels of education are less accurate than those reported by mothers with higher levels of education.

The analysis of overlap between pregnancy and lactation from the retrospective reports by the mother indicates considerable inaccuracy in breastfeeding duration and/or birth dates. Reports of the duration of breastfeeding may be over- or under-estimates, but overlap is clearly associated with overreporting of breastfeeding durations. On the other hand, Trussell et al. (1992) have shown that there appears to be underreporting of breastfeeding duration. Using data from WFS and DHS, they compared estimates of breastfeeding duration from current status data and from retrospective life-table measures. The latter were consistently lower than the current status measures. The average mean duration of breastfeeding for 21 DHS countries was 16.5 months based on the current status data and 15.7 months based on the retrospective lifetable measures. Trussell et al. (1992) concluded that this discrepancy was not due to very recent increases in breastfeeding and that 'there is a tendency for retrospective reports in DHS to be biased downward'. This conclusion is not necessarily inconsistent with our findings of unlikely proportion of overlap, probably due to overreporting of breastfeeding duration. Both overreporting and underreporting may occur, and the analysis by Trussell et al. suggests that underreporting is more common than overreporting.

## Feeding in the last 24 hours
For children who were still breastfed at the time of the survey, questions were asked about liquids and foods given during the preceding 24 hours. The DHS-I core questionnaire asked about water, juice, powdered milk, cow's or goat's milk, other liquids, and solid or mushy food. The surveys in many countries modified these questions and asked about specific foods and liquids commonly used for infants and young children. In most instances, these country-specific questions can easily be translated into one of the standard categories.

Although the DHS-I questionnaires inquired about the child's food intake during the 24 hours preceding the survey, the mother was not asked whether these foods and liquids were given regularly. Information was also *not* collected to determine if a child sometimes, though not every day, received anything other than breast milk. Hence, an individual child cannot be classified with complete certainty as exclusively breastfed. If the child sometimes received ritual foods, honey or sugar water etc., but not in the last 24 hours before the interview, he or she should be classified as 'almost exclusively' breast-fed. However, the DHS-I information gives a fairly good picture of the proportion of children who receive something other than breast milk. In addition, there are a few DHS-I surveys in which mothers were asked to recall the age when breastfeeding was supplemented by other liquids or solids on a regular basis.

The questions on the number of breastfeedings given during daytime and nighttime re-sulted in very high proportions of women answering 'on demand.' The analysis of the effect of breastfeeding on postpartum amenorrhoea suggested that 'on demand' may have very different meanings for different women and in different contexts (Rutstein, 1991).

### Implications for DHS-II
In addition to the DHS-I questions, mothers were asked to recall feeding information for all births in the last five years, i.e., the age in months at which the child received (on a regular basis) formula or milk other than breast milk, plain water, other liquids, and any mushy or solid food.

Data collected on the number of breastfeedings during day and night time (for lastborn breastfed children) indicate a very large proportion responding on demand. Since the meaning of on demand varies greatly between populations and individuals, the DHS-II questionnaire was adapted to make the respondent specify what she meant by on de-mand.

In DHS-II, the median duration of breastfeeding is calculated based on current status data only. Recalled data on the duration of breastfeeding are not used.

## Child anthropometry

Anthropometry provides an objective assessment of children's health and nutritional status. When interpreting such information, it is important to know whether the chil-dren in the sample are representative of the population of children from which the sam-ple was drawn, and whether the recorded measurements correctly reflect the child's true weight and height. Although it is possible to assess what proportion of the children earmarked for anthropometric assessment were actually measured for height and/or weight, it is more difficult to assess whether there is a systematic bias in the recorded measurements. The quality of child anthropometric data is summarized below. (Som-merfelt and Boerma, 1994)

### Sample of children
The height and weight of the survey respondents' young children were measured in nineteen surveys in the first phase of the DHS program. In most of the surveys, all chil-

dren in a specified age group were supposed to be measured. The exceptions were Northeast Brazil, Egypt, and Senegal, where only the children of a subsample of respondents were included.

When anthropometry was included in the survey, the 'standard' recommendation in the DHS-I program was to measure all the respondent's children 3 through 36 months of age.[1]

Eleven surveys followed this recommendation. Three of the earliest surveys obtained measurements only for children age 6 through 36 months (Dominican Republic, Ondo State in Nigeria, and Senegal); in the remaining five surveys the age group was extended beyond the 'standard'. Children were weighed and measured starting from birth in four surveys (Northeast Brazil, Morocco, Togo, and Uganda). In four countries the upper age limit was extended through 60 months of age (Northeast Brazil, Morocco, Uganda, and Zimbabwe).

## Missing values

The proportion of the eligible children whose height and/or weight were measured ranged from 79 percent in Trinidad and Tobago to 98 percent in Morocco. Over 90 percent of the children were measured for height and/or weight in eleven of the countries. Both measurements were obtained for almost all these children; however, in a few cases children were measured only for height or only for weight. The largest proportion of children with only one measurement is seen for Northeast Brazil, where 2 percent of children were weighed, but not measured for height.

Children who were reported as not living with their mother were less likely to have their height and weight measured. Similarly, children whose mothers were visitors and not regular residents in the household may not have accompanied their mother, and hence, may not have been included in the anthropometric assessment. Missing values were also more likely for older children under five years, which was mainly due to fostering status and residency.

There is also a definite trend toward more missing data among the next-to-last children than among last-born children in about two-thirds of the countries (median 14 percent versus 7 percent). However, it is noticeable that this trend is not seen in two of the four surveys that included all children 60 months and younger (Northeast Brazil and Morocco), whereas it is observed in the remaining two countries (Uganda and Zimbabwe), where a sizeable proportion of children do not live with their mother. Finally, missing values were more common in urban areas than in rural areas.

## Age reporting

To be able to compare the nutritional status of children from different population subgroups or from different countries and to assess changes in nutritional status over time, the WHO has recommended that children's height-for-age, weight-for-age, and weight-for-height be expressed as standard deviation units (or z-scores) from the median of the international reference population (usually the NCHS/CDC/WHO international reference population) (Dibley et al., 1987, WHO, 1981, and WHO, 1986). Accuracy and completeness of age information are crucial for the analysis of anthropometric data. The height and weight of each child is compared to the height and weight of children of the same age in months in the reference population. Only the third anthropometric indicator, weight-for-height, is independent of the child's age. Several possible systematic biases in the reporting of the child's age may affect the anthropometry results: completeness of reporting, missing data on birth date, field imputation of birth date by the interviewer, digit preference, or systematic over- or underreporting.

In three countries, a large proportion of children did *not* have a month and day of birth reported by their mothers. Mali had the highest proportion (40 percent), followed by Morocco (20 percent) and Togo (16 percent). Between 5 and 10 percent did not have a reported month and year of birth in Ghana and Egypt. It should be noted that in Morocco interviewers were allowed to record season instead of month of birth. Each season listed in the questionnaire was approximately three months long. Mothers reported the season, year, and age for 19 percent of all children eligible for height and weight measurement; only 1 percent had neither a month nor a season reported.

In the remaining countries mothers knew the date of birth for almost all children, but an unknown amount of field imputation of the birth dates may have been more common in some countries, i.e., the interviewer may have entered a month and year of birth even if the mother could not give exact information. The analysis of data on month of birth for children under five years raises concern regarding the quality of the data on the ages of children (Bicego and Boerma, 1994).

## Height and weight measurements

The accuracy of these measurements can only be definitively assessed in a validation study involving duplicate measurements where the heights and weights recorded by the enumerators are compared to a standard, e.g., measurements carried out by an expert. The identification of intra-observer variation also requires remeasurement of the same child. However, some properties of the quality of the data can be gleaned from an examination of the degree of heaping. Some surveys, such as the Dominican Republic and Morocco, show marked heaping of height and weight measurements on figures ending in .0 and .5. In most surveys, however, there is no heaping.

The height-for-age, weight-for-age, and weight-for-height z-scores have been calculated according to the guidelines developed by the CDC and recommended by WHO, and are included in the DHS recode data files. In cases where month and year of birth are not reported, z-scores are not calculated, and a 'missing' value will be shown for the height-for-age and weight-for-age variables. In Morocco, a z-score is calculated for children whose mother reported the child's age as well as the season and year of birth.

Improbably high or low z-scores are not shown; instead the variable is flagged. The guidelines provided by the CDC were followed. Height-for-age and weight-for-age z-scores above +6 and below -6 were flagged, as were weight-for-height scores above +6 and below -4. In addition, the following combinations of z-scores were flagged: height-for-age z-score below -3.09 and weight-for-height z-score above +3.09, and height-for-age z-score above +3.09 and weight-for-height z-score below -3.09.

The percentage of flagging was similar for all three indices within each country. Less than 1 percent of the z-scores was flagged in about half the countries. The lowest percentage was seen in Colombia (under 1 percent) and the highest in Guatemala (4 percent).

## Implications for DHS-II

In DHS-II, the age group for anthropometric measurements was expanded to include all children age 0–60 months. Maternal anthropometry was also introduced. The procedures for measuring weight were changed in most DHS-II surveys, i.e., the hanging spring balance scale was replaced by a digital bathroom scale having 100 grams of accuracy. The latter can be used for both mother and child.

## Causes of death in early childhood

In selected DHS surveys the probable causes of death were ascertained for dead children born during the preceding five years. The inclusion of a causes of death module in DHS surveys depended on the country's implementing agency. The questions used differed from survey to survey and are evaluated on a survey-by-survey basis (Boerma et al., 1993). The assessment of data quality is difficult. For example, consider a survey in which the results indicate that 20 percent of all deaths under five years of age were associated with diarrhoea. Although the results seem plausible on the basis of longitudinal epidemiological studies (e.g., Gray, 1991), the data may not be of good quality. In a population where 20 percent of the children had diarrhoea in the two weeks before the survey, it would be expected that 20 percent of the deceased children had diarrhoea during the illness preceding death, even if having diarrhoea does not increase the risk of death.

In this evaluation, the focus is on the types of questions used in the DHS surveys and how this affects the results. The countries involved are Bolivia, Ecuador, Egypt, Morocco, Senegal and Tunisia (all DHS-I surveys) and Cameroon (DHS-II survey). The following are our major conclusions:

• The cause of death section was embedded in the health section of the DHS questionnaire, where only information on children born in the five years before the survey was collected. Therefore, the cause of death data refer to all children born in the preceding five years, but not to children born more than five years ago. Consequently, there is under-representation of deaths at older ages among the under-fives.

- In general, the results on the causes of death in the seven DHS surveys analyzed here are disappointing, primarily due to inadequate questions asked in the earlier surveys, which led to a large proportion of deaths reported due to unknown causes and unlikely distributions for the leading causes of assigned deaths. The more extensive questionnaire was not very successful in Bolivia, but appears moderately successful in Cameroon. Overall, the quality of data is difficult to assess, and caution should be used in interpreting the results of the causes of death distribution. A conservative approach should also be used in evaluating the results from epidemiological studies (Gray, 1991), since validation studies are few.

- Classification into main and contributory causes is not feasible on the basis of a short questionnaire. However, the use of multiple causes gives a better picture of the causes of death pattern than the use of single causes. Therefore, multiple causes should be allowed, as was done for Cameroon, using the diagnostic criteria and without distinguishing between main and contributory causes.

- Based on the results of a few studies a recall period of 6–24 months has been recommended (Gray et al., 1990). The length of the recall period in the DHS surveys is 0–4 years. There was a moderate increase in the proportion of 'don't know' responses if the recall period was more than two years in three of the surveys, but no increase in three other surveys. This does not suggest that the length of the recall period is the major problem. However, information given for deaths more than two years ago may be less accurate, but this cannot be evaluated with the DHS datasets.

- Further improvements can possibly be made when more emphasis is placed on traditional names and classifications of causes of death. Such an effort has been shown to be worthwhile in several studies, but may take several weeks to months of research. Since DHS surveys are often carried out in multiple languages, such anthropological studies may not be feasible within the limited timespan of a DHS survey.

- Causes of neonatal mortality generally are more difficult to determine in verbal autopsy than causes of death among older children. DHS has made little effort to determine the causes of neonatal mortality, other than tetanus; however, an effort to determine these causes would certainly be worthwhile.

In sum, it remains to be seen whether it is possible to obtain reasonably accurate data on the leading causes of childhood deaths in large-scale cross-sectional surveys. With a well-developed questionnaire (more validation studies are required) it is possible to obtain a general picture of the causes of death, which can be used for advocacy purposes. If the objective is to assess cause-specific mortality trends (e.g., four of the World Summit for Children health goals are cause-specific mortality reductions) one must be more cautious for two reasons: misclassification and sampling errors. The results of validation studies show that misclassification of causes of death is common, and such studies are assumed to give the best possible picture (since only hospital deaths are used).

# Conclusions

The methods available to assess the quality of health data in DHS-I surveys are limited and in most cases it is not possible to judge the quality of the data. Nevertheless, the analyses presented in this report have given some insight into the quality of health data. In many areas the questionnaire appears to provide very useful data for health planners, policymakers, and researchers. The most important points that emerged from the data quality assessment include:

- The health section of the core questionnaire was clearly in a developmental stage during DHS-I. Some improvements were made during the first phase, and some countries opted for questions different from the core questionnaire. When interpreting the results, the way the information was gathered should always be taken into account.
- The health section focuses on all births in the five years preceding the survey. In populations where birth dates are not immediately known by the interviewer, who then must do substantial probing, a considerable number of births were displaced out of the birth history. In other words, there is a deficit of four-year-old children. This does not have serious implications for most health indicators. More important, however, is the evidence of displacement of births towards the interview date of more recent births. There appears to be displacement of births into the last year of life and also preference for months just before the survey month. The quality of the data on age in months has important implications on the analysis of anthropometric data and the use of current status measures, such as median duration of breastfeeding.
- Mothers with more than one child born in the five years preceding the survey have to answer the health section questions more than once. The analysis shows that missing values are more common for the next-to-last birth than for the last birth, but the difference is small. The difference is larger for second-to-last births (or before) compared with last birth: yet, the proportion of missing values is still small, even for the second-to-last births (or before). In general, it seems to be possible to collect information on all births in the last five years, although some interviewer fatigue occurs. However, there are not adequate instruments to evaluate the quality of data for more distant births and to compare the results to more recent births.
- A major finding in the assessment of the quality of maternity data is that missing values are rather common for deceased children, which affects certain analysis of such data. The same was found for reports on breastfeeding duration for deceased children. In addition, data on current pregnancy were not considered to be reliable. Apart from these problems, maternity care data appear to be of reasonably good quality.
- Many DHS-I surveys did not gather information about specific vaccinations from the mother, which complicated coverage estimation somewhat. The proportion of cards that were reported by the mother and were actually seen by the interviewer varied considerably between countries, and was well below 50 percent in several surveys. This clearly weakens the quality of the vaccination coverage estimate.

- The child morbidity data in DHS-I are generally not reliable. This is due to the general difficulties one encounters when measuring morbidity, especially to the lack of good questions available to measure morbidity in cross-sectional surveys. The questions on respiratory infections changed considerably during DHS-I and seemed to be more useful at the end of DHS-I. The treatment patterns need to be interpreted carefully, since this information depends on the reporting of morbidity and on mother's recall of type of treatment, which is particularly difficult for medicines.
- The data on breastfeeding give only a rough indication of duration. Heaping at multiples of six months is considerable. The analysis of the overlap of breastfeeding and pregnancy among women with at least two births in the last five years showed that, in many surveys, there is a tendency to overreport breastfeeding.
- Child anthropometric data generally appear to be of good quality, with minor problems of digit preference, flagged values, or missing values.
- Verbal autopsy modules were used in seven surveys and generally did not lead to satisfactory results, which was mostly due to poor questionnaire design. Only in the most recent survey (actually a DHS-II survey) in Cameroon was a more extensive questionnaire used that seemed to give more plausible results; the results might be useful for health planning.

In general, the DHS health data are a sound database for basic health indicators, which are essential for health planning and evaluation in developing countries. In several instances, DHS data also provide a useful basis for research on determinants of child health, although researchers need to be cognizant of the problems summarized above.

## Note

1  In the DHS-II program, all children from birth through 60 months of age are measured for height and weight.

## Acknowledgments

Thanks to the following people for reviewing the subject areas noted:
Noreen Goldman and Roy Miller, immunization;
Ron Gray, verbal autopsy;
Beverley Carlson and John Mason, anthropometry;
Kenneth Hill, maternity care;
Virginia Laukaren and Chessa Lutter, breastfeeding;
Stan Becker, demographic aspects; and,
Roy Miller, morbidity.

# References

Anker, M. 1991. Epidemiological and statistical methods for rapid health assessment: Introduction. *World Health Statistics Quarterly* 44(3): 94–97.

Arnold, F. 1990. Assessment of the Quality of Birth History Data in the Demographic and Health Surveys. In *An Assessment of DHS-I Data Quality.* DHS Methodological Reports, No. 1. Columbia, Maryland: Institute for Resource Development/Macro Systems Inc.

Baqui, A.H., R.E. Black, M.D. Yunus, A.R.A. Hoque, H.R. Chowdhury, and R.B. Sack. 1991. Methodological issues in diarrheal diseases epidemiology: Definition of diarrheal episodes. *International Journal of Epidemiology* 20(4): 1057–1064.

Becker, S. 1984. *A response bias in the reporting of month of birth in pregnancy history surveys.* IPD Working Paper 1984–85, Brussels, Belgium: Vrije Universiteit Brussel, Interuniversity Programme in Demography.

Bicego G.T. and Boerma J.T. Demographic aspects of the quality of data on births in the Demographic and Health Surveys. In: Macro International Inc. 1994. *An assessment of the quality of health data in DHS-I surveys.* DHS Methodological Reports no. 2, Calverton, Maryland: Macro International Inc. pp. 29-55.

Boerma J.T. and Bicego G.T. The quality of data on child immunization in DHS-I surveys. In: Macro International Inc. 1994. *An assessment of the quality of health data in DHS-I surveys.* DHS Methodological Reports no. 2, Calverton, Maryland: Macro International Inc. pp. 81-93.

Boerma, J.T., R.E. Black, A.E. Sommerfelt, S.O. Rutstein, and G.T. Bicego. 1991a. Accuracy and completeness of mother's recall of diarrhoea occurrence in preschool children in Demographic and Health Surveys. *International Journal of Epidemiology* 20(4): 1073–1080.

Boerma J.T. and Sommerfelt A.E. Assessment of the qualtity of breastfeeding data in DHS-I surveys. In: Macro International Inc. 1994. *An assessment of the quality of health data in DHS-I surveys.* DHS Methodological Reports no. 2, Calverton, Maryland: Macro International Inc. pp. 111-124

Boerma, J.T., A.E. Sommerfelt, and S.O. Rutstein. 1991b. *Childhood Morbidity and Treatment Patterns.* DHS Comparative Studies, No. 4, Columbia, Maryland: Institute for Resource Development/Macro International Inc.

Boerma, J.T., A.E. Sommerfelt, S.O. Rutstein, and G. Rojas. 1990. *Immunization: Levels, Trends and Differentials.* DHS Comparative Studies No. 1, Columbia, Maryland: Institute for Resource Development/Macro Systems Inc.

Boerma J.T., Sommerfelt A.E. and Van Ginneken J.K. Causes of death in childhood: an evaluation of the results of verbal autopsy questions used in seven DHS surveys. In: Macro International Inc. 1994. *An assessment of the quality of health data in DHS-I surveys.* DHS Methodological Reports no. 2, Calverton, Maryland: Macro International Inc. pp 145-158.

Boerma J.T. and Van Ginneken J.K. The quality of data on child morbidity and treatment in DHS-I surveys. In: Macro International Inc. 1994. *An assessment of the quality of health data in DHS-I surveys.* DHS Methodological Reports no. 2, Calverton, Maryland: Macro International Inc. pp 97-108.

Dibley, M.J., J.B. Goldsby, N.W. Staehling, P. Nieburgh, and F.L. Trowbridge. 1987. Development of normalized curves for the international growth reference: Historical and technical considerations. *American Journal of Clinical Nutrition* 46(5): 749–762.

Ferry, B. 1981. *Breastfeeding.* WFS Comparative Studies No. 13. Voorburg, Netherlands: International Statistical Institute.

Galazka, A. and G. Stroh. 1986. *Neonatal tetanus: Guidelines on the community-based survey on neonatal tetanus mortality.* EPI/Gen/86.8, Geneva: WHO.

Gray, R.H. 1991. Interview-based diagnosis of morbidity and causes of death. Paper presented at seminar, Measurement of Maternal and Child Mortality, Morbidity and Health Care: Interdisciplinary Approaches. Cairo, IUSSP, 4–7 November 1991.

Gray, R.H., G. Smith, and P. Barss. 1990. *The Use of Verbal Autopsy Methods to Determine Selected Causes of Death in Children.* Occasional Papers No. 10, Baltimore, Maryland: Institute for International Programs, The Johns Hopkins University.

Grummer-Strawn, L. and T.J. Trussell. 1990. Computing the mean duration of breastfeeding from current-status data. Princeton, New Jersey: Office of Population Research, Princeton University.

Haaga, J.G. 1988. Reliability of retrospective survey data on infant feeding. *Demography* 25(2): 307–314.

Henderson, R.H. and T. Sundaresan. 1982. Cluster sampling to assess immunization coverage: A review of experience with a simplified sampling method. *Bulletin of the World Health Organization* 60(2): 253–260.

Huttly, S.R.A., F.C. Barros, C.G. Victora, J.U. Beria and J.P. Vaughan. 1990. Do mothers overestimate breast feeding duration? An example of recall bias from a study in southern Brazil. *American Journal of Epidemiology* 132(3): 572–575.

Kroeger, A. 1983. Health interview surveys in developing countries: A review of methods and results. *International Journal of Epidemiology* 12(4): 242–254.

Lemeshow, S., A.G. Tserkovnyi, J.L Tulloch, S.K. Dowd, S.K. Lwanga, and J. Keja. 1985. A computer simulation of the EPI survey strategy. *International Journal of Epidemiology* 14(3): 473–481.

Lesthaeghe, R.J. and H.J. Page. 1980. The post-partum non-susceptible period: Development and application of model schedules. *Population Studies* 34(1): 143–169.

Peters, D.H., S. Becker, J. Logarta, R.H. Gray, and R.E. Black. 1991. Estimates of Availability and Use of Oral Rehydration Salts for the Treatment of Diarrhoea in Cebu, the Philippines, 353–368. In *Measurement of Maternal and Child Mortality, Morbidity and Health Care: Interdisciplinary Approaches.* Edited by J.T. Boerma, Liege: IUSSP/Derouaux-Ordina Editions.

Pison, G., E. van de Walle, and M. Sala-Diakanda. 1989. Les Jumeaux: Fréquence, statut social et mortalité. In *Mortalité et Société en Afrique au Sud du Sahara*. Paris: Presses Universitaires de France.

Ross, D.A. and J. P. Vaughan. 1986. Health interview surveys in developing countries: A methodological review. *Studies in Family Planning* 17(2): 78–94.

Rutstein, S.O. 1991. The impact of breastfeeding on fertility. In *Proceedings of the Demographic and Health Surveys World Conference* Vol. 2, pp. 897–924. Washington, D.C., August 1991. Columbia, Maryland: Institute for Research Development/Macro International Inc.

Sommerfelt A.E. and Boerma J.T. Anthropometric status of young children in DHS-I surveys: an assessment of data quality. In: Macro International Inc. 1994. *An assessment of the quality of health data in DHS-I surveys*. DHS Methodological Reports no. 2, Calverton, Maryland: Macro International Inc. pp. 127-142.

Stewart K., Boerma J.T. and Van Ginneken J.K. Assessment of the wuality of data on meternity care in the Demograophic and Health Surveys. In : Macro International Inc. 1994. *An assessment of the quality of health data in DHS-I surveys*. DHS Methodological Reports no. 2, Calverton, Maryland: Macro International Inc. pp. 61-77.

Trussell, T.J., L. Grummer-Strawn, G. Rodriguez, and M. Van Landingham. 1992. Trends and differentials in breastfeeding behavior: Evidence from the WFS and DHS. *Population Studies* 46: 285–308.

World Health Organization. 1981. *Development of indicators for monitoring progress toward Health for All by the Year 2000*. ("Health for All" Series No. 4). Geneva: WHO.

World Health Organization Working Group. 1986. Use and interpretation of anthropometric indicators of nutritional status. *Bulletin of the World Health Organization* 64: 929–941.

4

# Accuracy and completeness of mothers' recall of diarrhoea occurrence in pre-school children in demographic and health surveys

*J. Ties Boerma, R.E. Black, A. Elisabeth Sommerfelt, Shea O. Rutstein and George T. Bicego*

International Journal of Epidemiology, *vol. 20, no. 4, 1991, pp. 1073–1080.*

## Abstract

In the context of the Demographic and Health Surveys program (DHS), data were collected on diarrhoeal diseases in childhood and related treatment patterns. In this paper we assess the accuracy and completeness of mothers' recall of diarrhoea in 19 national DHS surveys and discuss the implications for health interview surveys in developing countries. It is concluded that there is under-reporting of diarrhoea if the recall period is longer than 2–3 days, whereas there may be over-reporting of very recent or current diarrhoea in most DHS surveys. Reporting errors appear to vary considerably between countries, which affects the comparability of survey results. A second and related issue, that is addressed in this paper, is the reporting of treatment practices by duration of diarrhoeal episode. There were no major differences in reported treatment patterns between children with diarrhoea that terminated in the last two weeks and children with current diarrhoea of at least two days' duration. The implications of the findings for retrospective surveys on childhood morbidity and treatment patterns are discussed.

## Introduction

Health interview surveys aim to ascertain the burden of important illnesses and the associated utilization patterns of health services.[1,2] The information is generally collected in a cross-sectional survey, in which respondents are requested to recall symptoms of illnesses that have occurred in the recent past. Health interview surveys have several methodological problems, particularly concerning lack of standardization in survey methodology and methods of analysis, that limit the comparability of results.[1] In addition, perceptions, recall and reporting of morbidity depend on cultural factors,[2] which may have a greater effect on morbidity data than on more uniform and objective child health indicators, such as child mortality or anthropometric measurements.[3]

Diarrhoea in children, being a leading illness in childhood, is one of the most frequently studied morbid conditions in health interview surveys. A two-week recall period for the occurrence of diarrhoea has been selected in most studies, since it has been considered to be the best balance between minimizing the problem of recall errors and a feasible sample size for household surveys.[1] But even within a two-week recall period memory lapse occurs. In Guatemala, the number of days ill with diarrhoea in a two-week interview period was estimated to be under-reported by 22% for pre-school children.[4] The level of under-reporting increased with the length of the interval between the occurrence of the diarrhoea and day of interview. In rural Bangladesh, a one-week recall period was used in a survey on diarrhoea in pre-school children.[5] It was found that reporting of diarrhoea episodes declined by one-third when the recall period exceeded 48 hours. The authors concluded that the decline was due to memory lapse for diarrhoea more than two days before the interview and not to over-reporting of recent diarrhoea. The latter possibility, however, should be considered in this particular study, since medical action (oral rehydration therapy, rectal swab, referral) was undertaken by the interviewer if diarrhoea was present on the day of the interview. In urban Ethiopia, daily morbidity interviews were compared with fortnightly interviews.[6] The interview with a two-week recall period produced a relative over-reporting of recent illness and an under-reporting of earlier events compared to the daily interview results. This may be due to memory loss for the earlier events. It may also be that illnesses that occurred within the recall period were transferred to the more recent past .[1] This transfer poses a methodological problem for morbidity studies, since it may also happen for illnesses that occurred before the recall period, and would thus affect two-week prevalence or incidence rates.

In this study, data on diarrhoea occurrence, ascertained by two-week recall, in children under five years of age are examined for 19 national surveys. These surveys were carried out as part of the Demographic and Health Survey Program (DHS) in the period 1986–1989. This programme, funded by the United States Agency for International Development (USAID), assists developing countries in the organization of nationally representative surveys, aiming to provide information for policy and programme decision-making and for scientific research. Survey data include information on fertility and childhood mortality levels, use of family planning, and various maternal and child health indicators. Survey respondents are women of childbearing ages. The prime objective of the childhood diarrhoea questions in DHS surveys was to assess treatment patterns.

Two main issues are addressed in this paper. The first concerns the estimation of diarrhoea prevalence from cross-sectional survey data. Specific attention is given to possible diarrhoea recall or reporting problems, including memory lapse, time misplacement and misinterpretation of the recall period. In addition, it will be assessed whether recall errors differ by the mothers' level of education. The second issue of this paper pertains to treatment practices. Data on treatment practices during child diarrhoea are analyzed cross-nationally according to whether the child was having diarrhoea at the time of the survey and according to the duration of the episode.

## Data and methods

In the standard DHS questionnaire, used in the first phase of the programme, diarrhoea prevalence was assessed as follows, for all children under five years age of the respondent:
- Has this child (name of child) had diarrhoea in the last 24 hours? The prevalence of diarrhoea in the last 24 hours is assumed to be equal to the proportion currently having diarrhoea, or equal to the point prevalence on the day of interview. Since the interview is on average held at the middle of the working day (12 noon), the reference period includes 12 hours of the previous day.
- If there was no diarrhoea in the last 24 hours the interviewer asked: has this child (name) had diarrhoea in the last two weeks? This question refers to the period from the second to the 14th day (referred to as 2–14 days) before the interview.

The sum of the affirmative answers to these two questions provides an estimate of the period prevalence of diarrhoea in the last two weeks. Diarrhoea was not defined in the DHS surveys, but it was left to the respondents to decide whether the child had (had) diarrhoea or not. The sample sizes of the surveys ranged from 1800 to 6000 children under five years.

In this study we will use the prevalence data to evaluate data quality. Durations of diarrhoea can be estimated from the proportions with diarrhoea in the last 24 hours and in the period 2–14 days before the survey. In a prospective study the two-week prevalence ($P_{14}$) equals the sum of the point prevalence (existing cases) at the beginning of the period ($P_1$) and the incidence during the remainder of the period ($I_{13}$).[7] For the retrospective data collected in DHS surveys, the diarrhoea prevalence in the last 24 hours is equal to $P_1$ and the diarrhoea cases that terminated 2–14 days before the survey is equal to $I_{13}$, if steady state conditions prevail.

Under these conditions (implying constant prevalence and incidence during the last month or so) the number of new occurrences is equal to the number of terminated cases during the same period.[8] The duration of a diarrhoeal episode (D) can be estimated from the relationship between prevalence (P) and incidence (I) as follows:

$$P = I*D/(1 + I*D)^{8,9}$$

which leads to $P = I*D$ for rare conditions.

Diarrhoea, however, is not a rare condition among children in many developing countries. Thus, $D = P/(I*(1-P))$, which for this study can be written as:

$$D = P_1/(I_1*(1-P_1))$$
$$= P_1/(I_{13}/13*(1-P_1))$$
$$= 13*P_1/(I_{13}*(1-P_1))$$

The ratio of diarrhoea prevalence in the last 24 hours to diarrhoea terminated at days 2–14 before the interview will be referred to as CT ratio (Current/Terminated = $P_1/I_{13}$).

In addition to the indirect estimate of duration of a diarrhoea episode, a 'direct' estimate is possible for some countries. Specific questions on the duration of diarrhoea episodes were used in five DHS countries.

For all five countries the mean duration-to-date of diarrhoeal episodes can be calculated. These data, however, cannot be used to estimate mean duration (by multiplying the mean duration to date by two), since there are relatively more long episodes in the

**Table 1** Diarrhoea prevalence for the two weeks preceding the survey (last 24 h, 2–14 days before survey, and total), ratio diarrhoea in last 24 h to diarrhoea 2–14 days ago (CT ratio) and indirect estimate of duration of diarrhoea episodes (weighted data) among children 1–59 months of age

| Country | Children No. | Per cent with diarrhoea | | | CT ratio | Duration (days) |
| | | Last 24 h | 2–14 days | Total last 2 weeks | | |
|---|---|---|---|---|---|---|
| **Africa** | | | | | | |
| Botswana | 2648 | 4.8 | 6.5 | 11.3 | 0.74 | 10.1 |
| Burundi | 3403 | 8.4 | 9.2 | 17.6 | 0.91 | 13.0 |
| Ghana | 3529 | 13.9 | 13.1 | 27.0 | 1.06 | 16.0 |
| Kenya | 6390 | 6.8 | 6.2 | 13.0 | 1.10 | 15.3 |
| Mali | 2736 | 20.2 | 15.7 | 35.9 | 1.29 | 21.0 |
| Togo | 2688 | 14.6 | 15.7 | 30.3 | 0.93 | 14.2 |
| Uganda | 3984 | 15.4 | 11.0 | 26.4 | 1.40 | 21.5 |
| Zimbabwe | 2906 | 9.5 | 11.8 | 21.3 | 0.81 | 11.6 |
| Morocco | 5505 | 17.7 | 11.4 | 29.1 | 1.55 | 24.5 |
| Tunisia | 4208 | 10.5 | 10.2 | 20.7 | 1.03 | 15.0 |
| **Asia** | | | | | | |
| Sri Lanka | 3820 | 2.2 | 3.8 | 6.0 | 0.58 | 7.7 |
| Thailand | 3416 | 6.3 | 9.8 | 16.1 | 0.64 | 8.9 |
| **Latin America and Caribbean** | | | | | | |
| Bolivia | 4753 | 16.9 | 13.6 | 30.5 | 1.24 | 19.4 |
| Brazil | 3141 | 7.6 | 9.6 | 17.2 | 0.79 | 11.1 |
| Colombia | 2527 | 10.0 | 9.2 | 19.2 | 1.09 | 15.7 |
| Dominican Rep | 3878 | 14.3 | 12.0 | 26.3 | 1.19 | 18.1 |
| Guatemala | 4170 | 10.4 | 6.3 | 16.7 | 1.65 | 24.0 |
| Peru | 2778 | 16.6 | 16.0 | 32.6 | 1.04 | 15.8 |
| Trinidad | 1819 | 2.1 | 4.1 | 6.2 | 0.51 | 6.8 |

sample of children with current diarrhoea. This is called 'length-biased sampling'.[10] In two DHS surveys (Bolivia and Tunisia) the mean duration of diarrhoea episodes could be computed from the terminated cases of diarrhoea.

In most DHS surveys sample weights have been used to obtain national estimates of population and health indicators. In this paper unweighted data will be used since the major objective is to assess the accuracy of responses. However, in Table 1 weighted data have been used to show the national levels of diarrhoeal prevalence by country.

# Results

### Indirect estimates of duration
Prevalence of diarrhoea among children under five years for the two weeks preceding the survey varied from less than 10% in Trinidad and Tobago and Sri Lanka to well

**Table 2** CT ratio by mothers' level of education

| Country | None | Primary schooling | Secondary schooling or more |
|---|---|---|---|
| **Africa** | | | |
| Botswana | 0.44 | 1.27 | 0.60 |
| Burundi | 0.91 | 0.72 | * |
| Ghana | 1.22 | 0.94 | * |
| Kenya | 1.47 | 1.07 | 0.75 |
| Mali | 1.37 | 1.48 | * |
| Togo | 1.11 | 0.94 | 0.63 |
| Uganda | 1.35 | 1.28 | 1.54 |
| Zimbabwe | 0.89 | 0.73 | 0.66 |
| Morocco | 1.62 | 1.05 | 1.79 |
| Tunisia | 1.02 | 1.36 | 0.48 |
| **Asia** | | | |
| Sri Lanka | 0.68 | 0.38 | 0.63 |
| Thailand | 0.71 | 0.62 | 0.84 |
| **Latin America and Caribbean** | | | |
| Bolivia | 1.57 | 1.18 | 1.44 |
| Brazil | 0.95 | 0.77 | 0.86 |
| Colombia | *1 | 1.12 | 1.02 |
| Dominican Rep | 3.17 | 1.30 | 0.95 |
| Guatemala | 1.78 | 1.43 | 0.60 |
| Peru | 1.57 | 1.07 | 1.10 |
| Trinidad | * | 0.47 | 0.55 |

* Implies N < 100.

over 30% in Mali and Peru (Table 1). The Current (C) to Terminated (T) ratio varied considerably between the countries: from 0.51 in Trinidad and Tobago to 1.65 in Guatemala. The last column of Table 1 shows the corresponding average durations of diarrhoeal episodes, derived from the CT ratio, as described in the methodology section. Trinidad and Tobago and Sri Lanka have the shortest calculated durations of about seven days. Thailand, Botswana, Zimbabwe and Brazil have durations from 8–11 days. All other countries have mean durations of diarrhoeal episodes of 12 days or more, and Guatemala, Mali, Morocco and Uganda even over 20 days.

Recall errors may vary by the educational characteristics of the respondent. For example, illiterate mothers may have misinterpreted (extended) the 24-hour recall period, and included diarrhoea episodes that ended more than 24 hours ago in their answers to the first survey question on diarrhoea (resulting in a higher CT ratio). Under-reporting may also be more common among illiterate mothers. Table 2 presents the CT ratio by mothers' level of education for children 6–35 months. This age group was selected, as the CT ratio tended to be higher for children under six months and lower for children 36–59 months, compared with children aged 6–35 months. In 14 of 17 countries women with no education had higher CT ratios than women with primary education; in ten of 14 countries women with secondary education had lower ratios than women with no education. There is no consistent difference between primary and secondary educa-

**Table 3**  Mean duration to date of current diarrhoeal episodes and mean duration of episodes terminated 2–14 days before the survey in children under 5 years

| Country | N | Mean duration to date | (Var) | Mean duration from terminated episodes | (Var) |
|---|---|---|---|---|---|
| Botswana | 119 | 4.4 | (19.9) | | |
| Kenya | 379 | 5.1 | (28.9) | | |
| Uganda | 537 | 5.3 | (18.9) | | |
| Tunisia | 577 | 4.1 | (10.0) | 4.7 | (10.2) |
| Bolivia | 839 | 4.3 | (26.4) | 3.8 | (12.6) |

tion. The countries, for which the inverse relationship between CT ratio and mothers' level of education is most apparent, are Kenya, Togo, Zimbabwe, Tunisia, Dominican Republic, Guatemala and Peru.

## Direct estimates of duration

Table 3 presents the data on durations from five countries. The mean duration-to-date was 4–5 days in all countries, but variance was larger in countries with more long episodes (Bolivia and Kenya). The estimated mean duration of a diarrhoeal episode will be less than two times the mean duration-to-date, since there is length-biased sampling in the sample of children with current diarrhoea. In Bolivia and Tunisia, mothers were asked about the duration of diarrhoeal episodes which had stopped in the two weeks before the survey. The mean duration of diarrhoea among these children was 3.8 days in Bolivia and 4.7 days in Tunisia. The estimates are considerably lower than the durations derived from the CT ratio.

In Figure 1 data on the onset of the current episode of diarrhoea are examined. Since the percentage distribution of current diarrhoea cases by the number of days since the diarrhoea started was very similar in all five countries, the data were pooled. A small proportion of diarrhoeal cases were reported to start on day 0, which represents only half a day. However, the proportion on day 1 was also lower than day 2 or 3 before the interview, possibly due to lower reporting rates for diarrhoea cases that have just started. There was considerable heaping on seven days prior to the survey in all countries (13.7% responses was at 7–8 days). A second smaller peak occurred at 14 days (4.4% of total at 14–15 days).

The DHS questionnaires in Bolivia and in the experimental DHS surveys in Peru and the Dominican Republic allowed the mother to respond in days, weeks or months to the questions on when the last episode of diarrhoea had occurred (Table 4). Among those children reported to have had diarrhoea 0–14 days or 1–2 weeks before the survey, more than half were said to currently have diarrhoea. A significant proportion of cases were recalled as one or two weeks ago, and not in days ago. In Bolivia and the Dominican Republic more than 10% of the answers were two weeks ago.

**Figure 1** Days since diarrhoea started for children under 5 years currently with diarrhoea

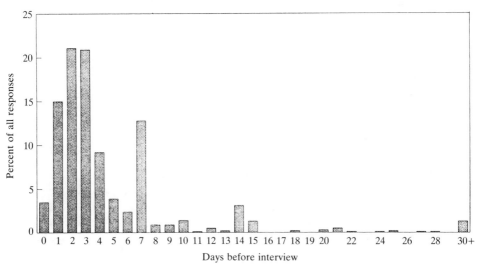

Botswana, Kenya, Uganda,
Tunisia and Bolivia DHS surveys

**Table 4** Time since last episode of diarrhoea occurred in children under 5 years: distribution of mothers' responses in days and weeks[1]

| Time ago | Bolivia | | Peru | | Dominican Republic | |
|---|---|---|---|---|---|---|
| | N | % | N | % | N | % |
| Current | 839 | 53.9 | 333 | 68.4 | 343 | 55.2 |
| Days | 248 | 15.9 | 93 | 19.1 | 149 | 24.0 |
| Weeks 1 | 241 | 15.5 | 41 | 8.4 | 60 | 9.7 |
| Weeks 2 | 230 | 14.8 | 20 | 4.1 | 69 | 11.1 |
| Total | 1558 | 100.0 | 487 | 100.0 | 621 | 100.0 |

1. Includes only responses of less than 18 days or less than 3 weeks.

## Recall lapse: Bolivia

Data from the Bolivia DHS survey can be used to study reporting of diarrhoea in the most recent and more distant period before the interview. Questions were asked both about the time elapsed since the childs' last diarrhoeal episode, and about the duration of that episode, and an estimate of daily prevalence and incidence of diarrhoea can be made (Figure 2). It is assumed that the mother referred to the end of the last episode. If the mother had said one week ago, this was distributed over the period 4–10 days before the survey. If the mother had responded two weeks ago this was distributed over the period 11–17 days before the survey. Daily prevalence in Bolivia dropped from over 150 per 1000 children on day 1 and 2 before the survey to prevalences rates of well below 100 per 1000 after four days or more before the survey. The incidence in Bolivia also peaked during the three days before the survey and had a small peak at day

**Figure 2**  Daily occurrence of diarrhoea in children under 5 years by day before the survey in Bolivia

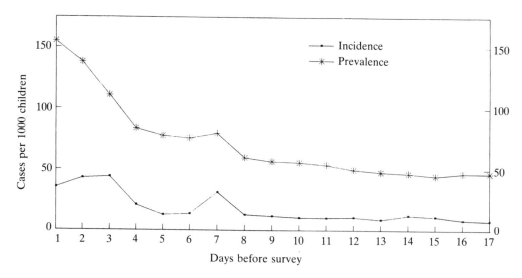

7 before the survey. For most of the days, however, incidence was only one-third of what it was during the three days prior to the interview.

## Treatment patterns

In Figure 3 the proportion of children with diarrhoea taken to a medical facility is plotted against the level of diarrhoea prevalence. There is a fairly consistent relationship between the two variables: the higher the level of diarrhoea prevalence in a country the lower the percentage visiting a medical facility ($R^2 = 0.60$). One of the major objectives of health interview surveys is to assess treatment patterns for current or recent illness episodes. Table 5 presents treatment patterns for under-fives with diarrhoea by status of diarrhoea (current or terminated) and by duration of current episodes for the five countries with data on duration. The upper part (A) of Table 5 shows the percentage of children taken to a medical facility, the middle part (B) the percentages having used oral rehydration packets and the lower part (C) the percentage having used home-made solution (with sugar and salt added to water).

The duration of the illness episode affected the reported treatment pattern. For current episodes of diarrhoea two days of duration appeared to be a good cut-off point. If diarrhoea had started at least two days before the interview, treatment patterns did not differ much from treatment patterns for the children whose diarrhoea had ended in the last two weeks.

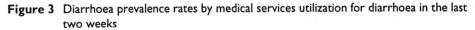

**Figure 3** Diarrhoea prevalence rates by medical services utilization for diarrhoea in the last two weeks

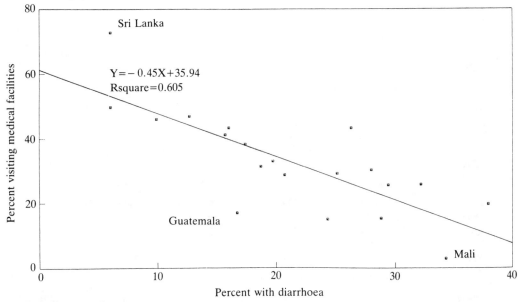

Children under 5 years

The cross-national analysis of DHS data on diarrhoea in the last 24 hours and during the last two weeks, and on duration of diarrhoeal episodes demonstrates the limitations of the use of retrospective morbidity data. There is evidence of considerable memory lapse within the two-week recall period in the DHS surveys. The indirect estimates of mean duration of a diarrhoeal episode, based on the CT ratios, were much higher in most DHS surveys (well over ten days in virtually all surveys) than mean durations reported by other (longitudinal) studies of diarrhoea in children, which are usually of the order of 5–6 days.[11,12] The direct estimates of mean duration of diarrhoeal episodes in the Bolivia and Tunisia DHS surveys were also considerably lower than the direct estimates. This discrepancy, due to a high CT ratio, may have been caused by under-reporting of diarrhoea cases that terminated 2–14 days before the interview. Additional evidence of omission of terminated cases of diarrhoea was found in the Bolivia DHS survey: data on daily prevalence and incidence of diarrhoea within the two-week recall period showed a rapid decline for the period more than 2–3 days before the interview. The decline in prevalence in the Bolivia DHS survey is larger than that observed in studies in Guatemala,[4] Bangladesh[5] and Ethiopia.[6] Another possible explanation, for the high CT ratios and corresponding indirect estimates of duration, is over-reporting of current/recent diarrhoea, as was also observed in Ethiopia.[6] The CT ratios may be high because of a tendency to report diarrhoea that ceased recently (but more than 24 hours ago) as diarrhoea cases in the last 24 hours, perhaps because the mother was unsure if the diarrhoea has ended, or in the belief that treatment would be provided. Such a time shift may occur to a greater extent if the reference period of 24 hours before the inter-

**Table 5**  Percentages of children with diarrhoea who were taken to a medical facility, receiving oral rehydration solution (ORS) packets, and receiving home-made sugar and salt solution

| Country | Diarrhoea in last 2 weeks | Currently diarrhoea All | < 2 days | ≥ 2 days | Diarrhoea terminated |
|---|---|---|---|---|---|
| | *Taken to medical facility* | | | | |
| Botswana | 48.1 | 44.9 | (19.2) | 53.1 | 50.6 |
| Kenya | 48.3 | 43.3 | 19.5 | 52.3 | 53.3 |
| Uganda | 31.5 | 28.2 | 15.1 | 30.9 | 35.6 |
| Tunisia | 15.0 | 14.1 | (4.3) | 15.2 | 15.9 |
| Bolivia | 25.0 | 20.8 | 21.2 | 20.7 | 30.5 |
| | *ORS packet used* | | | | |
| Botswana | 46.1 | 38.6 | (19.2) | 44.9 | 51.8 |
| Kenya | 20.7 | 18.1 | 11.7 | 20.1 | 23.5 |
| Uganda | 15.1 | 13.2 | 7.5 | 14.2 | 17.4 |
| Tunisia | 16.6 | 15.2 | (4.3) | 16.5 | 18.0 |
| Bolivia | 24.8 | 23.8 | 19.6 | 24.8 | 26.1 |
| | *Home-made sugar and salt solution used* | | | | |
| Botswana | 24.7 | 15.0 | (23.1) | 13.3 | 32.1 |
| Kenya | 47.6 | 44.0 | 35.1 | 48.4 | 51.3 |
| Uganda | 3.6 | 2.9 | 3.6 | 1.1 | 4.4 |
| Tunisia | 4.1 | 3.9 | (4.3) | 3.8 | 4.4 |
| Bolivia | 9.7 | 9.9 | 8.7 | 10.3 | 9.4 |

Percentage in parentheses means based on less than 50 children with diarrhoea, but more than 25. All other cells are based on more than 50.

view is not well understood by the respondent. This may be reflected by the fact that in about half of the countries the CT ratio was much higher for women without formal education. The relatively high proportion of diarrhoea cases reported by them in the last 24 hours may be due to difficulty in interpreting specific time periods.

An issue of special interest is differences in the magnitude of the recall errors by mothers' education. The socioeconomic differentials in childhood morbidity tend to be much less pronounced than for other child health status indicators (child mortality, nutritional status)[13] and this may in part be caused by differential reporting by mothers. Such differences have been observed by mothers' education for reporting of breastfeeding duration.[14] DHS data suggest that recall errors are more common among mothers with no education in most countries, as evidenced by the higher CR ratios among these women. This may be due to more under-reporting of past diarrhoea, or to more over-reporting of current diarrhoea. Part of the difference may be genuine: chronic diarrhoea could very well be more common among children of illiterate mothers.

For mothers it is difficult to recall the exact termination of more distant episodes of diarrhoea. In DHS surveys in Peru, the Dominican Republic and Bolivia, answers in weeks ago were recorded as such and not converted into days by the interviewer. A significant proportion of women responded by saying one or two weeks ago. What respondents mean by two weeks ago may vary between cultures. Assuming that the responses of two weeks ago refer to the period 11–17 days before the survey (1.5–2.5 weeks), diarrhoea prevalence in last two weeks will be over-estimated by about 2–7%, if all two weeks responses are included in the two-week recall period. Studies with one-week recall period would have similar problems.

The analysis of treatment practices by diarrhoea prevalence showed a surprisingly strong and inverse association between prevalence and proportion seeking medical assistance. Two explanations can be put forward. First, the relationship may be an effect of a common cause. A country with a poor overall development level has, for example, inadequate water supply and poor hygienic conditions for the majority of the population and diarrhoea is very common. Similarly, retarded development has led to a poor health services infrastructure and thus services are not available to most sick children. The second explanation may be that there are different reporting tendencies, which vary between countries and cultures. In countries with high levels of diarrhoea larger numbers of less severe cases are reported, as suggested by the lower levels of medical services utilization. On the other hand, one would think that in countries where diarrhoea is very common, mothers would be less likely to report mild episodes. These observations also suggest that retrospective morbidity data do not provide accurate estimates of diarrhoea prevalence.

The primary aim of the questions on diarrhoea in the DHS surveys, is to assess treatment patterns. As in most other studies a recall period of two weeks was selected, since it is considered the best balance between the quality of information that can be obtained on treatment (best for current or very recent illness) and the representativeness of that treatment information (possibly best for recent but not current episodes). The selection of a two-week recall period implies that treatment patterns are assessed jointly for a mixed group of sick children: diarrhoea which has terminated, diarrhoea which has just started, and diarrhoea which has been present for a while and still continues. DHS data show that there are no major differences in treatment patterns for children with terminated diarrhoea and children with current diarrhoea of at least two days duration. Both could be used to evaluate treatment practices.

However, the treatment patterns for children with current diarrhoea of less than two days duration are different and can be analyzed separately to assess home practices in the early stages of diarrhoea. It should also be taken into account that there appears to be under-reporting of diarrhoea in the first 1–2 days of illness, as was shown for five DHS countries This may be a recognition problem (by the mother), which has implications for health programmes: if the diarrhoea is not recognized as an illness it will not be treated as such.

The use of multiple questions on diarrhoea prevalence and duration has the advantage that data quality can be evaluated. However, it is obvious from the DHS survey results that reporting errors regarding disease prevalence vary considerably between surveys, both in magnitude and direction. No methods of correcting for recall errors are available, and this limits the comparability of the results. To assess diarrhoea prevalence it may be better to focus on point prevalence: children with diarrhoea at the time of the survey. In this case, however, over-reporting of diarrhoea should be taken into account in analysis of diarrhoea prevalence. To assess treatment practices a 24-hour recall period is adequate, if the duration of the episode is asked as well. Data quality concerning diarrhoea treatment of current episodes may be better than treatment patterns derived from a two-week recall period, in which selective under-reporting and inaccurate recall of treatment practices may occur. To limit health interview surveys to current episodes will, however, have implications for sample size requirements. The number of children with diarrhoea in the last 24 hours, which lasted at least two days, was about half of the number of children with diarrhoea in the last two weeks in the DHS surveys. Since the DHS surveys did not provide evidence of inaccurate recall of treatment for diarrhoeal episodes that terminated within the two-week recall period, there are no persuasive reasons for restricting the sample to children with current diarrhoea, since this would imply doubling the sample size. If the primary purpose of the survey is to assess treatment use two week recall periods are adequate.

## Acknowledgement

We wish to thank the staff of the WHO Control of Diarrhoeal Diseases Division, especially Dr J. Tulloch and Dr O. Fontaine, for their helpful comments on an earlier version of this paper.

## References

1 Ross D.A. and Vaughan J.P. Health interview surveys in developing countries: a methodological review. *Studies in Family Planning* 1986; 17: 78–94.
2 Kroeger A. Health interview surveys in developing countries: a review of methods and results. *Int. J Epidemiol* 1983: 12: 242–54.
3 Van Norren B., Boerma J.T., Sempebwa E.K.N. Simplifying the evaluation of primary health care programmes. *Soc Sci Med* 1989; 28: 1091–7.
4 Martorell R., Habicht J.P., Yarbrough C., Lechtig A., Klein R.E. Underreporting in fortnightly recall morbidity surveys. *Environ Child Health* 1976; 129–34.
5 Alam N., Henry F.J., Rahaman M.M. Reporting errors in one-week diarrhoea recall surveys: experience from a prospective study in rural Bangladesh. *Int J Epidemiol* 1989; 18: 697–700.
6 Freij L., Wall S. Exploring child health and its ecology: the Kirkos study in Addis Ababa. *Acta Paediatr Scand* 1977, Supplement 267.
7 Black R.E. Diarrhoeal diseases and child morbidity and mortality. In: Mosley W.H. and Chen L.C., Child survival: strategies for research, *Pop Dev Rev* 1984 suppl. vol 10: 141–62.
8 K. Kleinbaum D.G., Kupper L.L., Morgenstern H. *Epidemiologic research: principles and quantitative methods.* Belmont, California: Lifetime Learning Publications, 1982.
9 Rothman K.J. *Modern epidemiology.* Little, Brown and Company Publishers, Boston/ Toronto, 1986.
10 Freeman J., Hutchinson G.B. Prevalence, incidence and duration. *Am J Epidemiol* 1980; 112: 707–23.

11  Black R.E., Lopez de Romana G., Brown K.H., Bravo N., Balazar O.G., Creed-Kanashiro H. Incidence and etiology of infantile diarrhea and major routes of transmission in Huascar, Peru. *Am J Epidemiol* 1989; 129: 785–99.

12  Snyder J.D., Merson M.H. The magnitude of the global problem of acute diarrhoeal disease: a review of active surveillance data. Bulletin WHO 1982; 60: 605–13.

13  Boerma J.T., Sommerfelt A.E., Rutstein S.O. Childhood morbidity and Treatment patterns in the Demographic and Health Surveys. *DHS Comparahve Studies* No. 4, 1991.

14  Huttly S.R.A., Barros F.C., Victora C.G., Beria J.U., Vaughan J.P. Do mothers overestimate breastfeeding duration? An example of recall bias from a study in southern Brazil. *Am J Epidemiol* 1990; 132: 572—5.

5

# Comparison of substantive results from demographic and epidemiological survey methods

*J. Ties Boerma and Jeroen K. Van Ginneken*

*Boerma JT (editor),* **Measurement issues in maternal and child mortality, morbidity and health care: interdisciplinary approaches.** *IUSSP, Derouaux-Ordina Editions, Liège, 1992, pp. 27—60.*

## Introduction

Both demographic and epidemiological studies have made significant contributions to current knowledge of the determinants of child mortality. Demographic studies generally have focused on the socioeconomic and biodemographic determinants of child survival, while epidemiological studies have tended to concentrate on the biological processes of specific diseases (Mosley and Chen, 1984). Both scientific disciplines have become increasingly aware of the benefits of integrating their work. Together, they may provide the improved health information that is needed:

- to describe more accurately the magnitude of different health problems,
- to identify the determinants of child survival and development, and
- to evaluate the impact of health interventions (Gray, 1989).

During the last decade, several conceptual models have been developed which incorporate both biological and behavioural determinants of child survival (Mosley and Chen, 1984, Van Norren and Van Vianen, 1986). Using the Mosley-Chen conceptual framework, Gray (1989) showed how epidemiological methods can be applied to demographic surveys and can contribute to the knowledge of the determinants of child survival. For example, researchers can use diagnostic algorithms to determine the cause of death or use case-control methodology to study rare events like mortality. Likewise, demographic methods can be applied in the field of epidemiology. It has been suggested, for example, that the preceding birth technique could be used to estimate mortality trends among children of mothers attending maternal and child health clinics (Hill and Aguirre, 1990, Feachem et al., 1989).

Apart from exchanging methods and techniques, demographers and epidemiologists could integrate their disciplines by collaborating in joint research teams, as has been done in some longitudinal studies in the past. Also, studies focusing on the determinants of child survival in a single country or region could benefit from a review of both demographic and epidemiological sources of data. This was done to evaluate mortality trends at the national level in Kenya (Ewbank et al., 1986).

In addition to demographic and epidemiological surveys, a third type of population-based survey contributes to health knowledge in developing countries. Management-oriented surveys, mostly of the coverage of certain health interventions but also sometimes of child health status, are an additional source of health information. This type of survey has been developed by the World Health Organization and other international organizations to provide management data for child health programmes. The surveys are cross-sectional and collect information on a limited range of topics. They are, however, more commonly conducted than population-based epidemiological and demographic surveys.

This paper compares the substantive results of epidemiological and demographic studies, while exploring the key methodological issues that arise in making such comparisons. While there are a wide range of topics common to both disciplines, this review will be limited to just four areas: morbidity due to diarrhoea, morbidity due to lower respiratory infections, immunization coverage, and neonatal tetanus mortality.

## Focus of the comparison

### Morbidity: diarrhoea and ALRI

Two of the leading causes of death in childhood are diarrhoeal diseases and acute lower respiratory infections (ALRI), which, taken together, may account for as many as half of all childhood deaths in developing countries (UNICEF, 1990). Morbidity due to diarrhoea and respiratory infections is also relatively common, and it has important consequences for the nutritional status of children.

Population-based epidemiological surveys of child morbidity mostly focus on the relationship between common childhood diseases and malnutrition; on the identification of causal microbiological agents; and on the effects of feeding patterns, water supply and sanitation on diarrhoea or the effect of air quality on ALRI. Demographic surveys collect data on child morbidity primarily to ascertain treatment patterns. Such surveys have been widely used to measure morbidity and the utilization of health services, but they have several methodological problems. The lack of standardization both in survey methodology and in the methods of analysis limits the comparability of the results (Ross and Vaughan, 1986). Sociocultural factors also restrict their comparability (Kroeger, 1983).

Data on diarrhoea and its treatment are also available from management-oriented surveys carried out as part of the Control of Diarrhoeal Diseases programme (CDD) of the

World Health Organization (WHO). These surveys vary considerably in terms of data quality.[1]

Three issues will be addressed:
- How is the *diagnosis* of diarrhoea or acute respiratory infection made? The focus here is on how uniformly the diagnostic methods used in epidemiological studies are applied and on how feasible it is to collect morbidity information in cross-sectional surveys.
- What are the *incidence or prevalence levels of the disease*? Results from longitudinal studies and cross-sectional surveys (especially DHS surveys) are compared to assess the impact of different data collection methods on estimates of disease occurrence. Can demographic surveys yield valid estimates of morbidity?
- What is known about the socioeconomic *determinants of child morbidity*? In many demographic studies, mother's education and other aspects of socioeconomic status have a strong impact on childhood mortality. Given these relationships, it has been hypothesized that socioeconomic status also has an impact on morbidity in children below the age of five.

## Immunization

Data on immunization are of special interest, both because immunization is one of the intermediate variables through which socioeconomic factors could influence child morbidity and mortality and because it is probably one of the best indicators of the utilization of health services (especially the use of preventive services). Immunization programmes have received high priority in international and national health programmes in the 1980s, and most developing countries have reported immunization data on a regular basis. National estimates of coverage are based either on national coverage surveys, using a thirty-cluster sample methodology, or on health facility reports of the number of vaccinations given. This paper will compare coverage estimates from these sources of data with the results of demographic surveys.

## Neonatal tetanus mortality

Neonatal tetanus mortality is an important cause of death in many countries; it can easily be prevented by tetanus toxoid immunization during pregnancy and by clean cord-cutting and maintenance practices. Surveys are important to assess the magnitude of mortality due to neonatal tetanus, which often is underestimated by health planners (Stanfield and Galazka, 1984), and to show the impact of immunization programmes or programmes to train traditional birth attendants. Cross-sectional neonatal tetanus mortality surveys have been conducted in more than 40 countries (Steinglass et al., 1991). These surveys follow a two-step study design proposed by WHO. First, all live births in a specified time period before the survey (usually one year) are identified. Then, the cause of each neonatal death is determined.

Demographers generally consider the use of a short, fixed-recall period inadequate in mortality surveys. This paper will assess how great a discrepancy exists between estimates of neonatal mortality based on neonatal tetanus mortality surveys and estimates drawn from DHS surveys.

## Results

### Diarrhoea

*Measurement*
In 1982 Snyder and Merson (1982) reviewed 22 longitudinal studies on diarrhoea to assess the annual morbidity and mortality from acute diarrhoeal disease in the developing world. All but three of these studies were conducted before 1975. They concluded that children under 5 years of age had 2.2–3.0 new episodes of diarrhoea each year. There was great variation by age of the child, with a peak in prevalence at 6–23 months of age. The variability in the definitions of diarrhoea used in the various studies was remarkable.

Table 1 summarizes the characteristics of a number of more recent population-based *epidemiological surveys* on the occurrence of diarrhoea. Here also, there is considerable variation in the definition of diarrhoea. The most popular definition is at least three loose stools in a 24–hour period, and some studies add any loose stools with blood or mucus to that definition. Other studies, however, have a much less strict definition of diarrhoea. In Fortaleza, Brazil, for example, diarrhoea was defined as an increase in stool frequency or a decrease in consistency lasting at least one day (Schorling et al., 1990). This study reported 11 episodes per child per year, and 40 per cent of the episodes lasted only 1 or 2 days. In contrast, a study in Sudan did not consider episodes lasting less than one day to be diarrhoea and found such episodes to be rare, accounting for only 0.4 per cent of all episodes (El Samani et al., 1988).

A problem specific to longitudinal studies is how to define the end of an episode of diarrhoea. Most studies considered a diarrhoea-free period of 2–3 days adequate to distinguish between two episodes, although in some cases it was only one day. Pickering et al. (1987) showed that the choice of the length of the diarrhoea-free interval had a relatively small effect on the total number of episodes recorded or on the mean duration per episode. It did, however, have an effect on the prevalence of chronic diarrhoea.

A number of studies have relied on the mother's definition of diarrhoea; most demographic surveys have also taken this approach. If the correct term(s) for diarrhoea are not used, however, misreporting is likely. Some surveys are preceded by anthropological research. In Thailand, it was found that the regular term for diarrhoea did not cover diarrhoea in infants, because such episodes were thought to be natural and had a different name (Thongkrajai et al., 1990). In Bangladesh, four different illnesses can refer to diarrhoeal disease (Chowdhury et al., 1988). In the Gambia, diarrhoea was considered

**Table 1** Main characteristics of selected epidemiological. Studies on diarrhoea occurrence

| Study Location | Period of study | N of home visits/ 2 weeks | N of children | Age group (months) | Definition | Interval for end episode | Medical action | Reference |
|---|---|---|---|---|---|---|---|---|
| Bangladesh, Teknaf, rural | 1980-83 Three years | 2 | 390 | 6-23 | >= 3 loose stools in 24 hr. period | 48 hrs no symptoms | ORT, swab, referral | Alam et al. (1989a, 1989b) |
| Bangladesh, Dhaka, slums | 1984-85 3 months | 1 | 925 | 0-71 | >= 3 unformed stools in any 24 hr. period | No symptoms in 2 wks (previous round) | No | Clemens and Stanton (1987) |
| Bangladesh, Dhaka, slums | 1985 6 months | 1 | 1400 | 0-71 | >= 3 unformed stools in any 24 hr. period | No symptoms in 2 wks (previous round) | Control group | Stanton and Clemens (1987) |
| Bangladesh, Mirzapur, rural | 1984 9 months | 2 | 350 | 0-59 | >= 3 loose motions in in 24 hr. period | No symptoms for 2 days | Rectal swab | Huttly et al. (1989 |
| Bangladesh, Matlab, rural | 1978-79 One year | 7 | 197 | 2-59 | >= 4 liquid stools for at least one day | One day with fewer than 3 stools | Rectal swab | Black et al. (1982) |
| Bangladesh, Matlab, rural | 1978-79 One year | 2 | 207 | 0-59 | >= 3 abnormal stool movements or any grossly abnormal stool movement in 24 hrs. | Normal stool pattern returned for 48 hrs | None | Chen et al. (1981) |
| India, near Hyderabad, rural | ? One year | 4 | 721 | 0-59 | >= 3 loose stools or one watery motion in a day | NS | Referral | Mathar et al. (1985) |
| Papua NG, urban poor | 1987-88 One year | 7 | 479 | 0-59 | >= 3 loose stools on one day with or without blood or mucus | Diarrhoea-free period of three days | None | Bukenya and Nwokolo (1991) |
| Thailand, northeast, rural | 1985 4 months | 1 | 1364 | 0-59 | Mother's (two local terms) and >=3 loose stools in 24 hr. period | NS | None | Thongkrajai et al. (1990) |

**Table I** Main characteristics of selected epidemiological. Studies on diarrhoea occurrence (continued)

| Study Location | Period of study | N of home visits/ 2 weeks | N of children | Age group (months) | Definition | Interval for end episode | Medical action | Reference |
|---|---|---|---|---|---|---|---|---|
| Peru, Huascar peri-urban | 1982-84 | 6 | 153 | 0-11 | >=4 liquid stools for at least 1 day (>=6 for neonates, >=5 for children 1 mo. old) | More than 2 days, less than 3 (semi-) liquid stools | ORT, swab, stool sample, referral | Black et al. (1989); Lopez de Romana et al. (1989) |
| Brazil, Fortaleza, slums | 1984-86 Two years | 6 | 175 | 0-59 | Increase in stool frequency or decrease in consistency lasting at least 1 day | No symptoms for 3 days | Stool collection if diarrhoea reported (2nd yr) | Schorling et al. (1990) |
| Brazil, Pacatuba, urban and rural | 1978-80 | 2 | 54 | 0-59 | Change in stools: decreased consistency or increased frequency | No diarrhoea for 3 days | Stool specimen collection | Guerrant et al. (1983) |
| Mexico, Mexico, urban | 1984 | 2 | 284 | 0-35 | >=3 loose stools in a calendar day or any loose stool with blood/mucus | No symptoms for 2 days | Visit made by doctor and nurse | Sepulveda et al. (1988) |
| Sudan, El Faki Hashim, rural | 1983-84 | 1 | 258 | 0-59 | >=3 bowel movements on at least two consecutive days | Less than 3 movements per day for 3 days | None | El Samani et al. (1988) |
| Nigeria, Malumfashi, rural | 1979 | 2 | 343 | 6-35 | Mother's (local term) | NS | ORS packet | Tomkins (1981) |
| Nigeria, Ibadan, urban poor | 198? 16-24 months | 2 | 131 | 0-11 | Mother's (?) | NS | Stool specimen, referral | Oyejide and Fabbami (1988) |
| Gambia, Bakau, urban | 1982 4 months | 2 | 244 | 6-35 | Mother's | 3 days, no diarrhoea | None | Pickering et al. (1987) |
| Kenya, Machakos rural | 1976-77 One year | 1 | 3899 | 0-59 | Mother's | NS | Mostly not | Leewenburg et al. (1984) |

to have a clear and unequivocal translation, and therefore the mother's definition was used (Rowland, 1983).

A few studies have compared the mother's definition of diarrhoea with those adopted by researchers. In Sudan, 95 per cent of the children with reported diarrhoea had 3 or more stools per day (El Samani et al., 1988). The agreement between the researchers' definition of diarrhoea and the mother's reporting of diarrhoea was 97 per cent in Bangladesh (Black et al., 1982). In Kenya, mothers were thought to over-report diarrhoea by 15–40 per cent as compared with data based on criteria of the investigators (Leeuwenburg et al., 1984).

A validation study of the diagnosis of diarrhoea in the Philippines found that the diagnosis of diarrhoea (with or without other concomitant diagnoses) could be made based on reports of the occurrence of frequent loose or liquid stool (sensitivity 95–97 per cent and specificity 80 per cent, as compared to diagnoses from medical records) (Kalter et al., 1991). Additional questions on the number of stools (more than 6 per day) increased specificity to 95 per cent, but reduced sensitivity to less than 90 per cent. In Guatemala, sensitivity was 66 per cent and specificity was 99 per cent in a study comparing mother's reporting of diarrhoea with a physician's diagnosis of diarrhoea made on the same day (Martorell et al., 1975).

The frequency of household visits varies from 1 to 7 during a two-week period in the longitudinal studies (Table 1). Some studies used daily home records on the occurrence of diarrhoea, to be completed by the caretakers, to improve recall (Clemens and Stanton, 1987). Several epidemiological studies made only one visit every two weeks. In a longitudinal study in the Gambia, the interval between rounds was about 5 weeks (Rowland et al., 1988, not included in Table 1).

Most epidemiological studies include some medical action if diarrhoea is reported, such as a rectal swab, collection of a stool specimen, distribution of oral rehydration salts, medical examination, or referral to a clinic. These actions may cause both under-reporting and over-reporting, depending on the expectations and perceptions of the care-taker. In a survey in Lesotho, for example, diarrhoea with blood or mucus was heavily over-reported to the interviewing nurse, presumably because of treatment expectations. Over-reporting is perhaps more likely if the interviewer is a health worker. In a study in Nigeria, mothers received ORS packets if diarrhoea was reported. To reduce the risk of over-reporting to obtain more packets, the mothers were given an adequate supply of ORS packets (Tomkins, 1981).

In *cross-sectional surveys*, most studies have selected a two-week recall period as the best balance between minimizing the problem of recall errors and keeping a feasible sample size (Ross and Vaughan, 1986). Several studies, however, have shown that even during a two-week recall period, memory lapse occurs (Martorell et al., 1976, Alam et al., 1989, Freij and Wall, 1977, Boerma et al., 1991a). Under-reporting occurs

**Table 2** Number of episodes of diarrhoea per child per year by age in months, mean duration of diarrhoeal episodes, and calculated prevalence rates for last 24 hours and last 2 weeks (percentages)*

| Study area | Study period <=1 yr. | Number of episodes by age per year | | | | | Duration (days) 0-59 | Prevalence in last | |
|---|---|---|---|---|---|---|---|---|---|
| | | 0-5 | 6-11 | 12-23 | 24-59 | 0-59 | months | 24 hrs. | 2 wks. |
| Bangladesh, Dhaka | No | ← | → | → | → | 4.6 | - | 6.0 | 22.7 |
| Bangladesh, Teknaf | Yes | 6.5 | → | 4.1 | → | | | | |
| Bangladesh, Mirzapur | No | 2.4 | 4.4 | 5.0 | 3.5 | 3.8 | 5.0 | 4.9 | 18.4 |
| Bangladesh, Matlab | Yes | 7.3 | → | 6.3 | 5.1 | 5.6 | 5.0 | 7.1 | 27.0 |
| India, Hyderabad | Yes | - | 3.1 | | - | 1.6 | 3.6 | 1.5 | 7.2 |
| Papua NG, Port Moresby | Yes | 0.2 | 1.7 | 1.3 | 0.3 | 0.7 | | 0.9 | 3.4 |
| Thailand northeast | No | 2.8 | → | 1.6 | 0.7 | 1.3 | - | 1.7 | 6.4 |
| Peru, Huascar | Yes | 9.8 | → | | | - | 5.8 | | |
| Brazil, Fortaleza | Yes | 9.4 | 14.1 | 15.1 | 9.7 | 11.3 | 7.2 | 18.2 | 58.3 |
| Mexico, Mexico City | Yes | 4.4 | 5.3 | 3.9 | 2.0 | 3.9 | 3.0 | 3.1 | 17.0 |
| Sudan, El Faki | Yes | | | | | 3.4 | - | 4.4 | 16.5 |
| Gambia, Bakau | No | - | 9.3 | 9.4 | | | 4.4 | | |
| Kenya, Machakos | Yes | 4.1 | 6.4 | 4.1 | 1.3 | 2.7 | - | | |
| Nigeria, Malumfashi | No | - | ← | 5.6 | → | | 6.8 | | |
| Nigeria, Ibadan | Yes | 2.2 | 4.0 | 1.7 | - | - | 5.0 | 3.6 | 13.1 |

* The prevalence rates were calculated from the annual number of episodes (N(ill)) and the duration of episodes as follows:

$I(1) = N(ill) / 366,$

$P(1) = I(1) * D / (1 + I(1) * D) * 100$ and

$P(14) = 13 * I(1) * 100 + P(1),$ where

$I(1)$ is the one day incidence, and $P(1)$ and $P(14)$ are the prevalence rates in the last 24 hours and last two weeks, respectively.

- Indicates no data.

whenever the recall period is longer than 2 or 3 days. On the other hand, over-reporting of current diarrhoea (that is, within the last 24 hours) is a possibility in cross-sectional surveys (Boerma et al., 1991a, Huttly et al., 1987), due to misinterpretation of the recall period or to treatment expectations.

## Occurrence of diarrhoea

Most *epidemiological studies* involve rural or urban poor children, so that their results cannot be used to generalize about regional, national, or global numbers of episodes of diarrhoea per child per year. In addition, it must be remembered that, even though the number of observations is often large, the number of children is mostly small: the results are based on repeated observations of the same children.

In most longitudinal studies, the period of observation was at least 12 months, which eliminates the effects of seasonality or, at least, intra-annual variation. This is an advantage of longitudinal over cross-sectional approaches. Quite a few longitudinal studies, however, have lasted less than a year, and their results cannot be extrapolated to obtain annual estimates of disease load.

Table 2 presents data from longitudinal studies on the occurrence of diarrhoea. In most studies, the annual number of episodes of diarrhoea per child ranges from 2 to 5. Three urban studies report considerably more frequent episodes: 9.8 for infants in Peru (Black et al., 1989), 11.3 in Brazil (Schorling et al., 1990), and 2.8 episodes in a 15 week-period in the Gambia (Pickering et al., 1987). The age pattern of diarrhoea occurrence is fairly consistent: the incidence is highest at 6–11 and 12–23 months of age, followed by 0–5 months, and it declines after the second birthday. The average duration of diarrhoeal episodes reported by the studies varies from 3–7 days.

The data on the annual number of episodes per child and the duration of diarrhoeal episodes has been used to calculate diarrhoea prevalence rates (Table 2). This allows the results of the longitudinal studies to be compared with the results of cross-sectional surveys, which, for the most part, collect data on the prevalence of diarrhoea during the last two weeks or during the last 24 hours. Whenever data on duration were not available, it was assumed to be 5 days. Prevalence rates in the longitudinal studies range from 1 to 7 per cent for the last 24 hours and from 3 to 27 per cent for the last two weeks.

Table 3 presents age-specific data on diarrhoea prevalence within the last 24 hours and over the last two weeks in DHS and other cross-sectional surveys. The prevalence of diarrhoea in the last 2 weeks ranges from 6 to 36 per cent. While prevalence is generally somewhat higher than in the longitudinal surveys, the age-specific pattern of diarrhoea prevalence is quite similar in both types of surveys. More pronounced are the differences concerning the 24–hour recall period. In more than half of the DHS surveys, the prevalence of diarrhoea in the last 24 hours was more than 10 per cent; a rate

**Table 3**  Diarrhoea prevalence by age of the child (in months) for the two weeks preceding the survey and prevalence of diarrhoea in last 24 hours in selected DHS and other cross-sectional surveys

| Country | No. of children | <6 | 6–11 | 12–17 | 18–23 | 34–35 | 36–47 | 48–59 | Total | Last 24 hours |
|---|---|---|---|---|---|---|---|---|---|---|
| **DHS surveys** | | | | | | | | | | |
| Bolivia | 4753 | 24.9 | 39.9 | 44.5 | 41.9 | 31.5 | 23.4 | 17.6 | 30.5 | 16.9 |
| Burundi | 3403 | 21.5 | 35.0 | 32.6 | 18.4 | 14.4 | 8.5 | 6.8 | 17.6 | 8.4 |
| Ghana | 3529 | 18.3 | 38.5 | 43.1 | 42.7 | 28.3 | 18.8 | 12.5 | 27.2 | 13.9 |
| Guatemala | 4170 | 17.4 | 30.0 | 30.5 | 20.7 | 15.5 | 10.3 | 7.4 | 16.7 | 10.4 |
| Kenya | 6390 | 18.0 | 25.5 | 25.9 | 18.4 | 10.9 | 5.1 | 3.3 | 13.0 | 6.8 |
| Mali | 2736 | 33.2 | 44.5 | 42.5 | 48.7 | 44.9 | 27.2 | 19.2 | 35.9 | 20.2 |
| Peru | 2778 | 36.8 | 50.7 | 47.4 | 44.7 | 31.1 | 24.0 | 20.1 | 32.6 | 16.6 |
| Sri Lanka | 3820 | 11.1 | 11.3 | 10.6 | 8.8 | 5.0 | 2.6 | 1.9 | 6.0 | 2.2 |
| Tunisia | 4208 | 27.0 | 38.5 | 37.2 | 29.3 | 18.3 | 11.0 | 9.2 | 20.7 | 10.5 |
| **Other surveys** | | | | | | | | | | |
| Nigeria (Imo) | 2389 | 15.8 | 37.3 | ← 35.7 → | | ← 19.1 → | | | 24.0 | . |
| Zaire (Bas Z.) | 2870 | 11.0 | 34.0 | ← 24.0 → | | | ← 12.0 → | | 20.0 | . |
| Brazil (NE) | 6524 | | | | | | | | 15.1 | . |
| Ecuador | 4366 | ← 32.9 → | | ← 35.8 → | | ← 18.0 → | | | 24.9 | . |

Sources: Huttly et al., 1987 (Nigeria), Tsui et al., 1988 (Zaire), Barros et al., 1991 (Northeast Brazil), Monteith et al., 1991 (Ecuador) and Boerma et al., 1991 (DHS surveys).

that high was observed in only one longitudinal study, in Fortaleza, Brazil, where the incidence of diarrhoea was extremely high (Fortaleza, Brazil).

*Determinants*

Many *epidemiological studies* focus on intermediate variables affecting the incidence and duration of diarrhoea, particularly breastfeeding and supplementary feeding patterns, nutritional status, measles immunization, water supply, sanitation, and personal and domestic hygiene (Feachem, 1986). Quite a number of epidemiological studies have also tried to measure the impact of health interventions. In many of these studies, mortality has been used as the dependent variable, but there are others where morbidity measures were used. Demographic and socioeconomic variables often are not included in epidemiological studies, and, when they are, they are treated as confounding variables which have to be controlled. Rarely have they been considered as factors which in themselves could have an influence on morbidity or mortality.

For example, many studies use case-control methodology to assess the impact of water supply and sanitation on the occurrence of diarrhoea (Briscoe et al., 1986). A number of these studies have included socioeconomic variables to control for possible confounding. Generally, these controls did not affect the relationship between the water supply and sanitation variables and diarrhoea (Young and Briscoe, 1987, Baltazar et al., 1988, Daniels et al., 1990). Briscoe et al. (1988) suggested excluding confounders, since the costs in additional fieldwork may be higher than the potential benefits. However, few of these case-control studies have been designed to analyze the association between the occurrence of diarrhoea and socioeconomic or demographic variables.

One which did was a case-control study in Nicaragua, where it was found that the level of maternal education was significantly associated with diarrhoea morbidity (Gorter et al., 1991). No such effect was observed in another case-control study in Lesotho, however (Daniels et al., 1990). In a longitudinal study in Addis Ababa, Ethiopia, many socioeconomic variables had an impact on the prevalence of diarrhoea (Freij and Wall, 1977). Longitudinal data from urban Gambia indicated that the incidence of diarrhoea decreased with higher education, but the relationship was not significant (Pickering et al., 1989). In urban Bangladesh, there was no association between mother's level of education and the occurrence of diarrhoea, but both income and housing did have an effect (Stanton and Clemens, 1987). No effects of education were reported from two cross-sectional surveys in Imo State, Nigeria (Huttly et al., 1987) and from longitudinal studies in urban Papua New Guinea (Bukenya and Nwokolo, 1991) and Teknaf, Bangladesh (Alam et al., 1989).

In a *cross-sectional survey* in Zaire, there was no consistent relationship between the occurrence of diarrhoea and mother's age, birth order, or mother's level of education (Tsui et al., 1988). The authors, however, felt that selective under-reporting obscured the expected relationships. Women in the lower educational categories might have reported less morbidity than more educated women because education enhances health knowledge and the recognition of disease. No conclusive evidence of selective under-reporting, however, was presented in this study. Data from DHS surveys suggests that selective misreporting of diarrhoea does occur by mother's level of education (Boerma et al., 1991a).

A considerable amount of data on the correlates of diarrhoea morbidity are available from DHS surveys (Boerma et al., 1991b). Bivariate analysis of most DHS surveys shows only a weak effect of mother's education on diarrhoea occurrence, although the overall tendency is a lower prevalence among children of mothers with at least secondary education. DHS survey results also show weak relationships between diarrhoea and indicators of the level of hygiene, such as source of drinking water, use of toilet facilities, and presence of soap. The associations are in the expected direction in most countries. Mother's education had a significant effect on diarrhoea prevalence in a multivariate analysis of the 1989 Ecuador Maternal and Child Health survey (Monteith et al., 1991).

## Acute lower respiratory infections (ALRI)

### Measurement
Table 4 shows how the diagnosis of ALRI was made in selected population-based *epidemiological studies*, to explore how feasible these methods are for demographic

**Table 4** Main characteristics of selected epidemiological studies on occurrence of acute lower respiratory infections

| Study location | Period of study | N of home visits/ 2 weeks | Chil- dren | Age group (months) | Diagnosis | Reference |
|---|---|---|---|---|---|---|
| Bangladesh, Matlab, rural | 1978-79 One year | 7 | 197 | 2-59 | Physician; weekly visits to all households | Black et al. (1982) |
| China, Dong Ghuan, rural | 1981-83 2 years | 2 | 174 | 0-59 | Physician; visit to hospital if severely ill, and special ARI outpatient department for the study and fieldworkers (barefoot doctors) | Zhang et al. (1985) |
| Nepal, Kathmandu valley, rural | 1984 6 months | 1 | 1085 | 0-59 | Fieldworker with supervision of health assistant: cough, history of shortness of breath, rapid breathing, fever, chest indrawing, nasal flaring, auscultation | Pandey et al. (1985) |
| Papua NG, Asaro, rural | 1985-87 18 months | 4 | 156 | 0-59 | Physician or nurse (at health post): cough and respiratory rate >40/min. if not verified by health worker, history of cough + breathlessness | Smith et al. (1991) |
| Papua NG, Tari, rural | 1972-74 2 years | 1 | 1595 | 0-59 | Fieldworker referred children sick with cough. Doctor: cough or dyspnoea with respiratory distress symptoms and rapid breathing (>50 for infants, >40 if >=1 yr.) | Riley et al. (1981, 1983) |
| Peru, Huascar, peri-urban | 1982-84 | 6 | 153 | 0-11 | If symptoms of respiratory distress, child referred to physician: respiratory illness + fever + rapid breathing or dyspnoea = pneumonia and either ausculation or X-ray; resp. illness + bronchospasms = bronchiolitis | Lopez de Romana et al. (1989) |

**Table 4** Main characteristics of selected epidemiological studies on occurrence of acute lower respiratory infections  (continued)

| Study location | Period of study | N of home visits/ 2 weeks | Children | Age group (months) | Diagnosis | Reference |
|---|---|---|---|---|---|---|
| Burkina Faso, Bana, rural | 1983-4 6 months | 2 | 151 | 0-59 | Physician (about once a month a visit), parents' reports of symptoms (fever, nasal discharge, cough, auricular discharge) | Lang et al. (1986) |
| Gambia, Bakau, urban | 1981-2 2 years | 5 | 126 | 0-24 | Physician, visits to local clinics on monthly basis | Rowland et al. (1988) |
| Gambia, Basse, rural | 198? 2 years | 2 | 500 | 0-59 | Fieldworker: If rapid breathing and distress, referral to doctor: cough with RR >50/min., indrawing, wheeze/stridor.  Radiology. | Armstrong and Campbell (1991); Campbell et al. (1989) |
| Kenya, Machakos, rural | 1974-77 3 years | 1 | 3899 | 0-59 | Symptoms reported by mother: nasal discharge, cough, fever, ear discharge, respiratory distress (flaring nostrils, lower rib recession, etc.) | Van Ginneken (1990) |
| Philippines, Manila, urban poor | 1985-87 2 years | 2 | 1954 | 0-59 | Nurses or paramedical staff, at home; if cough with cyanosis, chest indrawing or RR >50/min., then ALRI; referred to physician for final diagnosis | Tupasi et al. (1990) |
| Thailand, Bangkok, urban poor | 1966-87 2 years | 4 | 674 | 0-59 | Home visit by fieldworker, revisits by researchers; referral to clinic; wheeze, rales, stridor, cyanosis, crepitation, RR >50/min. | Vathanophas et al. (1990) |
| Colombia, Cali, urban poor | 1987-89 17 months | 2 | 340 | 0-17 | Home visits by paramedical personnel; if any ARI symptom, referral to clinic.  Physician diagnosis: RR >50/min., rales, stridor, wheezing, cyanosis | Borrero et al. (1990) |

surveys. Reviews of acute respiratory infections, including data on ALRI mortality and upper respiratory infections, can be found elsewhere (Van Ginneken, 1990, Selwyn, 1990, and Pio et al., 1985).

In virtually all the studies in Table 4 the diagnosis was made by a physician, and, in addition to symptoms of respiratory illness and breathing abnormalities, specific signs at auscultation and sometimes radiology signs were used to diagnose ALRI. Only in the Kenya and Nepal studies were no physicians involved. Studies that use physicians may miss ALRI cases, since the children either must be brought to a health facility to be examined by a doctor or are visited by a physician much less frequently than by fieldworkers. In the Philippines, for example, only 63 per cent of the children referred to the health centre for suspected ALRI were actually seen at the centre (Tupasi et al., 1990).

Three of the studies in Table 4 were part of an inter-country study of epidemiology among young children (the BOSTID study). In this ten-country study focusing on urban children, lower respiratory tract infection was diagnosed if a child had at least one of six symptoms: rales or crepitations, wheezing, stridor, a respiratory rate of 50 or more per minute, cyanosis, or chest indrawing (Selwyn, 1990). An episode was considered new if the child had been free of symptoms of respiratory infection for a week. Apart from the BOSTID studies, only two of the studies in Table 4 specified the symptom-free interval required to distinguish between old and new episodes of ALRI. In Peru, a period of ten days without symptoms defined the end of an episode (Lopez de Romana et al., 1989), while in the Gambia a child was omitted from the study for two weeks after an episode to ensure that he or she had recovered (Armstrong and Campbell, 1991).

As with diarrhoea, the use of appropriate local terms is very important. For example, in Lesotho, a specific term is used for respiratory illness with breathing difficulties: *letsoejana*, 'little heart jumping' (Wilson and Kimane, 1989). In coastal Kenya, the term for illnesses with respiratory distress, *kushikwa mbavu*, 'one's ribs are being held,' is not very specific for pneumonia (Boerma and Baya, 1990). Studies in Guatemala, the Philippines, and Turkey suggest that local terminology for signs and symptoms of respiratory infections is very extensive (Black, 1990).

In *demographic surveys* generally it is not feasible to have physicians make the diagnosis of ALRI. Instead, the diagnosis is based on symptoms reported by the mother. Kalter et al. (1991) evaluated the validity of diagnoses of ALRI based on maternal health interviews in the Philippines, by comparing them with diagnoses found on medical records. A history of cough and dyspnoea (difficult breathing) with concomitant fever provided the optimal algorithm: sensitivity was 82 per cent and specificity was 79 per cent when compared to non-respiratory illnesses. Specificity dropped to 58 per cent if compared to upper respiratory tract infections. Specificity was slightly lower if the diagnosis of ALRI was made on the basis of cough and dyspnoea, irrespective of fever. If symptoms of respiratory distress were added (flaring of the nostrils or intercostal retractions), specificity increased to 83 per cent, but sensitivity fell to 68 per cent. Addition of information on the duration of the symptoms did not improve either specificity or sensitivity.

In the Gambia, information on clinical signs and symptoms was compared with radiological results (lobar consolidation) (Campbell et al., 1989). Intercostal indrawing and nasal flaring were not satisfactory predictors of pneumonia. High fever, vomiting, and refusal to breastfeed were the best predictors in infants, while the best predictors in children aged 1–4 were high fever and rapid breathing (more than 60 per minute). The diagnosis of pneumonia is more difficult in early infancy when cough and respiratory distress may not be as prominent as later in life: respiratory rates may be high under normal circumstances in awake infants, and specific symptoms, such as retractions or chest indrawings, are less specific for pneumonia (Berman, 1989).

More recent DHS surveys attempt to identify respiratory illnesses by two questions: the presence of cough and the presence of difficult breathing during the last two weeks. In addition, there is a question on the prevalence of fever during the same recall period.

*Occurrence of ALRI/pneumonia*
Table 5 presents the incidence and prevalence of ALRI by age of the child in a number of *epidemiological studies*. Most acute lower respiratory tract infections in young children are pneumonia, but two studies distinguished between pneumonia, bronchitis, and bronchiolitis. In both studies bronchitis was more frequently diagnosed than pneumonia, and it probably refers to milder forms of ALRI. The number of episodes with ALRI during the first year of life was between 0.3 and 0.8 in five studies, 1 in Peru, 2 in Colombia, and over 3 in Papua New Guinea. The incidence did not decrease much during the second year of life, with the exception of Papua New Guinea. In the Burkina Faso study, the incidence of episodes with coughing was computed from weekly reports by parents; there were more than 7 such episodes per child per year. In urban Thailand, 9 episodes of coughing per child per year were reported. In two studies in Table 5, the diagnosis based on clinical signs was compared with the diagnosis based on radiology. In both studies, about one-third of the clinical cases of ALRI were confirmed by radiology.

Prevalence of ALRI, as diagnosed by physicians, varied considerably between two studies in Sub-Saharan Africa, while prevalence was low in Peru and Bangladesh (Table 5). In Bana, Burkina Faso, a comparison of the prevalence of cough (as reported by parents) and the prevalence of ALRI (diagnosed by a doctor) showed that cough was about twice as prevalent as ALRI (22.5 versus 11.5 per 100 child days, respectively). In Machakos, Kenya, the prevalence of cough was markedly lower than in Burkina Faso, with 3.7 days with cough reported per 100 child days. Signs of respiratory distress were rarely reported in Kenya, with a prevalence of 0.06 per 100 child days. Very few studies report on the duration of ALRI episodes. In Peru, the episodes were short (3.3 days), but in Papua New Guinea where ALRI was very common, the mean duration of

**Table 5**    Incidence and prevalence of ALRI by age of the child in months in population-based epidemiological studies

| Study | Diagnosis or symptom | Episodes per child per year | | | | |
|---|---|---|---|---|---|---|
| | | 0–5 | 6–11 | 12–23 | 24–59 | 0–59 |
| Bangladesh, Matlab | Pneumonia | ◄— 0.57 —► | | | | |
| Peru, Huascar | Pneumonia | 0.11 | 0.22 | | | |
| | Bronchitis | 0.15 | 0.33 | | | |
| | Bronchiolitis | 0.09 | 0.18 | | | |
| | ALRI all | 0.35 | 0.73 | | | |
| Papua NG, Asaro | Pneumonia | 3.68 | 2.87 | 1.60 | 0.60 | 1.32 |
| Nepal, Kathmandu valley | ALRI all | ◄— 0.34 —► | | 0.55 | 0.20 | 0.30 |
| China, Dong Ghuan | Pneumonia | ◄— 0.08 —► | | ◄— 0.07 —► | | |
| | Bronchitis | ◄— 0.17 —► | | ◄— 0.22 —► | | |
| | Bronchiolitis | ◄— 0.04 —► | | ◄— 0.01 —► | | |
| | Asthma bronchitis | ◄— 0.00 —► | | ◄— 0.52 —► | | |
| | ALRI all | ◄— 0.29 —► | | ◄— 0.35 —► | | |
| Gambia, Basse | Pneumonia clinical | ◄— 0.70 —► | | 0.52 | 0.31 | 0.45 |
| | Pneumonia X-ray | ◄— 0.21 —► | | 0.17 | 0.16 | 0.17 |
| | Pneumonia clinical | ◄— 0.73 —► | | 0.39 | 0.09 | 0.28 |
| | Pneumonia X-ray | ◄— 0.26 —► | | ◄— 0.06 —► | | |
| Burkina Faso, Bana | Cough | ◄— 7.1 —► | | 8.0 | 7.4 | 7.5 |
| Philippines, Manila | ALRI | 0.6 | 0.9 | 0.8 | 0.4 | 0.5 |
| Thailand, Bangkok | ALRI | | | | | 0.07 |
| | Cough | | | | | 9.7 |
| Colombia, Cali | ALRI | 1.85 | 2.07 | 0.97 | | |
| Study | Diagnosis or symptom | Episodes per child per year | | | | |
| | | 0–5 | 6–11 | 12–23 | 24–59 | 0–59 |
| Bangladesh, Matlab | Pneumonia | | | | | 0.3 |
| Peru, Huascar | ALRI | ◄— 0.9 —► | | | | |
| Gambia, Bakau | ALRI | 2.3 | 5.7 | 3.8 | | |
| Burkina Faso, Bana | ALRI | ◄— 10.5 —► | | 14.0 | 11.0 | 11.5 |
| | Cough | ◄— 21.9 —► | | 23.1 | 22.7 | 22.5 |
| Kenya, Machakos | Cough | 3.8 | 5.0 | 4.1 | 3.0 | 3.7 |
| | Respiratory distress | 0.10 | 0.15 | 0.08 | 0.03 | 0.06 |

an episode was about 12 days. The latter, however, included the periods of cough and otitis media that often accompany ALRI episodes.

Table 6 presents results from recent *DHS surveys* on the prevalence of cough and dyspnoea in the two weeks preceding the interview.[2] prevalence rates are remarkably close for five of the six countries: they range from 41 to 49 per cent for cough and from 16 to 20 per cent for cough and dyspnoea. Only in Zimbabwe was the prevalence of cough with breathing difficulties considerably lower, but the questionnaire used in Zimbabwe was structured differently from the others. Questions about fever were asked in three of the surveys. In the Philippines (Kalter et al., 1991) the prevalence of cough with dyspnoea and fever proved to be the best algorithm for the diagnosis of ALRI. The preva-

**Table 6** Prevalence of symptoms of respiratory illness in the last two weeks among children under 5 years in DHS surveys, and prevalence of cough and dyspnoea by age in months

| Country | Year | N | Cough | Cough and dyspnoea | Cough and dyspnoea and fever | Cough and dyspnoea | | | |
|---|---|---|---|---|---|---|---|---|---|
| | | | | | | 0–5 | 6–11 | 12–23 | 24–59 |
| Egypt[1] | 1988 | 7912 | 43.4 | 20.2 | . | 18.0 | 28.9 | 23.1 | 18.2 |
| Sudan | 1989-90 | 5771 | 47.0 | 20.3 | 13.7 | 20.8 | 26.1 | 21.7 | 18.9 |
| Bolivia | 1989 | 5161 | 41.2 | 20.4 | . | 22.9 | 25.9 | 26.0 | 16.9 |
| Colombia | 1990 | 3641 | . | 15.8 | . | 20.3 | 20.1 | 16.2 | 14.1 |
| Paraguay | 1991 | 3715 | 44.0 | 17.8 | 12.3 | 10.5 | 25.4 | 22.1 | 16.1 |
| Zimbabwe[1] | 1988 | 2940 | 49.5 | 7.7 | 1.2 | 9.2 | 10.5 | 8.5 | 6.6 |

Missing values and don't know responses excluded.
1. Recall period 4 weeks.

lence of this combination of symptoms was 14 per cent in Sudan, 12 per cent in Paraguay, and 1 per cent in Zimbabwe. Age-specific data on the prevalence of cough with difficult breathing show that prevalence is somewhat lower after children's second birthday, but age patterns are much less pronounced than they are for diarrhoea.

The two-weekly prevalence rates for cough and dyspnoea are much higher in the DHS surveys than one would expect from the longitudinal studies. For example, one episode per child per year, assuming a mean duration of seven days per episode, would correspond with a two-week prevalence rate of 5.4 per cent (and a one day prevalence rate of 1.9 per cent). Even if fever is included, the prevalence of ALRI symptoms in DHS surveys still appears to be on the high side. Most likely, many of the children with cough and dyspnoea in DHS surveys have only upper respiratory tract infections.

*Determinants*
Paediatricians and epidemiologists have mentioned a number of specific risk factors (or determinants) for morbidity and mortality from acute respiratory infections. These include crowding in households, indoor air pollution, low birth weight, breastfeeding patterns, food availability, composition of the diet, and nutritional status of the child (Foster, 1984, Berman and McIntosh, 1985, and Pio et al., 1985). This section considers only demographic and socioeconomic determinants.

In two *longitudinal studies*, conducted in a rural area of Burkina Faso (Lang et al., 1986) and in an urban area of Ethiopia (Freij and Wall, 1977), various socioeconomic factors were not related to morbidity from respiratory infections. Birth order, however, did have an impact: morbidity was higher among children of high parity than among children of low parity. In the Ethiopian study, household size was included and also found to be related to morbidity.

Increasingly, research is conducted on the role indoor air pollution plays in acute respiratory infections in children. Two types of such pollution can be distinguished: smoke from cooking fires and smoke from cigarettes. Indoor air pollution is expected to be strongly related to socioeconomic status. A multi-country study found much higher levels of air pollutants from biofuels in traditionally built houses than in modern houses (Pandey et al., 1989). In studies in rural areas of Nepal and the Gambia, it was found that smoke from cooking fires and cigarettes did have an impact on morbidity due to acute respiratory infections in children (Pandey, 1985, Armstrong and Campbell, 1991).

Twelve *DHS surveys* provide information on the relationship between several demographic and socioeconomic factors and the indicators of acute respiratory infection (which may be cough, difficult breathing, or a combination of both) (Boerma et al., 1991b). In 6 of these surveys, ALRI prevalence tends to be higher among first-born children, and, in 8 of the 12 countries, children of younger mothers tend to have higher than average prevalence. In only a few of the 12 countries does mother's education have some impact on the prevalence of cough or breathing problems. In households with a radio, the prevalence of respiratory symptoms is generally lower than in households without a radio, but the differences are small. In a multivariate analysis of data from the 1989 Ecuador Maternal and Child Health Survey, severe acute respiratory infections were more common if the mother had at least 7 years of education, compared to children of less educated women (Monteith et al., 1991). The use of wood as cooking fuel was also associated with a greater prevalence of severe acute respiratory infections in this study.

## Immunization coverage

### Measurement

Immunization coverage rates are usually derived either from coverage surveys or from routine data collected by health facilities where vaccinations are given. Coverage surveys employ a standard survey methodology recommended by the Expanded Programme on Immunization (EPI) of the World Health Organization (Henderson and Sundaresan, 1982). The survey sample consists of 30 clusters selected with probability proportional to population size. In each cluster, the first household is randomly chosen and, to reduce survey costs, all subsequent households are selected from neighbouring households until at least seven children in a selected age group are identified. With this method, the level of immunization coverage can be estimated with a precision of about plus or minus 10 per cent (Lemeshow et al., 1985).

The EPI cluster sample coverage surveys are carried out in many countries, although two concerns have been raised regarding the reliability of their coverage estimates. First, the sample may be biased by overrepresentation of households located near health facilities. Secondly, the fact that interviews often are conducted by health workers may introduce another bias.

National coverage estimates can also be based on routinely reported clinic data. Data from these health information systems, however, are rarely complete and assumptions have to be made to extrapolate them to the national level. In addition, the denominator (the number of children eligible for vaccination) has to be estimated from other sources, such as population projections based on census data.

DHS surveys can be used to compare official estimates of immunization coverage based on either of the two methods, if the DHS survey covers the same time period. Since most EPI cluster coverage surveys focus on children 12–23 months of age, the comparison will be limited to this age group. As is done in EPI cluster sample surveys, information on vaccinations in DHS surveys is copied from the child health card if available. If no health card is presented, usually the mother is asked to recall specific vaccinations.[3]

*Levels of immunization coverage*
Table 7 presents data from 12 DHS surveys on immunization coverage for BCG, three doses of DPT and measles. Coverage estimates from all the EPI cluster sample surveys (available for Botswana, Kenya, Zimbabwe, Sudan, Ghana, and Nigeria) are close to the DHS figures. Coverage estimates based on clinic records, however, are much less consistent with DHS results. In Tunisia and Uganda, the health facility data agrees with the DHS estimates for the same time period; in Bolivia, health facility data for 1987–88 apparently underestimates coverage; and in Ghana, Nigeria, Paraguay, and Egypt, health facility data tends to overestimate immunization coverage relative to the DHS surveys.

*Determinants*
EPI cluster sample surveys are not designed to estimate coverage differentials. However, a few cross-sectional surveys other than DHS have explored the relationship between socioeconomic factors and immunization coverage. In surveys in urban areas of Cameroon and the Gambia, it was found, for instance, that coverage was lower for children of mothers with little or no education than for children whose mothers were more educated (Brown et al., 1982, Hanlon et al., 1988).

Data on correlates of coverage of BCG, DPT, and measles immunization are available from 19 DHS surveys. The results are derived from a bivariate analysis, limited to children 12–35 months old and based on information drawn from health cards. While the age of the mother and the sex of the child were not associated with immunization coverage, in many surveys first-born children were more vaccinated than children with a high birth order. Socioeconomic variables were more strongly related to coverage than demographic variables. Coverage in urban areas was much higher than in rural areas; children of mothers with no or a little education received fewer immunizations than children of mothers with higher education; and children in households with a radio had higher immunization levels than children in households without a radio (Boerma et al., 1991b).

**Table 7** Comparison of DHS and data reported to WHO on immunization coverage among children 12–23 months (percentages)

| Country | | BCG | DPT3 | Meas. | N | Remarks |
|---|---|---|---|---|---|---|
| Botswana | DHS Aug - Dec 1988 | 95 | 88 | 87 | 615 | Surveys in agreement with DHS |
| | Survey 1987 | 99 | 86 | 91 | 425 | |
| | Survey 1990 | 98 | 92 | 87 | NA | |
| Kenya | DHS Dec 1988 - May 1989 | 93 | 82 | 72 | 1315 | Large survey agrees well with DHS |
| | Survey 1987 | 86 | 75 | 60 | 2451 | |
| Zimbabwe | DHS Sep 1988 - Jan 1989 | 94 | 86 | 79 | 630 | Survey estimates close to DHS |
| | Survey 1988 | 97 | 79 | 83 | NA | |
| Sudan | DHS Nov 1989 - Jan 1990 | 76 | 60 | 61 | 1150 | Survey in line with DHS, 1990 |
| (Northern) | Survey early 1989 | 67 | 53 | 57 | 1260 | reported data appear overestimate |
| | Reported data 1990 | 94 | 81 | 71 | NA | |
| Ghana | DHS Feb - May 1988 | 69 | 42 | 51 | 782 | Survey data agree with DHS, but |
| | Survey 1987 | 71 | 37 | 40 | 209 | reported data overestimate |
| | Reported data 1988 | 94 | 45 | 67 | NA | |
| Nigeria | DHS Apr - Oct 1990 | 63 | 36 | 48 | 1356 | Survey 1989 in agreement with |
| | Survey 1989 | 58 | 44 | 46 | NA | DHS, but reported data for 1990 |
| | Reported data 1990 | 96 | 57 | 54 | NA | overestimate |
| Burundi | DHS Apr - Jul 1987 | 77 | 55 | 59 | 663 | Reported data are not consistent |
| | Reported data 1987 | 84 | 69 | 55 | NA | with high DPT3 |
| | Survey data 1989 | 53 | 47 | 39 | NA | |
| Bolivia | DHS Feb - Jul 1988 | 55 | 28 | 58 | 1108 | Reported data appear to |
| | Reported data 1987-88 | 27 | 39 | 44 | NA | underestimate coverage, although |
| | Reported data 1989 | 70 | 40 | 70 | NA | coverage may be increasing |
| Paraguay | DHS Apr - May 1990 | 66 | 52 | 57 | 815 | DHS in line with coverage year |
| | Reported data 1990 | 90 | 78 | 69 | NA | before, but 1990 reports |
| | Reported data 1989 | 58 | 68 | 59 | NA | overestimate |
| Egypt | DHS Oct 1988 - Jan 1989 | 70 | 66 | 76 | 1593 | Reported data appear serious |
| | Reported data 1988 | 80 | 87 | 84 | NA | overestimates, but DHS estimates |
| | Reported data 1989 | 83 | 90 | 93 | NA | also unreliable |
| Tunisia | DHS Jun - Oct 1988 | 95 | 88 | 78 | 759 | Reported data agree with DHS |
| | Reported data 1988 | 85 | 91 | 83 | NA | |
| Uganda | DHS Sep 1988 - Jan 1989 | 70 | 38 | 49 | 946 | Reported data in line with DHS |
| | Reported data 1988 | 77 | 40 | 49 | NA | |

Sources: WHO (1989, 1990), Boerma et al. (1990), and DHS country reports.

## Neonatal tetanus mortality

*Measurement*

In verbal autopsies, the diagnosis of neonatal tetanus is usually based on the following algorithm (Gray, 1989): death between the third and thirtieth day of life, a history of normal suckling and crying from birth through at least the first two days of life, trismus, and generalized stiffness or 'convulsions' with unremitting spasms. Algorithms of this kind have very high sensitivity.

Most cross-sectional surveys on neonatal tetanus mortality employ a 12–month recall period for neonatal deaths (Galazka and Stroh, 1986). The World Health Organization recommends interviewing mothers whose babies were born alive during a recent 12-month period. Whenever a neonatal death is mentioned, trained staff take a careful history of the circumstances of the death. The use of a 12–month recall period in a single round survey for estimating mortality is considered inaccurate in demography (Ewbank, 1984). There is a high risk that deaths and births will be omitted, and the method is also vulnerable to the misdating of events (both in and out of the reference period). Mortality rates are often underestimated by 30–40 per cent (Tabutin, 1984).

Surveys of neonatal tetanus mortality generally do not discuss the under-reporting of births and deaths. The only exception is a survey in Ivory Coast where a recall period of 20 months was used (WHO, 1983, Sokal et al., 1988). Massive under-reporting of neonatal deaths appeared to occur if the recall period was longer than 7 months. In response, some subsequent surveys even adopted a 6–month recall period (e.g. Maru et al., 1986). There also was, however, massive under-reporting of births in the Ivory Coast survey, which was thought to be due to the absence of women with older children who were working in the fields (Sokal et al., 1988), and no revisits were made. Thus, while under-reporting may increase with the length of the recall period, the Ivory Coast survey cannot be used as evidence of such a lapse within an 18–month recall period.

*Levels of neonatal tetanus mortality*

Mortality due to neonatal tetanus varies greatly between populations. For example, *longitudinal studies* in Niakhar, Senegal (Leroy and Garenne, 1987), and Matlab, Bangladesh (Bhatia, 1989), reported neonatal tetanus rates of 15.9 and 13.7 per 1,000 live births respectively – representing 31 and 20 per cent of all neonatal deaths. In both areas, tetanus toxoid coverage was quite low, and the majority of women delivered at home. On the other hand, a 1975–78 longitudinal study in Machakos, Kenya, found no deaths due to neonatal tetanus, even though three-quarters of the women delivered at home (Omondi-Odhiambo et al., 1990). Important factors affecting tetanus mortality are the proportion of women delivering in health facilities, tetanus toxoid coverage levels, environmental exposure to tetanus organisms, and traditional cord-cutting practices (Foster, 1984, Stanfield and Galazka, 1984).

Table 8 compares neonatal mortality rates from two sources: cross-sectional neonatal tetanus mortality surveys, using a 12–month recall period as outlined above, and DHS surveys. The DHS estimates are based on full birth histories. Data for corresponding time periods are available for seven countries. In Kenya, seven neonatal tetanus mortality surveys have been conducted during the period 1983–89 in areas where mortality is not expected to be lower than the national average (Melgaard et al., 1990, Steinglass et

**Table 8** Comparison of results of neonatal tetanus mortality surveys and DHS surveys in the same country: neonatal mortality rates (per 1,000 live births), neonatal tetanus mortality rates (per 1,000 live births) and percent of neonatal deaths due to neonatal tetanus

| Country/Area | Neonatal tetanus mortality surveys | | | | | | DHS surveys | | |
| --- | --- | --- | --- | --- | --- | --- | --- | --- | --- |
| | Year | N | Neonatal mortality rate | NTT mortality rate | Per cent NTT of neonatal deaths | | Area | Year | Neonatal mortality rate |
| **Kenya** | | | | | | | | | |
| Kisii | 1983 | 2301 | 9.6 | 5.6 | 59.1 | | National | 1983-88 | 41.7 |
| Meru | 1984 | 2132 | 15.9 | 11.3 | 70.6 | | | | |
| Tana River | 1985 | 2133 | 22.5 | 15.5 | 68.8 | | | | |
| Meru | 1985 | 2132 | 16.4 | 11.3 | 68.6 | | | | |
| Kisii | 1985 | 2301 | 9.6 | 5.6 | 59.1 | | | | |
| Meru | 1986 | 859 | 14.0 | 3.5 | 25.0 | | | | |
| Kilifi | 1989 | 2556 | 21.1 | 3.1 | 14.8 | | | | |
| **Tunisia** | | | | | | | | | |
| National | 1988 | 9478 | 12.3 | 1.2 | 9.4 | | National | 1983-88 | 27.8 |
| Rural | 1988 | 3167 | 20.8 | 2.8 | 13.6 | | Urban | 1978-87 | 26.3 |
| Urban | 1988 | 6311 | 8.1 | 0.3 | 3.9 | | Rural | 1978-87 | 32.7 |
| **Indonesia** | | | | | | | | | |
| Rural | 1979 | 1570 | 49.1 | 22.9 | 46.2 | | National | 1977-83 | 41.9 |
| 19 provinces | 1982 | 4971 | 20.9 | 10.7 | 51.0 | | Rural | 1977-86 | 39.9 |
| Urban | 1982 | 2310 | 17.3 | 6.9 | 40.0 | | Urban | 1977-86 | 24.5 |
| **Egypt** | | | | | | | | | |
| National | 1986 | 8286 | 13.0 | 7.0 | 53.7 | | National | 1984-88 | 38.5 |
| Rural | 1986 | | 18.0 | 10.0 | 54.0 | | Rural | 1979-88 | 57.6 |
| Urban | 1986 | | 5.0 | 2.0 | 53.0 | | Urban | 1979-88 | 33.2 |
| **Togo** | | | | | | | | | |
| Plateaux | 1984 | 4966 | 10.9 | 5.6 | 51.9 | | National | 1978-82 | 46.0 |
| | | | | | | | National | 1983-88 | 43.4 |
| **Ghana** | | | | | | | | | |
| National | 1989 | 2694 | 22.3 | 2.6 | 33.3 | | National | 1983-88 | 43.8 |
| **Sudan** | | | | | | | | | |
| National | 1981 | 9632 | 21.4 | 6.9 | 32.0 | | National | 1980-84 | 41.7 |
| Rural | 1981 | 5117 | 27.9 | 8.6 | 30.8 | | Rural | 1980-90 | 45.4 |
| Urban | 1981 | 4515 | 14.0 | 4.9 | 34.9 | | Urban | 1980-90 | 37.4 |

Sources: WHO (1991), DHS country reports and Sullivan et al. (1990).

al., 1989). The neonatal mortality rates vary from about 10 to 22 per 1,000 live births, which is about half the national estimate of neonatal mortality obtained from the DHS survey (41.7 per 1,000 live births). In Tunisia, the national neonatal tetanus survey in 1988 reported a neonatal mortality rate of 12.3 per 1,000 live births, which is also less than half the DHS estimate for the period 1983–88. Likewise, in Indonesia, neonatal tetanus surveys in Jakarta and 19 provinces (Arnold et al., 1986) showed considerably lower levels of neonatal mortality than did the DHS estimate for the period 1977–82.

The levels of neonatal mortality in national neonatal tetanus surveys were also about half the DHS estimates in Ghana, Egypt, and Sudan.

This comparison clearly shows that neonatal tetanus surveys using a 12–month recall period yield much lower neonatal mortality levels than do DHS surveys. The DHS results themselves are certainly not free from recall bias and may be an underestimate as well. The fact that neonatal tetanus surveys apparently miss about half of neonatal deaths may, however, have important implications for the estimates of the levels of neonatal tetanus mortality. The issue is whether neonatal tetanus deaths are subject to the same recall bias as other neonatal deaths. There are two reasons to suspect that neonatal tetanus deaths may be reported better than other neonatal deaths. First, neonatal tetanus deaths generally occur after three days of life, and under-reporting is less serious at 3–30 days than for first-and second-day deaths. Second, the identification of deaths due to neonatal tetanus is the subject of the survey, which reduces the likelihood of under-reporting. Zimicki (1990) suggested that a similar mechanism caused relative over-reporting of tetanus deaths during the neonatal period in Matlab, Bangladesh.

## Conclusions

This review of the methods and results of epidemiological and demographic studies on child morbidity, immunization, and neonatal tetanus mortality has demonstrated the importance of integrating the two disciplines. Such integration is necessary to obtain the full benefits of expensive longitudinal studies of child health, but it can also improve the scope and relevance of smaller studies, such as case-control studies. Likewise, demographic surveys can become useful instruments for the collection of epidemiological information, as evidenced by DHS surveys. They can also contribute significantly to the understanding of major determinants of child survival and thus to the development of health programmes.

A review of epidemiological studies of diarrhoea showed considerable diversity in definitions of diarrhoea, study designs, and the incidence of diarrhoea. Reporting of diarrhoea in demographic surveys generally relies on mother's reports, and misreporting of diarrhoea is thought to be common. Both epidemiological and demographic studies would benefit from the use of a standard set of questions, to be used by all studies, to determine the occurrence of diarrhoea. These questions would cover not only the mother's definition of diarrhoea, but also a diagnostic algorithm like the one proposed by Kalter et al. (1990). Further validation studies of instruments to measure diarrhoea morbidity under field conditions are required.

The determinants of diarrhoea morbidity can only be studied if a satisfactory and standardized algorithm for the diagnosis of diarrhoea has been used. Currently, socioeconomic and demographic variables are conspicuously absent in many epidemiological studies, while demographic surveys have not been able to show consistent evidence of differentials in the prevalence of diarrhoea, except in analyses by the age of the child. Questions on the occurrence of diarrhoea in management-oriented surveys and in demographic surveys are often primarily aimed at assessing treatment patterns. Their assessments of treatment patterns will also be less reliable if the occurrence of diarrhoea is not measured accurately.

The situation regarding ALRI is even more complicated than that for diarrhoea. The diagnosis of ALRI morbidity in epidemiological studies largely depends on examinations by physicians, and demographic surveys do not have such staff in the field. Furthermore, ALRI is a relatively rare event, so its incidence is more difficult to determine. The current questions on the prevalence of cough and difficult breathing (with fever) used in DHS surveys appear to be the most feasible approach to identifying ALRI, although specificity is likely to be low. Knowledge of the socioeconomic and demographic determinants of ALRI morbidity is limited, and, in this respect, the situation is similar to that for diarrhoea.

The review of data on immunization coverage compared the results of thirty-cluster sample surveys, which are recommended by WHO, with data from DHS surveys. The comparison showed that estimates of both sources were in the same range for most countries. Reported data based on health information systems, however, have to be approached with scepticism and, at present, cannot be considered a good substitute for population-based surveys. Demographic surveys also can make an important contribution to the knowledge of the determinants of childhood immunization.

To assess the quality of the data gathered by special neonatal tetanus mortality surveys with a 12–month recall period, their neonatal mortality rates were compared with those reported by demographic surveys relying on birth histories. Under-reporting of neonatal deaths in neonatal tetanus surveys was extremely high, and, on average, half of the neonatal deaths were missed. It is unclear to what extent this affects the estimates of neonatal tetanus mortality produced by such surveys. It is likely that these surveys overestimate the problem of neonatal tetanus mortality, at least when it is expressed as the proportion of neonatal deaths caused by tetanus to all neonatal deaths.

## Notes

1  The focus of the CDD surveys is on treatment patterns, although there are also modules to estimate morbidity and mortality levels associated with diarrhoea. For treatment questions, the surveys use a 24-hour recall period for diarrhoea occurrence; however, they ask for *incidence* during the last two weeks (which is unusual for a cross-sectional survey). Most CDD surveys focus on children under 5 years of age, but there is no information on the age of the children. A recently published example of a well-documented survey of this kind is Barros et al. (1991).

2  Questions on respiratory symptoms have changed considerably since the first years of the DHS project, when most surveys did not distinguish between cough and dyspnoea. Table 6 only includes

those surveys with separate questions on cough and difficult breathing. The 1990 Colombia survey permits estimations of the prevalence levels of cough, but the data were not available when this table was produced.

3   In some DHS surveys, data on specific vaccinations was limited to children for whom a health card was presented to the interviewer. For children without a health card, the mother was asked whether the child had ever been vaccinated, but no data on specific vaccinations were asked. The procedure used to obtain vaccination coverage estimates for all children is outlined in Boerma et al. (1990). Of the surveys listed in Table 7, this procedure was used for Botswana, Kenya, Zimbabwe, Burundi, Egypt and Uganda. The remaining 6 DHS surveys in this table included data on specific vaccinations from mothers' reports.

## References

Alam N, Henry FJ, Rahaman MM (1989). Reporting errors in one-week diarrhoea recall surveys: experience from a prospective study in rural Bangladesh. *Int J Epidemiol* 18: 697–700.

Alam N, Wojtyniak B, Henry F and Rahaman MM (1989). Mothers' personal and domestic hygiene and diarrhoea incidence in young children in rural Bangladesh. *Int J Epidemiol* 18: 242–247.

Armstrong JRM and Campbell H (1991). Indoor air pollution exposure and lower respiratory infections in young Gambian children. *Int J Epidemiol* 20: 424–429.

Arnold RB, Soewarso TI and Karyadi A (1986). Mortality from neonatal tetanus in Indonesia: results from two surveys. *Bull World Hlth Organ* 64: 259–262.

Baltazar J, Briscoe J, Mesola V, Moe C, Solon F, Vanderslice J and Young B (1988). Can the case-control method be used to assess the impact of water supply and sanitation on diarrhoea? A study in the Philippines. *Bull World Hlth Organ* 66: 627–35.

Barros FC, Victora CG, Forsberg B, Maranhao AGK, Stegeman M et al. (1991). Management of childhood diarrhoea at the household level: a population-based survey in north-east Brazil. *Bull World Hlth Organ* 69: 59–65.

Berman S (1990). Overview of pneumonia in early infancy. In: Gadomski A (ed.) Acute lower respiratory infections and child survival in developing countries: understanding the current status and directions for the 1990s. Proceedings of a workshop, Washington DC, pp. 39–52.

Berman S and McIntosh K (1985). Selective primary health care: strategies for control of disease in the developing world. XXI Acute respiratory infections. *Rev Inf Dis* 7: 674–691.

Bhatia S (1989). Patterns and causes of neonatal and postneonatal mortality in rural Bangladesh. *Stud Fam Plann* 20: 136–146.

Black RE (1990). Household management of diarrhea and acute respiratory infections. Report of a scientific meeting. Johns Hopkins University, Occasional Paper No.12, Baltimore, Maryland.

Black RE, Brown KH and Becker S (1984). Malnutrition is a determining factor in diarrheal duration, but not incidence, among young children in a longitudinal study in rural Bangladesh. *Am J Clin Nutr* 37: 87–94.

Black RE, Brown KH, Becker S and Yunus M (1982). Longitudinal studies of infectious diseases and physical growth of children in rural Bangladesh I. Patterns of morbidity. *Am J Epidemiol.* 115: 305–314.

Black RE, Huber DH and Curlin GT (1980). Reduction of neonatal tetanus by mass immunization of non-pregnant women: duration of protection provided by one or two doses of alumimium-absorbed tetanus toxoid. *Bull World Hlth Organ* 58: 927–930.

Black RE, Lopez de Romana G, Brown KH, Bravo N, Bazalar OG, Creed-Kanashiro H (1989). Incidence and etiology of infantile diarrhoea and major routes of transmission. *Am J Epidemiol* 129: 785–799.

Boerma JT and Baya MS (1990). Maternal and child health in an ethnomedical perspective: traditional and modern medicine in coastal Kenya. *Hlth Pol Plann* 5: 347–357.

Boerma JT, Black RE, Sommerfelt AE, Rutstein SO and Bicego GT (1991a). Accuracy and completeness of mothers' recall of diarrhoea occurrence in pre-school children in Demographic and Health Surveys. *Int J Epidemiol* 20: 1073–1080.

Boerma JT, Sommerfelt AE and Rutstein SO (1991b). Childhood Morbidity and Treatment Patterns in Demographic and Health Surveys. *DHS Comparative Studies* #4, Institute for Resource Development, Columbia, Maryland.

Boerma JT, Sommerfelt AE, Rutstein SO and Rojas G (1990). Immunization: levels, trends and differentials in the Demographic and Health Surveys. *DHS Comparative Studies* #1, Institute for Resource Development, Columbia, Maryland.

Borrero IH, Fajardo LP, Bedoya A, Zea A, Carmona F and De Borrero MF (1990). Acute respiratory tract infections among a birth cohort of children from Cali, Colombia, who were studied through 17 months of age. *Rev Inf Dis* 12 Suppl 8: S950–S956.

Briscoe J, Baltazar J and Young B (1988). Case-control studies of the effect of environmental sanitation on diarrhoea morbidity: methodological implications of field studies in Africa and Asia. *Int J Epidemiol* 17: 441–447.

Brown J, Djogdom P, Murphy K, Kesseng G and Heymann D (1982). Identifying the reasons for low immunization coverage: a case study of Yaounde (United Republic of Cameroon). *Rev Epidem Sante Publ* 30: 35–47.

Bukenya G and Nwokolo N (1991). Compound hygiene, presence of standpipe and the risk of childhood diarrhoea in an urban settlement of Papua New Guinea. *Int J Epidemiol* 20: 534–539.

Campbell H, Byass P, Lamont AC, Forgie IM, O'Neill KP, Lloyd-Evans N and Greenwood BM (1989). Assessment of clinical criteria for identification of severe acute lower respiratory tract infections in children. *Lancet* 1: 297–299.

Chen LC, Huq E and Huffman SL (1981). A prospective study of the risk of diarrheal diseases according to the nutritional status of children. *Am J Epidemiol* 114: 284–292.

Chowdhury A, Mushtaque R, and Vaughan JP (1988). Use and safety of home-made oral rehydration solutions: an epidemiological evaluation from Bangladesh. *Int J Epidemiol* 17: 655–665.

Clemens JD and Stanton BF (1987). An educational intervention for altering water-sanitation behaviors to reduce childhood diarrhea in urban Bangladesh. *Am J Epidemiol* 125: 284–291.

Daniels DL, Cousens SN, Makoae LN and Feachem RG (1990). A case-control study of the impact of improved sanitation on diarrhoea morbidity in Lesotho. *Bull World Hlth Organ* 68: 455–463.

Duboz P (1984). Mortalite et morbidite infantile et juvenile en Republique du Congo. *Cah ORSTOM ser Sci Hum* XX: 157–169.

El Samani EFZ, Willett WC and Ware JH (1988). Association of malnutrition and diarrhea in children aged under five years. A prospective follow-up study in a rural Sudanese community. *Am J Epidemiol* 128: 93–105.

Ewbank DC, Henin R and Kekovole J (1986). An integration of demographic and epidemiologic research on mortality in Kenya. In: United Nations, *Determinants of mortality change and differentials in developing countries: the five country case study project.* Depart. of International Economic and Social Affairs, Population Studies 94.

Ewbank DC (1984). Uses of mortality data for evaluating the success of specific health and development programmes. In: United Nations, *Data bases for mortality measurement.* Department of International Economic and Social Affairs, Population Studies #84.

Feachem RG, Graham WJ and Timaeus IM (1989). Identifying health problems and health research priorities in developing countries. *J Trop Med Hyg* 92: 133–191.

Feachem RG (1986). Preventing diarrhoea: what are the policy options? *Hlth Pol Plann* 1: 109–117.

Foster SO (1984). Immunizable and respiratory diseases and child mortality. In: WH Mosley and LC Chen (eds.), Child survival: strategies for research. *Pop Dev Rev* suppl to vol 10, pp. 119–140.

Freij L and Wall S (1977). Exploring child health and its ecology: the Kirkos study in Addis Ababa. *Acta Paed Scand* Suppl 267.

Galazka A and Stroh G (1986). Neonatal tetanus: guidelines on the community-based survey on neonatal tetanus mortality. Unpublished document EPI/GEN/86.8, WHO, Geneva.

Gorter AC, Sandiford P, Smith GD and Pauw JP (1991). Water supply, sanitation and diarrhoeal disease in Nicaragua: results from a case-control study. *Int J Epidemiol* 20: 527–533.

Gray RH (1989). The integration of demographic and epidemiologic approaches to studies of health in developing countries. In: Ruzicka L, Wunsch G and Kane P (eds.), *Differential mortality: methodological issues and biosocial factors*, Clarendon Press, Oxford, pp. 36–63.

Guerrant RL, Kirchhoff LV, Shields DS, Nations MK, Leslie J et al. (1983). Prospective study of diarrheal illnesses in Northeastern Brazil: patterns of disease, nutritional impact, etiologies, and risk factors. *J Inf Dis* 148: 986–997.

Hanlon P, Byass P, Yamuah M, Hayes R, Bennett S and M, Boge BH (1988). Factors influencing vaccination compliance in peri-urban Gambian children. *J Trop Med Hyg* 91: 29–33.

Henderson RH and Sundaresan T (1982). Cluster sampling to assess immunization coverage: a review of experience with a simplified sampling method. *Bull World Hlth Organ* 60: 253–260.

Hill AG and Aguirre A (1990). Childhood mortality estimation using the preceding birth technique: some applications and extensions. *Pop Stud* 44: 317–340.

Huttly SRA, Hoque BA, Aziz KMA, Hasan KZ, Rahaman MM, and Feachem RG (1989). Persistent diarrhoea in a rural area of Bangladesh: a community-based longitudinal study. *Int J Epidemiol* 18: 964–969.

Huttly SRA, Blum D, Kirkwood RR, Emeh RN and Feachem RG (1987). The epidemiology of acute diarrhoea in a rural community in Imo State, Nigeria. *Trans Roy Soc Trop Med Hyg* 81: 865–870.

Kalter HD, Gray RH, Black RE and Gultiano SA (1991). Validation of the diagnosis of childhood morbidity using maternal health interviews. *Int J Epidemiol* 20: 193–198.

Kroeger A (1983). Health interview surveys in developing countries: a review of methods and results. *Int J Epidemiol* 12: 242–254.

Lang T, Lafaix C, Fassin D, Arnaut I, Salmon B, Baudon D and Ezekiel J (1986). Acute respiratory infections: a longitudinal study of 151 children in Burkina Faso. *Int J Epidemiol* 15: 553–561.

Leeuwenberg J, Gemert W, Muller AS and Patel SC (1984). The incidence of diarrhoeal disease. In: JK Van Ginneken and AS Muller (eds). *Maternal and Child Health in Rural Kenya: An Epidemiological Study*, Croom Helm, London, pp. 109–117.

Lemeshow S, Tserkovnyi AG, Tulloch JL, Dowd SK, Lwanga SK and Keja J (1985). A computer simulation of the EPI survey strategy. *Int J Epidemiol* 14: 473–481.

Leroy O and Garenne M (1987). La mortalite par tetanos neonatal: la situation a Niakhar au Senegal. In: Proceedings of IUSSP seminar on mortality and society in Africa south of the Sahara, Yaounde, 19–23 October.

Lopez de Romana G, Brown KH, Black RE and Creed-Kanashiro H (1989). Longitudinal studies of infectious diseases and physical growth of infants in Huascar, an underprivileged peri-urban community in Lima, Peru. *Am J Epidemiol* 129: 769–784.

Martorell R, Habicht JP, Yarbrough C, Lechtig A, Klein RE (1976). Under-reporting in fortnightly recall morbidity surveys. *Env Child Hlth* 1976: 129–134.

Maru M, Getahun A and Hosana S (1988). A house-to-house survey of neonatal tetanus in urban and rural areas in the Gondar region, Ethiopia. *Trop Geogr Med* 40: 233–236.

Mathur R, Reddy V, Naidu AN, Ravikumar and Krishnamachari KAVR (1985). Nutritional status and diarrhoeal morbidity: a longitudinal study in rural Indian preschool children. *Hum Nutr: Clin Nutr* 39C: 447–454.

Melgaard B, Mutie DM and Kimani G (1988). A cluster survey of mortality due to neonatal tetanus in Kenya. *Int J Epidemiol* 17: 174–177.

Monteith R, Stupp P, Montana E and Oroczo L (1991). Risk factors for cause-specific child mortality and morbidity in Ecuador. Paper presented at PAA Annual meetings, Washington DC, March 20–23.

Mosley WH and Chen LC (1984). An analytic framework for the study of child survival in developing countries. In: WH Mosley and LC Chen (eds.), Child survival: strategies for research. *Pop Dev Rev* suppl to vol 10, pp. 25–45.

Omondi-Odhiambo, Van Ginneken JK and Voorhoeve AM (1990). Mortality by cause of death in a rural area of Machakos District, Kenya in 1975–78. *J biosoc Sci* 22: 63–75.

Oyejide CO and Fagbami AH (1988). An epidemiological study of rotavirus diarrhoea in a cohort of Nigerian infants: II. Incidence of diarrhoea in the first two years of life. *Int J Epidemiol* 17: 908–912.

Pandey MR, Boleij JSM, Smith KR and Wafula EM (1989). Indoor air pollution in developing countries and acute respiratory infection in children. *Lancet* 1: 427–429.

Pandey MR, Shrama PR and Nuepane RP (1985). Preliminary report of a community study of childhood ARI in Nepal. In: Douglas RM and Kerby-Eaton E (eds.), *Acute respiratory infections in childhood*. Dept of Community Medicine, University of Adelaide, pp.131–135.

Pickering H, Hayes RJ, Tomkins AM, Carson D and Dunn DT (1987). Alternative measures of diarrhoeal morbidity and their association with social and environmental factors in urban children in The Gambia. *Trans Roy Soc Trop Med Hyg* 81: 853–859.

Pio A, Leowski J and ten Dam HG (1985). The magnitude of the problem of acute respiratory infections. In: Douglas RM and Kerby-Eaton E (eds.), *Acute respiratory infections in childhood*. Dept of Community Medicine, Univ. of Adelaide, pp.3–16.

Riley ID, Carrad E, Gratten H, Gratten M, Lovuru K et al. (1983). The status on acute respiratory infections in children in Papua New Guinea. *Ped Res* 17: 1041–1043.

Riley ID, Everingham FA, Smith DE and Douglas RM (1981). Immunization with a polyvalent pneumococcal vaccine. *Arch Dis Childhood* 56: 354–357.

Ross DA and Vaughan JP (1986). Health interview surveys in developing countries: a methodological review. *Stud Fam Plann* 17: 78–94.

Rowland MG, Rowland SG and Cole TJ (1988). Impact of infection on the growth of children from 0 to 2 years in an urban West African community. *Am J Clin Nutr* 47: 134–138.

Rowland MGM (1983). Epidemiology of childhood diarrhoea in the Gambia. In Chen LC and Scrimshaw NS (eds.), *Diarrhea and malnutrition: interactions, mechanisms and interventions*, New York, Plenum Press, pp. 87–98.

Schorling JB, Wanke CA, Schorling SK, McAuliffe JF, de Souza MA and Guerrant RL (1990). A prospective study of persistent diarrhoea among children in an urban Brazilian slum. *Am J Epidemiol* 132: 144–156.

Selwyn BJ (1990). The epidemiology of acute respiratory tract infection in young children: comparison of findings from several developing countries. *Rev Inf Dis* 12 Suppl 8: S870–S888.

Sepulveda J, Willett W and Munoz A (1988). Malnutrition and diarrhoea. *Am J Epidemiol* 127: 365–376.

Smith TA, Lehman D, Coakley C, Spooner V, Alpers MP (1991). Relationships between growth and acute lower-respiratory infections in children aged 5 y in a highland population in Papua New Guinea. *Am J Clin Nutr* 53: 963–970.

Snyder JD and Merson MH (1982). The magnitude of the global problem of acute diarrhoeal disease: a review of active surveillance data. *Bull World Hlth Organ* 60: 605–613.

Sokal DC, Imbouo-Bogui G, Soga G, Emmou C and Jones TS (1988). Mortality from neonatal tetanus in rural Cote d'Ivoire. *Bull World Hlth Organ* 66: 69–76.

Stanfield JP and Galazka A (1984). Neonatal tetanus in the world today. *Bull World Hlth Organ* 62: 647–69.

Stanton BF and Clemens JD (1987). Socio-economic variables and rates of diarrhoea-disease in urban Bangladesh. *Trans Roy Soc Trop Med Hyg* 81: 278–282.

Steinglass R, Brenzel L and Percy A (1991). Tetanus. In: Jamison DT and Mosley WH (editors), Disease control priorities in developing countries. New York: Oxford University Press for the World Bank, forthcoming.

Steinglass R, Mutie DM, Kimani G, Mjomba M, Orinda V and Bjerregaard P (1989). Neonatal tetanus mortality in Kilifi district, Kenya: preliminary results of a community survey, 1989. Paper presented at the Kenya Paediatric Association Annual Scientific Conference, Nairobi, May 3.

Sullivan JM, Bicego GT and Rutstein SO (1990). Assessment of the quality of data used for the direct estimation of infant and child mortality in the Demographic and Health surveys. In: Institute for Resource Development, Assessment of DHS-I data quality. *DHS Methodological Reports* No. 1, Columbia, Maryland.

Tabutin D (1984). Comparison of single and multi-round surveys for measuring mortality in developing countries. In: Vallin J, Pollard JH and Heligman L (eds.), Methodologies for the collection and analysis of mortality data. Proceedings of a seminar at Dakar, Senegal, July 7–10, 1981, Liege: Ordina Editions, pp.11–25.

Thongkrajai E, Stoeckel J and Thongkrajai P (1990). Nutritional status and the incidence and duration of diarrhoeal disease among children in Northeast Thailand. *Soc Sci Med* 30: 773–776.

Tomkins A (1981). Nutritional status and severity of diarrhoea among pre-school children in rural Nigeria. *Lancet* 1: 860–862.

Tsui AO, DeClerque J and Mangani M (1988). Maternal and sociodemographic correlates of child morbidity in Bas-Zaire: the effects of maternal reporting. *Soc Sci Med* 26: 701–713.

Tupasi TE, De Leon LE, Lupisan S, Torres CU, Leonor ZA et al. (1990). Patterns of acute respiratory tract infection in children: a longitudinal study in a depressed community in metro Manila. *Rev Inf Dis* 12 Suppl 8: S940–S949.

UNICEF (1990). *The State of the World's Children* 1990. Oxford University Press.

Van Ginneken JK (1990). Behavioural factors affecting transmission and treatment of acute respiratory infections. In: What we know about health transition: the cultural, social and behavioural determinants of health. Proceedings of workshop, Canberra, May 1989, volume II, Health Transition Centre, Australian National University, Canberra, pp. 843–863.

Van Norren B and Van Vianen HAW (1986). The malnutrition-infections syndrome and its demographic outcome in developing countries. Programming Committee for Demographic Research Publication No.4, The Hague.

Vathanophas K, Sangchai R, Raktham S, Pariyanonda A, Thangsuvan J et al. (1990). A community-based study of acute respiratory tract infection in Thailand. *Rev Inf Dis* 12 suppl 8: S957–S965.

Wilson RP and Kimane I (1990). Mothers' perception of ALRI: a case study in Lesotho. In: Gadomski A (ed.) Acute lower respiratory infections and child survival in developing countries: understanding the current status and directions for the 1990s. Proceedings of a workshop, Washington DC, pp. 153–60.

World Health Organization (1991). EPI Information System. Unpublished document: EPI/CEIS/91.1, WHO, Geneva.

World Health Organization (1989). CDD Household Survey Manual. Diarrhoea Case Management, Morbidity and Mortality. Unpublished Document CDD/SER/86.2 Rev 1., WHO, Geneva.

Young G and Briscoe J (1988). A case study of the effect of environmental sanitation on diarrhoea morbidity in Malawi. *J Epidemiol Comm Hlth* 42: 83–88.

Zhang Z, Gao L, Wang Z, Cao Y, Wu G, Zhu Z (1985). Acute respiratory infections in childhood in Beijing. Part 1. Epidemiological studies at Dong Guan Brigade. In: Douglas RM and Kerby-Eaton E (eds.), *Acute respiratory infections in childhood*, Dept of Community Medicine, University of Adelaide, pp.115–121.

Zimicki S (1986). Old and new approaches to assessment of the cause structure of mortality: a case study from Bangladesh. In: Vallin J, D'Souza S and Palloni A (eds.), *Measurement and analysis of mortality: new approaches*. Clarendon Press, Oxford, pp. 99–122.

6

# Validation study of verbal autopsy method for causes of childhood mortality in Namibia

*Cynthia C. Mobley, J. Ties Boerma, Stephen Titus, Britte Lohrke, K. Shangula, Robert E. Black*

## Abstract

Verbal autopsy, a method used in developing countries, uses caretaker interview to determine the cause of death. We conducted a study of the major causes of death in Namibia to determine the validity of this method. A questionnaire, including signs and symptoms of the diagnoses of interest was administered to the caretaker in 135 deaths that were identified from hospital records. The 243 diagnoses included malnutrition (77), diarrhoea (73), pneumonia (36), malaria (33), and measles (24). Sensitivity and specificity of various algorithms of reported signs and symptoms were compared to the medical diagnoses. An algorithm for malnutrition (very thin of swelling) had 73% sensitivity and 76% specificity. An algorithm for cerebral malaria (fever, loss of consciousness or convulsion) had 72% sensitivity and 85% specificity while for all malaria deaths, the same algorithm had low sensitivity (45%) and high specificity (61%). Cough with dyspnoea or tachypnoea had 72% sensitivity and 64% specificity. An algorithm for measles (age $\geq$ 120 days, rash) had 71% sensitivity and 85% specificity. The study results suggest verbal autopsy data can be useful to ascertain the leading causes of death in childhood, but may not be adequate for health impact evaluation.

## Introduction

The need for accurate infant and childhood mortality data in developing countries is great, as this information is essential in establishing priorities for health care programs, planning intervention strategies and evaluating their effectiveness.[1] However, this information can be difficult to ascertain in developing countries where childhood deaths frequently occur at home and vital statistic data are often unreliable.[2] Demographers have developed techniques for obtaining estimates of infant and child mortality rates in developing countries, but simple methods for obtaining cause-specific mortality rates are also needed.

One such method of obtaining cause-specific mortality rates is through the use of the verbal autopsy, an interview-based method of diagnosis which involves questioning the caretaker of the deceased child about illness prior to death.[3] Although this method is increasingly used in national cross-sectional health surveys in developing countries to determine causes of death in childhood, few validation studies of the method have been performed. One was conducted by Kalter et al. in the Philippines[4] for four causes of death (diarrhoea, acute lower respiratory infection, measles, and neonatal tetanus). A study by Snow et al.[5] compared verbal autopsy with medical diagnosis in Kenya, including malaria and malnutrition. Since the results of verbal autopsy validation studies may be influenced by causes of death in childhood was conducted in Namibia. Included were five leading causes of death: diarrhoea, malnutrition, pneumonia, malaria, and measles.

## Methods

The validation study was conducted during the period March 30 through May 9, 1992. Childhood deaths selected for the study were obtained through examination of death registries and ward logbooks at three rural hospitals in northwest Namibia, a region inhabited by the Ovambo. Children who had died under the age of 5 years with one or more of the five diagnoses of interest (malnutrition, diarrhoea, pneumonia, malaria, and measles) were identified. Originally, the study also included neonatal tetanus deaths, but too few neonatal tetanus deaths occurred to permit validation. Deaths selected had occurred between January 1, 1989 and March 15, 1992 at two hospitals and between June 1, 1991 and March 15, 1992 at one hospital. Two of the hospitals were mission hospitals and one was a large district referral state hospital. Two of the hospitals were mission hospitals and one was a large district referral state hospital. In addition to serving a large area in northwest Namibia, the hospitals also served people from southern Angola, who belong to the same ethnic group.

A total of 517 childhood deaths included at least one of the diagnoses of interest. Of these deaths, medical records were obtainable and diagnoses were confirmed for 281 (54%), according to pre-determined criteria. Medical record abstraction was performed by the first author, a paediatrician. Information abstracted included the following, where available; place of residence; identification of relative and headman; gender; dates of birth, admission, and death; admission; history of present illness; laboratory and other diagnostic studies; hospital course and treatment; admission, intercurrent and death certificate diagnoses. Some records contained incomplete medical information.

Access to medical records, quality and quantity of medical record documentation, and availability and diagnostic test varied among the hospitals. However, deaths in the three hospitals were similar regarding maternal age, education level, and parity.

Deaths were selected if the child had at least one of the five diagnoses of interest on admission or developed any of the diagnoses during hospitalization, based on the medical record information. Minimum criteria were established to determine each diagnosis, as follows:

- *Malnutrition* – physician diagnosis of kwashiorkor *or* admission weight-for-age less than or equal to 3 standard deviations below the mean;
- *Diarrhoea* – documentation of diarrhoeal stools during hospitalization *or* history of diarrhoea and diagnosis of dehydration;
- *Pneumonia* – physician diagnosis of pneumonia *and* either a positive chest X-ray or auscultation of rales;
- *Malaria* – physician diagnosis of malaria and positive blood smear for malaria parasites *or* physician diagnosis of cerebral malaria and documentation of unconsciousness of seizure;
- *Measles* – physician diagnosis of measles during the three months prior to death, at an age of greater than 4 months, *and* observation of the typical measles rash or desquamation.

In the determination of wasting, three standard deviations below the mean was selected as the weight-for-age cut-off because it is commonly used in defining severely malnourished individuals who are also at increased mortality risk. To minimize the possibility of over-diagnosis of wasting in those children admitted with concurrent dehydration, a conservative weight adjustment was performed by adding ten percent to the admission weight. However, in the final analysis, the admission weight was used, as there was little difference in the results when compared to the adjusted weight.

The study questionnaire was developed based on the questionnaire used in the Philippines verbal autopsy validation study and on previous experience with the Cameroon DHS survey. It was translated into the local language (Oshiwambo) and modifications were made based on discussions held with hospital staff, Ministry of Health and Social Services staff, and other key informants. Emphasis was placed on obtaining the most accurate translation for specific keywords and phrases and included translation of some keywords and phrases into both of the two major dialects of Oshiwambo. There are seven dialects of Oshiwambo but most residents of the study region spoke at least one of these two major dialects. The questionnaire was translated back into English for verification. Households of the deceased children were located by two interviewer teams. The interviewers were Namibia secondary school graduates who spoke both Oshiwambo and English. Interviewers were provided with information necessary to locate household of the child, but not the child's cause of death.

Selection of the respondent took place upon arrival at a study household. First choice for the respondent was the primary caretaker of the child during the illness prior to death. If unavailable, another adult who was present during the illness prior to death. If unavailable, another adult who was present during and knowledgeable about the child's illness prior to death was interviewed. If a caretaker could not be located, the death was excluded from the study.

Of the 281 abstracted medical records, caretakers of 135 (48%) children were located and interviewed. The relationship of the respondent to the child was mother (61%), grandmother (28%), aunt (8%), father (2%), and other relative or unrelated (2%). One caretaker declined the interview.

The questionnaire was administered after verbal consent was obtained. Following some basic demographic data and open-ended questions, the questionnaire included at least one filter question for each of the five diagnoses of interest. With an affirmative response to any of the filter questions, the interviewer was directed to the corresponding disease-specific module that included more closed-ended and a few open-ended questions.

Questionnaire and medical record abstraction data were entered data analyzed using Epi Info Version 5.01b. The disease-specific filter questions and their corresponding modules of questions were analyzed to determine the sensitivity and specificity of individual questions and various combinations of questions in predicting the medical diagnosis. Unless specified, the comparison group for determination of specificity included all other deaths that did not have the disease of interest as a diagnosis.

## Results

Among the 135 deaths, 82 (61%) had multiple diagnoses of interest and 51 (38%) had one diagnosis. The total 243 diagnoses of interest included malnutrition (77), diarrhoeal disease (73), pneumonia (36), malaria (33), and measles (24) (Table 1). Of those with multiple diagnoses, one child had five diagnoses, two had four diagnoses, 21 had three diagnoses and 58 had two diagnoses.

Of the interviews completed, 53% of the deaths were male and 47% were female. The mean age at death was approximately sixteen months. Those with malaria were the oldest (25 months). The mean interval between death and administration of the interview for all children was about 18 months. The mean duration of hospitalization during the illness that led to death was 10 days. According to the respondents, the children were ill for an average of 3 days (range 1–16 days) before treatment was sought for the illness with which the child eventually died.

### Diarrhoea
The presence of reported loose or liquid stool had 89% sensitivity and 61% specificity (Table 2). With the addition of 3 or more loose or liquid stools, the sensitivity decreased to 82% and specificity stayed the same. However, with increasing stool frequency, the sensitivity decreased while the specificity increased. Similarly, with loose

**Table 1** Death by cause with age at death, timing of interview and duration of stay in hospital (mean in days with standard deviation in parentheses)

| Diagnosis | Number of deaths | Mean age at death | Mean death-interview interval | Mean hospital duration |
|---|---|---|---|---|
| Malnutrition | 77 | 472 (233) | 585 (255) | 13 (13) |
| Diarrhoea | 73 | 475 (266) | 576 (263) | 13 (13) |
| Pneumonia | 36 | 327 (307) | 605 (238) | 8 (10) |
| Malaria | 33 | 766 (577) | 398 (200) | 9 (12) |
| Measles | 24 | 510 (262) | 669 (200) | 14 (15) |
| All deaths | 135 | 488 (381) | 534 (279) | 10 (12) |

**Table 2** Sensitivity and specificity of reported symptoms in diagnosis of diarrhoea associated deaths (n=73) compared to no-diarrhoea associated deaths (n=62)

| Reported signs/symptoms | Sensitivity (%) | Specificity (%) |
|---|---|---|
| Loose or liquid stool | 89 | 61 |
| > - 3 loose or liquid stools per day | 82 | 61 |
| > - 4 loose or liquid stools per day | 75 | 68 |
| > - 5 loose or liquid stools per day | 56 | 74 |
| > - 6 loose or liquid stools per day | 36 | 90 |
| Loose or liquid stool, thirst or sunken eyes | 75 | 71 |

**Table 3** Sensitivity and specificity of reported signs and symptoms in diagnosis of dehydration (n=45) compared to no-reported dehydration (n=20) among children with diarrhoea associated deaths and reported loose or liquid stool

| Reported signs/symptoms | Sensitivity (%) | Specificity (%) |
|---|---|---|
| Thirsty | 73 | 30 |
| Dry mouth | 67 | 35 |
| Weak | 67 | 50 |
| Sunken eyes | 64 | 60 |
| No tears if crying | 16 | 80 |
| Decreased urine amount | 11 | 85 |
| > - 2 of the above signs | 84 | 35 |
| > - 3 of the above signs | 67 | 50 |
| > - 4 of the above signs | 40 | 75 |

or liquid stools combined with either thirst or sunken eyes, sensitivity was 75% and specificity was 71%.

Also examined were various signs and symptoms of dehydration reported in children with diarrhoea, dehydration and caretaker report of loose of liquid stools compared to children with diarrhoea, no dehydration, and caretaker report of loose of liquid stools (Table 3). None of these individual signs or symptoms had both high sensitivity and specificity. When two or more signs or symptoms were present, the sensitivity was 84% and specificity was 35%, and the addition of other signs or symptoms decreased the sensitivity but increased the specificity. Algorithms with various combination had sensitivity and specificity that were substantially better than other combination, the results of one such algorithm is included here. With the report of loose or liquid stools, thirst and sunken eyes, the sensitivity was 75% and specificity was 71%.

## Malnutrition
Of the 77 malnutrition associated deaths, 51 (66%) had only wasting, 22 (29%) had both wasting and kwashiorkor, and four (5%) had only kwashiorkor. As kwashiorkor may occur in the absence of wasting and visa versa, and the clinical manifestations are different, validation of the questions and combinations of questions was performed for each separately. For kwashiorkor, the sensitivity of swelling was 76% and the specificity was 75% (Table 4). The addition of swelling duration longer than two weeks resulted in a substantial loss in sensitivity (50%) and increase in specificity (93%). For wasting, very thin had 60% sensitivity and 79% specificity.

When wasting or kwashiorkor-associated deaths were considered together, sensitivities of reported very thin alone (60%) or swelling alone (47%) were low with specificities of 81% and 86%, respectively. However, with the use of very thin *or* swelling, the sensitivity (73%) was greater than either alone and the specificity (76%) was somewhat lower.

Comparison of algorithms using the adjusted (for dehydration) and non-adjusted weight-for-age resulted in little difference in sensitivity and specificity (results not shown).

## Pneumonia
Cough alone had 78% sensitivity and 55% specificity (Table 5). The presence of cough until death had a sensitivity of 69% and specificity of 66%, as cough with dyspnoea. Another algorithm, that cough with dyspnoea or tachypnoea, had a 72% sensitivity and 64% specificity. The addition of other questions relating to cough duration or dyspnoea duration had little effect on sensitivity and specificity dropped slightly. Similarly, fever, dyspnoea or specific signs of dyspnoea lowered sensitivity with little improvement in specificity.

**Table 4** Sensitivity and specificity of reported signs and symptoms in diagnosis of malnutrition compared to no-reported malnutrition associated deaths

| Reported signs/symptoms | Compared with | Sensitivity (%) | Specificit y (%) |
|---|---|---|---|
| Swelling anywhere | K | 77 | 75 |
| Swelling anywhere, orange/red hair | K | 64 | 81 |
| Swelling anywhere, feet swollen | K | 62 | 83 |
| Swelling anywhere, > - two weeks | K | 50 | 93 |
| Very thin | W | 60 | 79 |
| Very thin > - two weeks | W | 56 | 84 |
| Very thin | K/W | 60 | 81 |
| Swelling anywhere | K/W | 47 | 86 |
| Very thin or swelling anywhere | K/W | 73 | 76 |

K - Kwashiorkor (n - 26) W - Wasting (n - 73) K/W Kwashiorkor or wasting (n - 77).

**Table 5** Sensitivity and specificity of reported signs and symptoms in diagnosis of pneumonia (n=36) compared to non-pneumonia associated deaths (n=99)

| Reported signs/symptoms | Sensitivity (%) | Specificity (%) |
|---|---|---|
| Cough | 78 | 55 |
| Cough, dyspnoea | 69 | 67 |
| Cough until death | 69 | 66 |
| Cough, dyspnoea or tachypnoea | 72 | 64 |
| Cough, fever | 67 | 65 |
| Cough, fever, dyspnoea or tachypnoea | 61 | 71 |

## Measles

An algorithm of signs and symptoms related to measles (Table 6) resulted in a 71% sensitivity and 85% specificity for an age greater than 120 days and presence of rash. Addition of rash and/or fever for three or more days decreased sensitivity but only increased specificity slightly.

## Malaria

Of the 33 malaria associated deaths, 18 were diagnoses of cerebral malaria and the other 15 diagnoses were based on blood smears positive for malaria parasites. Ten cases of cerebral malaria also had positive blood smears. Of the 25 total positive blood smears, 11 were described as highly positive or had greater than 1% infected red blood cells and 14 were described as positive or had less than 1% infected cells. The mean haemoglobin of all malaria deaths was 7.7 gm% (SD=2.7) compared to 9.7 gm% (SD=2.7) for non-malaria associated deaths. Among malaria deaths, the mean haemo-

**Table 6** Sensitivity and specificity of reported signs and symptoms in diagnosis of measles (n=24) compared to non-measles associated deaths (n=111)

| Reported signs/symptoms | Sensitivity (%) | Specificity (%) |
|---|---|---|
| Age at death > - 120 days, rash | 71 | 85 |
| Age at death > - 120 days, rash, fever > - 3 days | 67 | 90 |
| Age at death > - 120 days, rash > - 3 days, fever > - 3 days | 54 | 90 |

**Table 7** Sensitivity and specificity of reported signs and symptoms in diagnosis of all malaria associated deaths (n=33) and cerebral malaria (n=18), each compared to non-malaria associated deaths (n=102 and n=117 respectively)

| Reported signs/symptoms | Malaria compared to non-malaria | | Cerebral malaria compared to non-cerebral malaria | |
|---|---|---|---|---|
| | Sensitivity (%) | Specificity (%) | Sensitivity (%) | Specificity (%) |
| Fever | 94 | 26 | 94 | 24 |
| Fever, pallor | 67 | 41 | 72 | 40 |
| Fever, shaking of the body | 46 | 78 | 39 | 53 |
| Fever, convulsions | 42 | 91 | 65 | 90 |
| Fever, loss of consciousness | 41 | 89 | 56 | 86 |
| Fever, convulsions of loss of consciousness | 45 | 87 | 72 | 85 |

globin was 7.3. gm% (SD=2.3) in cases with cerebral malaria and 8.1 gm % (SD=3.1) in the blood smear based cases. This compared to 9.8 gm% (SD=2.1) for non-malaria deaths. Among malaria deaths, the mean haemoglobin was 7.3 gm% (SD=2.3) in cases with cerebral malaria and 8.1 gm% (SD=3.1) in the blood smear based cases. This compared to 9.8 gm% (SD=2.1) for non-malaria deaths.

Algorithms were developed using malaria related signs and symptoms on all malaria associated deaths (Table 7). However, because the signs and symptoms of cerebral malaria may be more distinct, analysis was also performed on only cerebral malaria associated deaths. For all malaria deaths and cerebral malaria deaths, fever alone has good sensitivity (94% and 94%, respectively) but poor specificity (26 and 24%, respectively). Considering all malaria deaths, the specificity for the algorithm with fever and convulsions *or* loss of consciousness was 87% but the sensitivity was low (45%). Using only cerebral malaria deaths, the specificities of fever with convulsions (90%) and fever with loss of consciousness (86%) were high; however, the sensitivities were 65% and 56%, respectively. When fever was combined with convulsions *or* loss of consciousness, the sensitivity was 72% and specificity is 85% for the cerebral malaria deaths.

# Discussion

Data on cause-specific mortality in childhood are needed to establish the relative public health importance of various causes of death and to assess the impact of health interventions.[6] The precision required for a ranking of leading causes of death is lower than for evaluation of cause-specific mortality trends. The latter is receiving increased attention in the context of the outcome of the World Summit for Children. Among 26 indicators for monitoring health goals of the Summit, at least four pertain to cause-specific mortality reductions (diarrhoea, acute respiratory infections, measles, and neonatal tetanus).[7]

In areas where good death certification systems are lacking, verbal autopsy methods are potentially the best source of data regarding levels of and trends in cause-specific mortality. An important application of the verbal autopsy is the incorporation of disease-specific modules in large-scale demographic and health surveys in order to obtain national data on causes of death. Verbal autopsy validation studies are instrumental in assessing the potential quality of cause of death data collected in such surveys. This validation study was conducted just prior to a national Demographic and Health Survey (DHS) in Namibia and, based on the study results, recommendations were made regarding inclusion of specific questions in the childhood mortality module of the DHS questionnaire.

Verbal autopsy has been widely used for the diagnosis of diarrhoea. Among diarrhoea deaths, we found loose or liquid stool to have high sensitivity (89%), but a specificity of 61%. This compares to Kalter et al. who found 78% sensitivity and 79% specificity in diarrhoea deaths (only those with concomitant diagnoses) in study in the Philippines (4) and Snow et al. who had 36% sensitivity and 96% specificity for gastroenteritis deaths in a study in coastal Kenya.[5]

In the diagnosis of pneumonia, we found cough and dyspnoea to have lower sensitivity (69%) as compared to Kalter et al. in whom these symptoms had 86% sensitivity in diagnosing acute lower respiratory infection associated deaths. However, cough and dyspnoea had higher specificity (76%) than that of Kalter et al. (47%).

For measles associated deaths, our best algorithm, which included age greater than 4 months and rash, had fair sensitivity (71%) and specificity (85%). When fever more than three days was added to this algorithm, sensitivity and specificity were 67% and 90%, respectively, as compared to that of Kalter et al. which had sensitivity and specificity of 98% and 90%, respectively. Snow et al. had 90% sensitivity and 96% specificity in the diagnosis of measles.

In the determination of the diagnosis of malnutrition, several algorithms were evaluated. The best algorithm included the presence of very thin or swelling and had a fairly good sensitivity (75%) and specificity (72%). Although wasting and kwashiorkor and diagnoses with two different etiologies and physical manifestations, it is generally recognized that there is a substantial degree of overlap in the presence of the deficiencies in a malnourished individual. Practically speaking, in most situations where verbal autopsy in used, it is not of great importance to be able to distinguish between them. In our study, only 5% of malnutrition deaths had kwashiorkor without wasting, as compared to 60% in the study by Snow et al. in Kenya. Therefore, nearly all malnutrition deaths in our study would have been detected by verbal autopsy with questions relating only to wasting. However, in areas where there is a high proportion of kwashiorkor without wasting, a verbal autopsy that included only questions directed at signs and symptoms of wasting, may fail to diagnose many malnutrition deaths. Therefore, in those areas, to increase sensitivity of an algorithm, questions directed at both wasting and kwashiorkor should be included.

Diagnosis of malaria by verbal autopsy method is difficult. This study did not determine an algorithm for all malaria deaths that had both high sensitivity and specificity. The results compare to those of Snow et al. who had a 46% sensitivity and 89% specificity in the validation of verbal autopsy for all malaria deaths. However, in our study, when cerebral malaria was considered alone, the sensitivity and specificity of the questions improved. The best algorithm had 72% sensitivity and 85% specificity, compared to that of Snow et al. who had 65% sensitivity for cerebral malaria deaths.

The differences between the results of these two studies may be due to the use of different criteria in determining the malaria deaths. It may also be due in part to differences in malaria transmission. In coastal Kenya, malaria is hyperendemic and transmission is high throughout the year. In northwest Namibia malaria is much more seasonal with a peak occurring during and after the rainy season. Although the proportion of malaria that expresses itself as cerebral malaria may vary among populations and over time, deaths due to cerebral malaria may be the best proxy for malaria mortality when conducting health surveys. In some malarious areas, as possibly demonstrated in this study, cerebral malaria may be the predominant mode of death as opposed to parasitemia with severe anaemia. For those malaria deaths in our study not associated with cerebral complications we did not demonstrate the presence of severe anaemia from the hospital data. This may indicate that, although parasitemia was present, malaria was not important as a contributory cause during the illness that lead to death.

The sensitivity and specificity of algorithms developed for some of the diagnoses of interest (diarrhoea, pneumonia, and measles) were somewhat lower than results obtained in other studies and several factors may have contributed to these differences. The death to interview interval was substantial longer in this current study with a mean recall period of 18 months, with the longest period just beyond 3 years. The study by Kalter et al. had a shorter interval (mean of four months, maximum of one year) and in the study by Snow et al. 75% had an interval of less than four months. Another important factor may be the substantial number of deaths (61%) in our study that had multiple causes as compared to that of Kalter et al. (43%) and Snow et al. (25%). The presence of multiple concomitant diseases during the illness that lead to death, may decrease the caretaker's ability to recall various signs and symptoms of the diagnoses of interest.

Performing a validation study such as this bears challenges independent of those inherent in the verbal autopsy method itself. As with any validation study, one must be confident of the 'gold standard' that is the basis for comparison. Even in ideal circumstances, the ability to make a correct medical diagnosis varies with each disease. Misdiagnosis by a clinician who determines the diagnosis of a large proportion of study deaths has the potential to introduce a bias that may alter the results dramatically. Similarly, there may be great variation in the completeness of hospital record documentation and availability and quality of diagnostic tests, as occurred in this study. Although the specific criteria used by Snow et al. are not included in their study article, in our study we included only those deaths that had adequate documentation to meet our stringent criteria.

As suggested by others and similarly demonstrated in this study, the verbal autopsy method is more effective in diagnosing certain diseases than for other diseases. Several factors are likely to contribute to the variation in the ability of algorithms to assist in the diagnosis of specific diseases, including the recognizability of signs and symptoms of the disease, overlap of signs or symptoms with those of other diseases, severity and acuteness of the illness, prevalence of the disease in the population. One should be cautious about attempting to generalize the results of a validation study to different population groups, even within the same geographic region, as differences in cultural, socioeconomic, and linguistic features among population groups may also influence the results of the verbal autopsy.

Additionally, since verbal autopsy validation studies are usually based on hospital deaths only, it is likely that these studies result in the 'best' sensitivities and specificities. Regarding deaths occurring at home, the caretakers may be less likely to have observed certain signs and symptoms than for deaths among children who died in a hospital.

The results of this validation study indicate that the verbal autopsy method may be used to determine the relative public health importance of leading causes of death. The level of misclassification is, however, substantial and indicates that assessment of trends in cause-specific mortality is more problematic.

## Acknowledgements

The investigator, a consultant for Macro International, was a Preventive Medicine Resident at Johns Hopkins University during the study. Financial assistance was provided by the World Bank through a grant from Japan.

The authors are grateful to the following for their assistance in conducting this study:

Dr. Nestor Shivute, Dr. Michael Rabbow, and Mr. Puumue Katjiuanjo at the Ministry of Health and Social Services, Republic of Namibia; Dr. Barbara Potschka, Oshikuku St. Martin's Hospital.

## References

1  Gray RH. Report of a Workshop on Health Impact Evaluation. Institute for International Programs, Johns Hopkins University. Occasional Paper 1, 1986, pp.1-24.

2  Sirken MG, Rosenberg HM, Cevarley FM, Curtin LR. The quality of cause-of-death statistics. American Journal of Public Health 1986; 77: pp.137-9.

3  Greenwood BM, Greenwood AM, Bradley AK, Tulloch S, Hayes R, Oldfield FSJ. Deaths in infancy and childhood in a well vaccinated, rural, West African population. Annals of Tropical Pediatrics 1987; 7: pp. 91-9.

4  Kalter HD, Gray RH, Black RE, Gultiano SA. Validation of post-mortem interviews to ascertain selected causes of death in children. Int Journal of Epidemiology 1990; 19: 380-86.

5  Snow RW, Armstrong JRM, Forster D, et al. Childhood deaths in Africa: uses and limitations of verbal autopsies. Lancet 1992; 340: pp.351-55.

6  Ross DA. Monitoring cause-specific infant and child mortality rates in areas where death certification systems are weak. Unpublished document.
WHO/ESM/UNICEF/CONS/WP/2. Geneva, 1992.

7  UNICEF-WHO. Progress report on development of health-related indicators and monitoring. Twenty-ninth session of UNICEF-WHO Joint Committee on Health Policy. JCHP 29/93.4.

# 7

# Causes of death in childhood: an evaluation of the results of verbal autopsy questions used in seven DHS surveys

*J. Ties Boerma, A. Elisabeth Sommerfelt, Jeroen K. van Ginneken*

**DHS Methodological Reports** *no. 2., Macro International Inc., Calverton, Maryland, USA, 1994, pp. 145–157.*

Analyzing the medical causes of death in childhood can be useful in identifying priority areas for health programs and evaluating the impact of health interventions. Since registration data are often lacking and hospital data are highly selective, increasing use is made of interview-based diagnosis of the cause of death. This approach to determining the causes of death is often called the verbal autopsy or postmortem interview technique.

There is very little experience with the use of verbal autopsy at the national level. Most population-based studies are based on small populations and carried out in the context of longitudinal epidemiological surveys. Only recently have efforts been made to standardize the methods used in verbal autopsy surveys (e.g., Gray et al., 1990). These efforts include the development of questionnaires and the use of diagnostic algorithms.

In selected DHS surveys the probable causes of death were ascertained for deceased children born during the five years preceding the survey. Whether or not a 'causes of death' module was included in a DHS survey depended on the country's implementing agency. The type of questions used differed from survey to survey. The different questions used are evaluated in this chapter, on a survey-by-survey basis. Assessing the data quality is difficult. For example, consider a survey the results of which indicate that 20 percent of all deaths under 5 years of age were associated with diarrhoea. The results seem plausible on the basis of longitudinal epidemiological studies (e.g., Gray, 1991). However, the data may not be of good quality. In a population where 20 percent of the children have diarrhoea in the last two weeks before the survey, one may expect to find that 20 percent of the children had diarrhoea during the illness preceding death, even if no children died due to diarrhoea.

In this evaluation the focus is on the type of questions used in the DHS surveys and the implications this choice had on the results. For each of seven surveys with cause-of-death questions, the questions used are reviewed and a table enumerating the leading causes of death by age of the child is presented. The age groups are neonatal (0 months), postneonatal (1–11 months), and child mortality (12–59 months). If the number of deaths in one of the latter two age groups was less than 100, both age groups were combined.

The cause of death section was embedded in the health section of the DHS question-naire, where only information on children born in the five years preceding the survey was collected. Therefore, the cause of death data refer to all children born in the last five years. Deaths of children born more than five years ago were not included in this cause of death section. Consequently, there is under-representation of deaths at older ages among the under fives.

 The assessment commences with two Latin American surveys (Bolivia and Ecuador), followed by three surveys in North Africa (Egypt, Morocco, and Tunisia) and two sur-veys in Sub-Saharan Africa (Cameroon and Senegal). The Cameroon survey was car-ried out during DHS-II.

## Bolivia

Two types of information were used to assess the likely cause of death. First, the re-spondent was asked to give the main disease or accident causing the death, which was entered by the interviewer in the questionnaire and later coded, using a list of causes of death provided by the Ministry of Health. Second, for deaths not caused by an accident, inquiries were made into the presence and duration of several specific symptoms and signs during the two-week period preceding the death. These symptoms included diarrhoea, diarrhoea with blood, difficult breathing, common cold/cough, rash, and fe-ver. The mother was also asked whether the baby had been sucking normally during the first days of life.

The mother was asked whether the child had died at home or in a health facility, and whether medical care had been sought for the illness preceding the death. If diarrhoea was one of the signs and symptoms present before death, it was determined whether oral rehydration therapy had been used.

Twenty-six percent of the respondents said they had a death certificate for the deceased child, but in only 2 percent of the cases was the certificate actually shown to the inter-viewer. Therefore, the death certificates could not be used to assess the causes of death.

Fever, diarrhoea, and breathing difficulties were the most common symptoms preced-ing death (Table 1). On average three of the eight symptoms probed were present. Diar-rhoea and fever were very common after the neonatal period (more than half of the deaths). Difficult breathing was twice as frequent as cough during the neonatal period, while both symptoms were reported with equal frequency after the neonatal period.

**Table I** Symptoms before death and causes of death by age in months among children under 5 years, Bolivia DHS, 1989

| | Age at death (months) | | | |
| --- | --- | --- | --- | --- |
| | 0–59 | 0 | 1–11 | 12–59 |
| **Symptoms** | | | | |
| Diarrhoea | 36.0 | 9.3 | 39.1 | 70.3 |
| Diarrhoea with blood | 9.3 | 1.3 | 8.2 | 23.1 |
| Cough | 24.0 | 15.8 | 25.9 | 33.1 |
| Dyspnoea | 30.5 | 35.6 | 28.2 | 26.8 |
| Rash | 11.7 | 5.5 | 8.3 | 26.8 |
| Convulsions | 3.6 | 2.7 | 4.2 | 4.0 |
| Fever | 48.1 | 22.8 | 57.9 | 68.4 |
| Other | 29.6 | 28.2 | 31.8 | 27.7 |
| **Causes of death according to mother** | | | | |
| Birth problems | 13.3 | 32.9 | 3.8 | 0.5 |
| Prematurity | 2.7 | 7.7 | .0 | .0 |
| Tetanus | 3.3 | 5.7 | 2.0 | 1.9 |
| Congenital anomaly | 0.8 | 1.0 | 1.1 | .0 |
| Diarrhoea | 35.7 | 13.1 | 39.1 | 63.8 |
| Respiratory illness | 20.5 | 17.2 | 25.7 | 15.9 |
| Measles | 1.2 | 0.2 | 2.1 | 1.2 |
| Other infections | 2.0 | 3.1 | 1.3 | 1.7 |
| Other diseases | 4.0 | 4.0 | 4.4 | 3.1 |
| Accidents | 7.4 | 7.9 | 8.4 | 4.8 |
| Unknown | 9.2 | 7.4 | 12.1 | 6.8 |
| **Probable diagnosis based on symptoms** | | | | |
| Diarrhoea | 33.4 | 7.6 | 37.1 | 65.1 |
| Respiratory infection | 8.8 | 3.3 | 11.2 | 11.4 |
| Measles | 3.1 | .0 | 2.6 | 8.7 |
| **Probable diagnosis based on symptoms and mother's report** | | | | |
| Diarrhoea | 26.7 | 4.5 | 30.0 | 54.6 |
| Respiratory infection | 1.8 | 1.2 | 2.1 | 2.3 |
| Measles | 0.3 | .0 | 0.8 | .0 |
| Number of deaths | 567 | 199 | 234 | 134 |

The duration of these symptoms was also asked, particularly to be able to exclude cases in which the symptoms started shortly before death and were not a likely cause of death. Most symptoms did not start until at least one day before death and most of these started well before. For difficult breathing a significant proportion of children (15 percent) had dyspnoea starting on the day of death. An additional 19 percent started one day before death. Most likely, these children did not have pneumonia but had breathing difficulties associated with general weakness, fever, etc. Therefore, it is very important to collect data on the duration of the dyspnoea symptoms as reported by the mother.

Mothers reported a cause of death for 91 percent of the deceased children. The proportion of deaths where the cause was either unknown or poorly defined by the respondent did not increase with the length of the recall period and was the same for both the first and the fourth years before the survey. Among infant deaths of unknown cause, 14 percent occurred the year before the survey, 12 percent the second year before the survey, 12 percent the third year, and 13 percent the fourth year.

The main causes of death as reported by the mother according to the age of the child are summarized in Table 1. In the neonatal period, problems associated with delivery, primarily traumatic delivery and neonatal asphyxia, were mentioned by almost one-third of the respondents. Respiratory illness was the next most frequently cited cause of death (17 percent), followed by diarrhoea (13 percent). Eight percent mentioned prematurity, and 6 percent tetanus. An unusually high proportion (8 percent) also mentioned accidents as a cause of neonatal death. This is likely to be due to the structure of the questionnaire and its interpretation by both interviewers and respondents. In several cases, deaths due to birth trauma were classified as accidental deaths, and there was not always sufficient detail to distinguish perinatal causes of death (mainly birth problems) from accidents.

In addition, the mother's assessment of the neonate's size at birth – available for all live births during the five years preceding the survey – was used to estimate the impact of low birth weight on mortality. Subjective assessments of the relative size of the infant at birth have been shown to be reasonable indicators of actual size at birth (Moreno and Goldman, 1990). Almost 10 percent of all neonates (deceased or surviving) were considered 'very small' by the respondents, and 20 percent were 'smaller than average'. For 25 percent of the neonatal deaths, the baby was reportedly very small at birth, and low birth weight can be considered an associated cause of death.

During the postneonatal period, diarrhoea was reported to be the leading cause of death (cited in 39 percent of the 234 deaths), followed by respiratory infection (26 percent). According to the mothers' reports, measles was not a leading cause of death.

From the list of symptoms and mother's report on the cause of death a probable diagnosis of the cause of death can be made (multiple causes possible). This was done for four leading causes of death – neonatal tetanus, diarrhoea, pneumonia, and measles – to show some of the difficulties in making a probable diagnosis. The results of application of these procedures for the last three diseases are found in Table 1.

Initially, three criteria were used to identify deaths due to neonatal tetanus: death occurring between 2 and 30 days after birth, normal sucking during the first days after birth, and convulsions. However, in Bolivia, the question on the presence of seizures was not very clear and a number of children who had convulsions may have been missed. No deaths met all three criteria. Omitting the question on convulsions and restricting the age range at death to 4–14 days, the period during which most neonatal tetanus deaths occur, 40 deaths were found, which is 20 percent of all neonatal deaths. In five of these cases (2.5 percent of neonatal mortality), the mother had also mentioned tetanus as the cause of her child's death. Using the mothers' diagnoses, 5.7 percent of all neonatal deaths were due to tetanus.

Diarrhoea was considered a probable cause if the child had diarrhoea (with or without blood in the stool) for at least two days. For 33 percent of the deaths among children under five years and for 65 percent of the deaths at ages 1–4 years, diarrhoea was a probable cause, based on the symptoms. In most of these cases the mothers had also spontaneously mentioned diarrhoea as the cause of death (Table 1). Diarrhoea was generally not associated with either pneumonia or measles. In only 6 percent of all deaths after the neonatal period did diarrhoea cause or contribute to the child's death in combination with pneumonia or measles.

If the child had a cough for at least four days and breathing difficulties for at least two days before death, pneumonia was listed as a cause (Kalter et al., 1990). Based on mothers' reports of their children's symptoms, lower respiratory tract infections caused fewer deaths than diarrhoeal diseases: pneumonia was a probable cause for 9 percent of all deaths. Respiratory infection was mentioned by the mother as the cause of death for only 2 percent and the symptom-based diagnosis was pneumonia.

Measles was considered a cause if the age at death was at least four months, a rash was present for at least three days, and the child had fever for at least three days. Measles, as defined above and occurring during the last two weeks before death, was a probable cause of 3 percent of the deaths and was associated with 9 percent of all deaths at age 12 months and over. However, mothers had mentioned measles as the cause of death for only two of these cases.

The long-term effects of measles on child mortality – children who have had measles are more likely to die from other causes, such as pneumonia, diarrhoea, or tuberculosis, in the months afterwards due to reduced resistance to these diseases – have been described in several studies (Koenig et al., 1990). Therefore, mothers were asked whether the dead child had had rash and fever in the six months before death. If so, they were asked the duration of the episode and the time elapsed between this illness and the child's death.

The proportion of deaths preceded by a presumed measles infection was estimated using questions about an illness consisting of rash and fever during the six months preceding the interview (data not shown). Using the same criteria for the diagnosis of measles as above, that is, an illness with a rash lasting three days or longer and with a fever for at least three days, 14 percent of children had a history of measles in the four weeks preceding death, 19 percent in the three months preceding death, and 21 percent in the six months preceding death. For children who died of respiratory diseases, according to the mother's report, 22 percent had had measles in the three months before death. The corresponding figure for diarrhoeal deaths was 15 percent. This suggests that measles may be more important as a cause of death than the data in Table 1 show.

Although the verbal autopsy questionnaire was more extensive in Bolivia than in most other DHS surveys before 1989, it cannot be shown that this has led to more valid and reliable results. However, the results do provide an indication of the quality of the data. The duration of breathing difficulties is a very important addition, and data on the duration of other symptoms enabled a more careful assessment of the probable cause of death using diagnostic algorithms. Unfortunately, mother's reported cause of death and the diagnosis based on the symptoms often are inconsistent. The inconsistencies may be due to errors in both methods.

The proportion of women responding 'don't know' to the open question on the cause of death in Bolivia is remarkably lower than in most other DHS surveys. In Bolivia, the interviewer wrote down what the mother said and the cause was coded in the office; in other surveys a short coding list was provided to the interviewer (in the questionnaire). This suggests that the large proportion of don't know responses is caused by the interviewers' problems with ascertaining the cause of death. It is, however, also possible that office editors had very loose instructions for coding the causes of death, and considerable room was left for the coders' interpretations.

## Ecuador

In Ecuador the interviewer coded the cause of death following one question to the mother:

*'Which symptoms did (NAME) have in the two weeks preceding death?'*

The questionnaire provided the following instructions to the interviewer:
- Tetanus: stopped sucking 7–10 days after birth, stopped crying 3 days before death, rigid body, convulsions
- Malaria: fluctuating fever, cold shivers, shaking of the body
- Acute respiratory infection (ARI): cough; fever; nasal discharge; difficult, rapid, or noisy breathing
- Measles: exanthema on the whole body, nasal discharge, cough, fever, red eyes
- Whooping cough: persistent and severe cough
- Acute diarrhoea: diarrhoea and vomiting, sunken eyes, sunken fontanel, very thirsty
- Various: traffic accident, burns, drug or food poisoning
- Others (specify).

Table 2 shows the results of these questions for 202 deaths for children under five years by age period. Forty percent of the deaths could not be classified by the interviewer in one of the eight categories of causes. It cannot be assessed whether the respondent did not know what the symptoms were or whether the interviewer did not know what diag-

**Table 2**   Causes of death among children under 5 years, by age in months, Ecuador DHS, 1987 (percentages)

| Cause | All | Age at death (months) | |
|---|---|---|---|
| | | 0 | 1–59 |
| Diarrhoea | 11.9 | 6.4 | 18.3 |
| ARI | 11.4 | 11.9 | 10.7 |
| Tetanus | 5.4 | 9.2 | 1.1 |
| Malaria | 4.5 | 3.7 | 5.4 |
| Measles | 2.5 | 2.8 | 2.2 |
| Pertussis | 1.5 | 0.9 | 2.1 |
| Accidents | 5.9 | 4.6 | 7.6 |
| Other | 16.8 | 21.1 | 11.8 |
| Don't know | 40.1 | 39.4 | 40.8 |
| Total | 100.0 | 100.0 | 100.0 |
| Number of deaths | 202 | 109 | 93 |

nosis to make from the symptoms recalled by the respondent. The proportion of don't know responses increased with the length of the recall period as follows: 30 percent of infant deaths in the first and second years, respectively, before the survey and 52 percent in the third and fourth years, respectively, before the survey.

For the remaining 60 percent of deaths, diarrhoeal diseases were the most common cause of death, especially after the neonatal period. During the neonatal period ARI and tetanus were the leading causes. Accidents, which were common in all age groups, were associated with 7 percent overall; deaths due to accidents were not likely to be classified as unknown. Presumably, this cause of death was the simplest to ascertain for the interviewer. However, it is possible that birth trauma has been reported or interpreted as an accident, since 5 percent of neonatal deaths were attributed to accidents.

Measles is conspicuously uncommon as a leading cause of death, accounting for only 2.5 percent of all deaths under five years of age. Under-reporting or misclassification by the interviewer are likely explanations.

Generally, the method used in Ecuador does not appear to provide useful results or a reasonably accurate picture of the causes of death in childhood. The proportion of deaths with unknown cause is large, but more importantly, the causes of death are highly sensitive to interviewer interpretation and biases.

# Egypt

In Egypt, no symptoms checklist was used, but a limited number of questions were asked to determine whether the child had died from a few important causes of death:

- Diarrhoea: Did the child have diarrhoea during the seven days before death? If yes, did the child also have watery stools?
- Acute lower respiratory infections: Did the child have a cough and difficulty breathing in the seven days before death (two separate questions)?
- Measles: Did the child have measles during the last seven days before death? [It often is argued that measles is the main cause of death, if it occurred within three months before the death (e.g., Koenig et al., 1990).]
- Other illness: Did the child have any other illness during the last seven days?
- Accident: Did the child have an accident during the last seven days?
- Neonatal tetanus: Did the child have convulsions and had it been nursing normally until it became ill?

The mother was also asked whether the child had been examined by a doctor during the period of illness before death.

There were no coding categories for don't know responses. Missing values occurred for 21 of 723 deaths in children under five years (2.9 percent), apparently because the interviewer skipped the whole section. Twenty percent of the mothers mentioned other illnesses as the cause of death; the most frequently mentioned conditions were severe diarrhoea, tetanus, and fever (Table 3). On the basis of this list of symptoms and diseases, it is possible to arrive at an estimate of the magnitude of the four leading causes of death.

Diarrhoeal diseases are very commonly reported (for one third of the deaths). Ninety percent of the children with diarrhoea in the terminal illness had watery diarrhoea. Diarrhoea can be considered a likely primary or contributory cause of death if the child had diarrhoea during the last week or if the mother spontaneously mentioned that the child had severe diarrhoea. Under these assumptions, more than 50 percent of the postneonatal and child deaths in Egypt are associated with diarrhoea.

Pneumonia is a probable cause of death for about one fourth of the child deaths if the diagnosis is based on the presence of cough with difficult breathing. It is notable that difficult breathing was more common than cough, especially among neonatal deaths and child deaths. For a very young infant with pneumonia, it is possible that the sick child cannot mount a cough response, but for a child 1-to 4-years-old this is less common. In addition, terminal breathing difficulties among children who are very sick while dying from causes other than pneumonia are likely to be reported as difficulty breathing, which may explain the high prevalence of breathing difficulties.

The diagnosis of measles could only be based on the mother's report of measles, since no symptoms were asked. Using the criterion that measles deaths can only occur in a

**Table 3** Causes of death and symptoms occurring before death among children under 5 years, by age in months, Egypt DHS, 1988 (percentages)

| | Age at death (months) | | | |
|---|---|---|---|---|
| | 0–59 | 0 | 1–11 | 12–59 |
| **Symptoms** | | | | |
| Diarrhoea | 32.5 | 7.5 | 55.6 | 48.9 |
| Watery stools | 29.3 | 6.8 | 51.5 | 40.7 |
| Cough | 20.7 | 8.0 | 31.2 | 31.6 |
| Difficult breathing | 27.9 | 20.7 | 31.4 | 40.3 |
| Measles | 4.0 | 0.7 | 4.4 | 12.6 |
| Other | 20.1 | 14.9 | 26.7 | 19.4 |
|    Severe diarrhoea | 12.7 | 2.7 | 23.4 | 16.2 |
|    Fever | 3.5 | 2.9 | 3.8 | 4.7 |
|    Tetanus | 5.7 | 9.2 | 2.6 | 2.8 |
| Convulsions | 13.9 | 30.3 | 0.0 | 0.0 |
| Nursing normal | 15.0 | 32.7 | 0.0 | 0.0 |
| Saw doctor | 61.8 | 42.1 | 78.6 | 78.2 |
| Missing | 3.1 | 3.4 | 2.8 | 2.6 |
| **Probable diagnosis** | | | | |
| Diarrhoea | 34.4 | 8.9 | 58.5 | 50.0 |
| Pneumonia | 16.1 | 6.3 | 23.9 | 25.7 |
| Measles | 3.3 | 0.0 | 3.2 | 12.6 |
| Neonatal tetanus | 6.2 | 13.6 | 0.0 | 0.0 |
| Number of deaths | 723 | 331 | 274 | 117 |

child at least four months old, 4 percent of the postneonatal deaths and 13 percent of deaths among children 1–4 years were reportedly due to measles.

Neonatal tetanus was spontaneously mentioned by 9 percent of mothers for neonatal deaths, and convulsions and nursing problems a few days after birth were each mentioned for about 30 percent of the neonatal deaths. If the diagnosis of neonatal tetanus is based on the presence of both symptoms and death between 3 and 28 days of life, then 14 percent of the neonatal deaths were due to tetanus.

In general, it appears that focusing on very few causes of death (diarrhoea, pneumonia, and measles for deaths after the neonatal period) leads to overestimation of the proportion of deaths caused by diarrhoea and ARI. Also, it is not possible to distinguish between main and associated causes of death. In addition, the mix of asking a few questions on symptoms preceding death and asking for a disease itself, namely measles, does not appear to lead to useful results. It is difficult to assess whether the two questions on convulsions and feeding for neonatal deaths provide an estimate of the importance of neonatal tetanus mortality.

## Tunisia and Morocco

Tunisia and Morocco used the same questionnaires to determine the causes of death in children under five years. They included:
- Questions on the presence of 17 symptoms or conditions during the illness that led to the child's death
- A question on the mother's opinion of the cause of death, with 10 coding categories.

The mother responded don't know to the latter question for 45 percent of the deaths in Tunisia and for 33 percent in Morocco (Table 4). About one quarter of the answers were classified as other. In Tunisia, the proportion of mothers responding don't know did not increase with the length of the recall period. Such responses were recorded for 43, 42, 43, and 36 percent among infant deaths for the first, second, third, and fourth years before the survey, respectively. In Morocco, there was a small increase when the recall period exceeded three years. The proportions responding don't know for the cause of infant deaths were 31, 31, 33, and 39 percent for the first, second, third, and fourth years before the survey, respectively.

Considering the main causes of death the following can be noted in Table 4:
- Diarrhoea: as a symptom very commonly reported in Morocco (more than 50 percent after the neonatal period) and also frequent in Tunisia (38 percent for postneonatal deaths). The mother reported diarrhoea as the cause of death for about 32 percent of the deaths after the neonatal period in Morocco and for 26 percent of the postneonatal deaths in Tunisia. It appears that in Morocco diarrhoea was mild or a secondary cause for about one fifth of all deaths, where, according to the mother, diarrhoea was not the cause of death but was present as a symptom.
- Acute respiratory infection: in both surveys difficult breathing was more common than cough. The difference was particularly large in Morocco. Overall, pneumonia, based on cough with difficult breathing, is less common than may have been expected. Mothers rarely gave respiratory illness as a cause of death.
- Measles: skin rash was not commonly reported in either country, but was reported for neonates. The lack of a specific term for a measles-associated skin rash may have contributed. Mothers also did not often mention measles as the cause of death.
- Neonatal tetanus: neonatal tetanus was not reported at all in Tunisia, but in Morocco it was mentioned for 5 percent of all neonatal deaths. Based on the symptoms, i.e., inability to open the mouth and convulsions, spasms, or body stiffness, the probable diagnosis of tetanus was made for neonatal deaths between 3 and 31 days. In this case 4 and 10 percent of the neonatal deaths are caused by tetanus in Tunisia and Morocco, respectively. In Morocco, the diagnosis of tetanus based on the symptoms agreed for only 29 percent with mother's report of tetanus.
- Malnutrition: extreme thinness of the child and, to a lesser extent, swollen body are potential symptoms of protein calorie malnutrition, and were reported frequently. If either of these two symptoms is taken as evidence of malnutrition then about one third of all deaths are associated with malnutrition in both countries. Extremely thin

**Table 4** Symptoms and causes of death, by age in months, for deaths among children under 5 years, Tunisia DHS 1988 and Morocco DHS 1987 (percentages)

| | Tunisia | | | Morocco | | |
|---|---|---|---|---|---|---|
| | Age at death (months) | | | Age at death (months) | | |
| | 0–59 | 0 | 1–59 | 0–59 | 0 | 1–59 |
| **Symptoms** | | | | | | |
| Body swollen | 15.4 | 13.7 | 17.3 | 9.0 | 4.0 | 12.5 |
| Extreme thinness | 28.6 | 25.6 | 31.8 | 28.4 | 14.5 | 42.2 |
| High fever | 22.9 | 10.3 | 36.4 | 31.2 | 15.7 | 46.8 |
| Diarrhoea | 20.3 | 3.4 | 38.2 | 34.0 | 11.7 | 55.6 |
| Vomiting | 16.7 | 5.1 | 29.1 | 34.4 | 14.9 | 53.6 |
| Mouth closed | 11.9 | 11.1 | 12.8 | 10.8 | 13.7 | 7.9 |
| Cough | 8.8 | 4.3 | 13.6 | 10.6 | 6.0 | 16.0 |
| Dyspnoea | 11.9 | 7.7 | 16.3 | 21.0 | 23.4 | 19.0 |
| Ictere | 12.3 | 6.8 | 18.2 | 4.0 | 5.6 | 2.2 |
| Skin rash | 7.9 | 5.1 | 10.9 | 4.0 | 2.0 | 5.2 |
| Convulsions | 6.2 | 4.3 | 8.1 | 8.0 | 5.2 | 10.7 |
| Stiff body | 8.8 | 5.1 | 12.7 | 4.0 | 6.0 | 2.1 |
| Muscular contractions | 4.4 | 3.4 | 5.5 | 6.8 | 9.3 | 4.5 |
| Accidents | 0.9 | 0.0 | 1.9 | 1.4 | 1.2 | 1.5 |
| Intoxication | 0.9 | 0.9 | 0.9 | 0.8 | 0.4 | 1.0 |
| Other | 37.9 | 47.9 | 27.3 | 25.6 | 38.3 | 13.9 |
| **Cause of death according to mother** | | | | | | |
| Diarrhoea | 12.8 | 0.9 | 25.5 | 19.6 | 7.3 | 31.6 |
| Tuberculosis | 2.6 | 4.3 | 0.9 | 0.2 | 0.0 | 0.5 |
| Respiratory disease | 6.2 | 4.3 | 8.2 | 5.0 | 7.3 | 2.8 |
| Meningitis | 2.6 | 0.9 | 4.5 | 0.6 | 0.0 | 1.3 |
| Whooping cough | 0.9 | 0.0 | 1.9 | 1.4 | 0.0 | 3.2 |
| Tetanus | 0.9 | 0.0 | 1.8 | 3.0 | 4.8 | 1.2 |
| Measles | 1.3 | 0.0 | 2.7 | 2.2 | 0.0 | 3.5 |
| Diphtheria | 0.9 | 1.7 | 0.0 | 1.6 | 0.4 | 2.6 |
| Other | 24.2 | 32.5 | 15.5 | 28.8 | 40.7 | 17.7 |
| Missing | 1.8 | 2.6 | 0.9 | 4.2 | 3.6 | 4.8 |
| Don't know | 45.4 | 53.0 | 37.2 | 33.4 | 35.9 | 30.7 |
| **Probable cause of death** | | | | | | |
| Malnutrition | 38.3 | 35.9 | 40.9 | 33.2 | 17.3 | 47.7 |
| Pneumonia | 4.0 | 1.7 | 6.4 | 4.2 | 2.8 | 5.8 |
| Pneumonia with fever | 3.1 | 0.9 | 5.5 | 2.4 | 1.2 | 3.8 |
| Diarrhoea with fever | 11.9 | 2.6 | 21.9 | 19.4 | 5.6 | 33.0 |
| Measles | 2.2 | 0.0 | 4.6 | 1.4 | 0.0 | 2.4 |
| Tetanus | 2.2 | 4.3 | 0.0 | 4.2 | 8.5 | 0.0 |
| Accidents | 1.8 | 0.9 | 2.7 | 2.2 | 1.6 | 2.4 |
| Malaria | 0.9 | 0.0 | 1.8 | 1.6 | 0.0 | 8.1 |
| Pertussis | 4.8 | 2.6 | 7.2 | 5.0 | 1.2 | 8.9 |
| Number of deaths | 227 | 117 | 110 | 500 | 248 | 252 |

for neonates probably refers to low birthweight babies. It is not clear how reliable the reports are. If it is malnutrition, the symptoms would have to be present for at least a month or so, but such information was not collected.

The leading probable causes of death that result from combining information on the list of symptoms and mothers' reports are listed in Table 4. It can be concluded that the checklist of symptoms in Tunisia and Morocco provides some insight into the leading causes of death in childhood, but many questions remain. Diarrhoea appears to be over-estimated and respiratory infections, measles, and neonatal tetanus underestimated. The questionnaires also included symptoms that were not well specified and causes of death that were not useful (e.g., diphtheria and typhoid).

## Senegal

Three questions were asked in Senegal to determine the probable cause of death:
- Did the child have one of the following symptoms during the disease that led to the child's death? (The presence of 12 signs and symptoms were probed; see Table 5.)
- Did the child have one of the following symptoms just before death? (Five symptoms were probed.)
- What was the principal cause of death? (There were coding categories for six conditions and for other causes.)

The results are shown in Table 5. The list of symptoms during the disease leading to death does not include the important symptoms of diarrhoea and difficult breathing. For 18 percent of the deaths the mother did not know what symptoms the child had had. This was a particularly common situation if it concerned a neonatal death: 38 percent don't know responses. The proportion of deaths with unknown cause according to the mother increased with the length of the recall period: 40 percent of the infant deaths in the year before the survey, 40 percent in the second year before the survey, 55 percent in the third, and 51 percent in the fourth year before the survey. High fever was a symptom for more than 70 percent of the postneonatal and childhood deaths. Dehydration was also very frequently reported for these children: about 45 percent. Most likely mothers understood the term dehydration. There were three symptoms referring to cough: cough, cough and vomiting, and attacks of coughing. Cough and vomiting, and attacks of coughing were more frequently reported than cough, which is inconsistent.

Muscular spasms, dehydration, and stiff body were all reported as symptoms occurring just before death (but may have been present longer) for about one in five deaths. Ten percent had convulsions. These questions do not provide useful information.

For 42 percent of the under-five deaths the mother could not give a cause of death. For neonatal deaths the value was 66 percent. Diarrhoea, measles, malaria, and other condi-

**Table 5** Symptoms and causes of death among children under 5 years by age in months, Senegal DHS 1986 (percentages)

| | Age at death (months) | | | |
|---|---|---|---|---|
| | 0–59 | 0 | 1–11 | 12–59 |
| **Symptoms present during terminal illness** | | | | |
| Could not drink | 27.8 | 33.7 | 33.5 | 18.5 |
| Could not cry | 14.0 | 16.3 | 15.5 | 10.8 |
| High fever | 58.7 | 32.1 | 72.0 | 72.5 |
| Skin rash | 12.8 | 4.6 | 16.8 | 17.1 |
| Cough | 9.7 | 5.1 | 14.3 | 10.4 |
| Red eyes | 14.3 | 6.1 | 19.3 | 18.0 |
| Cough and vomiting | 28.8 | 8.7 | 40.4 | 38.3 |
| Attacks of coughing | 5.5 | 2.0 | 9.3 | 5.9 |
| Dehydration | 32.6 | 5.6 | 45.3 | 47.3 |
| Red hair | 6.6 | 0.0 | 6.8 | 12.2 |
| Swollen feet | 3.6 | 1.0 | 0.6 | 8.1 |
| Accidents | 1.0 | 0.5 | 1.2 | 1.4 |
| Don't know | 18.3 | 37.8 | 5.6 | 10.4 |
| **Symptoms present just before death** | | | | |
| Muscular spasms | 19.3 | 15.8 | 23.6 | 19.4 |
| Convulsions | 10.0 | 7.1 | 9.9 | 12.6 |
| Dehydration | 24.9 | 4.1 | 32.3 | 37.8 |
| Stiff body | 21.2 | 17.3 | 20.5 | 25.2 |
| Paralysis | 5.7 | 4.6 | 6.2 | 6.3 |
| **Cause of death according to mother** | | | | |
| Tetanus | 4.0 | 6.6 | 5.6 | 0.5 |
| Whooping cough | 1.7 | 0.5 | 3.1 | 1.8 |
| Diarrhoea | 16.2 | 2.0 | 24.8 | 22.5 |
| Measles | 11.1 | 1.0 | 12.4 | 18.9 |
| Malaria | 4.8 | 0.5 | 6.2 | 7.7 |
| Influenza | 2.6 | 1.0 | 3.7 | 3.2 |
| Other | 16.2 | 20.9 | 15.5 | 12.6 |
| Don't know | 42.3 | 66.3 | 27.3 | 32.0 |
| **Probable causes of death** | | | | |
| Diarrhoea | 16.2 | 2.0 | 24.8 | 22.5 |
| Malaria | 14.9 | 0.0 | 22.4 | 22.5 |
| ARI | 11.9 | 4.1 | 18.6 | 14.0 |
| Measles | 8.1 | 0.0 | 9.9 | 14.0 |
| Whooping cough | 1.7 | 0.5 | 3.1 | 1.8 |
| Neonatal tetanus | 4.8 | 14.3 | 0.0 | 0.0 |
| Total | 579 | 196 | 161 | 222 |

tions were the most commonly reported causes. Pneumonia and accidents were not on the list of possible answers.

The last part of Table 5 shows probable causes of death which, taking into account the limitations of the Senegal questionnaire, are based on the following criteria:
- Diarrhoea: based on mother's report (about 25 percent of postneonatal and childhood deaths).
- Malaria/meningitis: based on mother's report of malaria or on the symptoms of high fever with muscular spasms or convulsions in a child at least 1 month old. Since Senegal is in the 'meningitis belt', meningitis is also probable and it is virtually impossible to distinguish between the two with the DHS questions.
- Acute respiratory infection: based on symptoms of cough (cough only, cough with vomiting, or attacks of coughing) with high fever.
- Measles: high fever and skin rash in a child at least 4 months old or diagnosis from mother's report.
- Whooping cough: mother's report of whooping cough, with cough and vomiting as reported symptoms.
- Neonatal tetanus: unable to drink, and just before death symptoms of muscular spasms or convulsions or stiff body, in a neonate aged 3–31 days. For 14 percent of the neonatal deaths tetanus could be considered a probable diagnosis.

In general, the Senegal questions on the causes of death have several inconsistencies and omissions and the results on the leading causes of death should be interpreted very carefully.


## Cameroon

The DHS-II survey in Cameroon was conducted in 1991 and built upon the experience of the other DHS surveys and verbal autopsy studies. Therefore, the data will be analyzed somewhat more extensively than for the other surveys.

For deaths not caused by an accident, two types of information were used to assess the probable cause of death. First, the respondent was asked to give the main cause of death, which was recorded by the interviewer on the questionnaire and later coded in the office, using a list of causes of death. Two causes could be coded. Second, inquiries were made into the presence, severity, and duration of selected symptoms and signs during the illness that led to the child's death. These symptoms, which included diarrhoea, diarrhoea with blood, cough, difficult/rapid breathing, rash, fever, convulsions, very thin, and swollen legs and/or face, were used to make a probable diagnosis (based on diagnostic algorithms). In order to distinguish between neonates, who were normal at birth, and those who were not, the mother was also asked whether the baby had been sucking normally during the first days of life. The latter group of babies includes those

**Table 6**  Cause of death according to the mother: Percent of deaths attributed to different causes by age in months for children born in the last five years, Cameroon DHS, 1991

| Cause of death[1] | Age at death (months) | | All |
|---|---|---|---|
| | 0 | 1–59 | |
| Prematurity | 11.6 | 0.0 | 4.3 |
| Birth problems | 9.2 | 0.0 | 3.4 |
| Tetanus | 9.3 | 1.9 | 4.7 |
| Congenital malf. | 0.5 | 1.4 | 1.0 |
| Malaria | 8.8 | 15.7 | 13.2 |
| Measles | 1.2 | 18.9 | 12.3 |
| Respiratory illness | 13.6 | 11.2 | 12.1 |
| . Pneumonia | 4.7 | 6.6 | 5.9 |
| . Asthma | 1.9 | 0.7 | 1.1 |
| . Pertussis | 0.7 | 2.1 | 1.6 |
| . ARI symptoms | 6.2 | 1.8 | 3.4 |
| Diarrhoea | 1.2 | 17.4 | 11.4 |
| Fever | 2.4 | 4.5 | 3.7 |
| Malnutrition | 0.0 | 4.2 | 2.6 |
| Anemia | 0.0 | 1.6 | 1.0 |
| Other infections | 0.0 | 1.6 | 1.0 |
| Accidents | 1.4 | 1.8 | 1.7 |
| Other | 11.6 | 9.6 | 10.3 |
| Don't know | 23.9 | 9.3 | 14.7 |
| Missing | 5.5 | 0.7 | 2.5 |
| Total | 100.0 | 100.0 | 100.0 |
| Number of deaths | 111 | 188 | 299 |

1. One cause per child.

traumatized during delivery and premature, as well as those with congenital malformations. The loss of the ability to suckle a few days after birth is typical of neonatal tetanus.

## Causes of death according to mother

The data on the main cause of death as reported by the mother for neonatal deaths and deaths at 1–59 months are summarized in Table 6. For all under five deaths there were 2.5 percent missing values and 15 percent don't know responses. These were more common for neonatal deaths: 6 percent missing and 24 percent don't know. The proportion of infant deaths with don't know responses increased with the length of the recall period: from 11 percent for deaths in the year before the survey, to 12, 21, and 21 percent in the second, third, and fourth years before the survey, respectively.

During the neonatal period, respiratory illnesses were the most frequently cited cause of death (14 percent), followed by prematurity (12 percent), tetanus (9 percent), birth problems (9 percent), and malaria (9 percent). The reliability of mothers' reports on the

**Table 7**  Symptoms during the illness that led to death: percent with symptom present, with symptom being severe, and with symptom lasting until death, by age at death, Cameroon DHS, 1991

| Symptom | Neonatal deaths (N = 111) | | | Deaths 1–59 months (N = 188) | | |
|---|---|---|---|---|---|---|
| | Symptom present | Symptom severe | Lasted until death | Symptom present | Symptom severe | Lasted until death |
| Diarrhoea | 6.0 | 2.0 | 4.8 | 41.6 | 31.9 | 32.7 |
| Diarrhoea with blood | 1.9 | 1.2 | 0.0 | 4.8 | 3.5 | 4.8 |
| Cough | 14.0 | 11.2 | 12.4 | 28.9 | 17.9 | 23.6 |
| Dyspnoea | 31.5 | 27.9 | 29.9 | 43.6 | 36.8 | 40.1 |
| Fever | 20.3 | 15.2 | 14.6 | 58.4 | 44.4 | 50.8 |
| Convulsions | 11.5 | 10.7 | 7.1 | 19.6 | 14.4 | 18.4 |
| Rash | 2.5 | 0.8 | 2.5 | 17.2 | 15.6 | 14.0 |
| Very thin | 7.1 | 5.1 | 7.1 | 40.6 | 34.1 | 35.5 |
| Swollen legs | 6.1 | 2.4 | 3.5 | 12.4 | 9.8 | 10.7 |

Note: Children who died of accidents are included in the denominator.

causes of death is not clear. Malaria may have been over-reported, since it is not common before six weeks of age.

After the neonatal period, measles is the leading cause of death (19 percent, as reported by the mother), followed by diarrhoea (17 percent), malaria (16 percent), and respiratory diseases (11 percent). Malnutrition was reported as the main cause of death for 4 percent of the deaths, and accidents accounted for 2 percent.

A secondary cause of death was also recorded if the mother reported more than one cause. This occurred for only 4 percent of all deaths and was attributed mostly to malaria or anaemia (not included in Table 6).

## Prevalence of symptoms before death
The percentages of children for whom each of the symptoms occurred during the terminal illness are shown in Table 7. Among neonatal deaths dyspnoea was very common (32 percent), while fever, cough, and convulsions were also reported for more than 10 percent of the deaths. Among the deaths at 1–59 months, fever (58 percent), dyspnoea (44 percent), diarrhoea (42 percent), and being very thin (41 percent) were commonly reported. Each of the remaining symptoms, with the exception of diarrhoea with blood, were reported for more than 10 percent of the deaths.

To be able to distinguish between symptoms that are very common in childhood (such as diarrhoea or thinness), but perhaps unrelated to the child's death, and symptoms that contribute to the death, it was asked whether the symptom or sign was severe. Table 7 shows that, for example, about three quarters of the respondents thought the diarrhoea was severe.

It was also asked whether the symptom lasted until death, and, if not, how long before death it stopped. These data would enable a distinction between causes that lasted until death (main or associated causes) and causes that stopped before death (contributory causes of death). Table 7 shows that in the large majority of cases the symptom lasted until death. If not, it usually stopped just a few days before death (data not shown). Therefore, the distinction between main, associated, and contributory causes of death will not be made here.

## Cause of death derived from symptoms

Table 8 presents the probable causes of death based on various diagnostic algorithms. Among neonatal deaths low birth weight was common: 19 percent of the deaths had either a reported birth weight of less than 2500 grams or, if no birth weight was available, the mother reported her child was very small at birth. Most of the deaths caused by low birth weight appeared to be associated with premature delivery: 17.5 percent of all neonatal deaths were reportedly delivered prematurely and had low birth weight, while only 1.5 percent were delivered on time, but had low birth weight, most likely due to intrauterine growth retardation. Some of the premature babies might in fact have been small-for-date babies due to intrauterine growth retardation.

Neonatal tetanus deaths typically occur between 3 and 30 days of life (about 90 percent occur at 4–14 days). In Cameroon, slightly more than one-fourth of the neonatal deaths occurred between 3–30 days and were associated with normal sucking during the first days of life (Table 8). This proportion may include all tetanus deaths, but also includes deaths due to nontetanus causes. If the reported convulsions, which probably also include spasms of the body in tetanus cases, are included, 5 percent of the neonatal deaths can be considered due to probable tetanus.

Diarrhoea was not common during the neonatal period, but was very common among deaths of older children. More than one third of the children dying after the neonatal period had at least two days of diarrhoea, 27 percent had at least two days of severe diarrhoea, and 5 percent had diarrhoea with blood (the latter is an indicator of dysentery).

If the diagnosis of respiratory illness in neonates was based on the presence of either at least one day of cough or at least two days of difficult breathing, then 25 percent of the neonatal deaths were associated with respiratory illness. The criteria used for the diagnosis of pneumonia (acute lower respiratory infection) in older children were cough for at least four days and difficult breathing for at least two days. The duration of breathing difficulties appears to be especially important, since many mothers report terminal breathing difficulties for their deceased children. About one in six deaths after the neonatal period was due to pneumonia.

A child was considered to have died from measles if the death occurred at the age of four months and older, with rash and fever for at least three days; this accounted for 6 percent of the deaths after the neonatal period. If fever is omitted from the criteria, the

**Table 8**  Presence of symptoms during the disease that led to death: percent with selected combinations of symptoms, Cameroon DHS, 1991

| Possible diagnosis | Symptoms | Age at death (months) | | |
|---|---|---|---|---|
| | | Neonatal | 1–59 | All |
| Low birth weight | Low birth weight | 19.0 | 5.7 | 10.6[1] |
| | With prematurity | 17.5 | 2.8 | 8.3 |
| | Delivery on time | 1.5 | 2.9 | 2.4 |
| Neonatal tetanus | Death at 3–30 days with normal sucking at birth | 27.4 | – | 10.2[1] |
| | With convulsions | 4.5 | – | 1.7 |
| Diarrhoeal diseases | Diarrhoea ≥ 2 days | 4.8 | 35.9 | 24.4 |
| | Diarrhoea severe, ≥ 2 days | 2.0 | 26.7 | 17.6[1] |
| | Diarrhoea with blood, ≥ 2 days | 1.9 | 4.9 | 3.8 |
| Pneumonia | Cough ≥ 1 day &/or dyspnoea ≥ 2 days | 25.0 | – | 9.3[1] |
| | Cough ≥ 4 days & dyspnoea ≥ 2 days | – | 16.3 | 10.3[1] |
| Measles | Death at 4 months and older with rash ≥ 3 days | – | 15.0 | 9.4 |
| | With fever ≥ 3 days | – | 5.6 | 3.5[1] |
| Malaria | Fever severe, ≥ 2 days | 9.9 | 37.1 | 27.1 |
| | Without rash, diarrhoea, or difficult breathing | 6.9 | 15.8 | 12.5[1] |
| Malnutrition | Very skinny, severe ≥ 1 month | – | 11.2 | 7.0 |
| | Swollen legs or face, severe, ≥ 1 month | – | 3.6 | 2.3 |
| | Either very skinny or swollen legs/face | – | 13.1 | 8.3[1] |

Note: Children who died of accidents are included in the denominator.
1. These diagnostic criteria were used to determine the probable cause of death in Tables 9 and 10.

proportion is 15 percent. Information was not obtained about deaths that occurred as a complication of measles after the clinical symptoms of measles had subsided (so-called post-measles deaths).

Malaria is difficult to diagnose. Serious fever for at least two days was reported for 37 percent of the deaths after the neonatal period. Of these, about 16 percent were without rash, diarrhoea, or difficult breathing. The latter two symptoms may occur in conjunction with malaria, but excluding them probably makes the diagnosis of malaria on the basis of serious fever more specific.

The diagnosis of malnutrition was made if the child was reportedly very thin for at least 1 month before death (wasting, marasmus), or had swollen legs or face for at least 1 month (kwashiorkor). Among deaths after the neonatal period, 13 percent were associated with malnutrition.

## Comparison of mother's reported cause and symptom-based diagnosis
For the five most common illnesses leading to death after the neonatal period, mother's reported cause of death was compared to the symptom-based diagnosis. In Table 9, the third column shows the percent of deaths for each diagnosis, derived from either the

**Table 9** Mother's reported cause of death and diagnosis based on reporting of probed symptoms for leading causes among deaths 1–59 months: percent from mother's report, from reported symptoms, from either source, and from both sources (in which both sources agree), Cameroon DHS, 1991 (N = 188 deaths)

| Disease | From mother's report | From symptoms | Either mother or symptoms | Both mother and symptoms |
|---|---|---|---|---|
| Diarrhoea | 17.4 | 26.7 | 32.7 | 11.4 |
| Malaria | 15.7 | 15.8 | 23.2 | 8.5 |
| Respiratory infection | 11.2 | 16.3 | 22.7 | 7.3 |
| Measles | 18.9 | 5.6 | 19.0 | 3.3 |
| Malnutrition | 4.2 | 13.1 | 14.5 | 2.8 |

mother's reported cause or the symptoms. The fourth column only includes cases in which mother's cause of death agreed with the diagnosis based on the symptoms. The proportions derived from each of the sources can be found in columns one and two of Table 9.

Diarrhoea was a mother-reported or a symptoms-based diagnosis for 33 percent of the deaths, but both sources were in agreement for only 11 percent of the deaths. For diarrhoea, malaria, and respiratory infection the proportion based on both sources is about one-third of the proportion based on either source. For measles and malnutrition the difference is much larger.

## Probable causes of death: a synthesis

Table 10 presents the probable causes of death, based on mother's report and on the symptoms as in Table 8. How the final diagnosis was made is indicated and multiple causes of death were allowed.

Low birth weight is the leading cause of death for neonatal mortality (19 percent), and is particularly prominent during the first days of life. Most of these deaths appear to be associated with reported prematurity. Birth problems, such as prolonged labour leading to asphyxia and other obstetric complications, account for 9 percent of neonatal mortality. Respiratory illness is a probable cause of death for 7 percent, and tetanus accounts for another 7 percent. The diagnosis of neonatal tetanus was based on the combination of age at death (3–30 days), normal sucking at birth, and mother's report of tetanus. Accidents are associated with 1 percent of the neonatal deaths. No cause of death is established for more than half of the neonatal deaths, including deaths for which only malaria/fever was mentioned, since malaria is unlikely for neonates, and fever only does not provide a diagnosis. This is due to the lack of knowledge among mothers about symptoms preceding neonatal death (e.g., 25 percent responded don't know to the open question on the cause of death), the lack of detailed questions on symptoms associated with causes of neonatal death, and the disagreement between mothers' diagnosis and symptoms reported for some deaths. In addition, the assessment of neonatal causes of death may be more difficult using the verbal autopsy technique.

**Table 10** Probable causes of death, based on mother's report on the main cause of death, and diagnostic algorithms, Cameroon DHS, 1991

**Neonatal mortality (N = 111)**

| Cause of death | Criteria for diagnosis | Percent |
|---|---|---|
| Low birth weight | Symptoms | 19.0 |
| Birth problems | Mother | 9.2 |
| Congenital anomalies | Mother | 0.5 |
| Tetanus | Mother, death 3–30 days, normal sucking first days | 7.0 |
| Respiratory illness | Mother & symptoms | 7.0 |
| Diarrhoea | Symptoms | 2.0 |
| Accidents | Mother | 1.4 |
| No cause identified | | 59.5 |

**Postneonatal and child mortality (N = 188)**

| Cause of Death | Criteria for Diagnosis | Percent |
|---|---|---|
| Diarrhoea | Symptoms (severe ≥ 2 d.) | 26.7 |
| Respiratory infection | Symptoms (cough & dyspnoea) | 16.3 |
| Measles | Mother or symptoms | 19.0 |
| Malaria | Mother or symptoms | 23.2 |
| Malnutrition | Mother or symptoms | 14.5 |
| Anaemia | Mother | 1.6 |
| Accidents | Mother | 1.8 |
| No cause identified | | 21.0 |

**All children under five years (N = 299)**

| Cause of death | Criteria for diagnosis | Percent |
|---|---|---|
| Diarrhoea | Symptoms (severe, ≥ 2 d.) | 17.6 |
| Respiratory infection | Symptoms (cough & dyspnoea) | 12.9 |
| Measles | Mother or symptoms | 12.0 |
| Malaria | Mother or symptoms | 14.6 |
| Malnutrition | Mother or symptoms | 9.1 |
| Anaemia | Mother | 1.6 |
| Accidents | Mother | 1.8 |
| Low birth weight | Symptoms | 7.1 |
| Birth problems | Mother | 3.4 |
| Tetanus | Mother & symptoms | 3.7 |
| No cause identified | | 35.3 |

Note: Multiple causes of death allowed.

After the neonatal period, diarrhoeal diseases are the leading cause of death with 27 percent, followed by malaria (23 percent), measles (19 percent), pneumonia (16 percent), and malnutrition (15 percent). Anaemia and accidents each accounted for less than 2 percent. The accidents included two deaths due to traffic accidents, one fall, one burn, and one classified as other. There was also one death due to poisoning. The causes of death may occur in combination with each other. Although one can argue about the accuracy of the estimates of the relative importance of the most prominent causes of death in childhood, it is clear from the Cameroon DHS survey that preventable causes of death are the most common killers in childhood.

In sum, the cause of death questions used in Cameroon appeared to have resulted in more plausible results than any of the preceding six DHS surveys discussed in this chapter with causes of death modules. The proportion of deaths that were classified as unknown was considerably smaller than in other surveys and reached acceptable levels for deaths after the neonatal period. Malaria and malnutrition also appeared on the list of leading causes of death. This in itself may present a more genuine picture of the leading causes of death, compared to verbal autopsy studies that focus only on diarrhoea, pneumonia, and measles. It is, however, very uncertain how accurate the estimates of mortality due to malaria and malnutrition are.

## Conclusion

In general, the results on the causes of death in the seven DHS surveys analyzed here are disappointing. Primarily, this is due to inadequate questions asked in the earlier surveys, which led to large proportions of deaths with unknown causes and unlikely distributions of the leading causes of death. The more extensive questionnaires were not very successful in Bolivia but were perhaps moderately successful in Cameroon. The quality of data is, however, difficult to assess and one has to rely on common sense to assess the resulting causes of death distribution. The same approach had to be used to evaluate data quality from epidemiological studies (Gray, 1991), since validation studies are few.

Classification into main and contributory causes is not feasible on the basis of a short questionnaire. However, the use of multiple causes gives a better picture of the causes of death pattern than the use of single causes. Therefore, multiple causes should be allowed, as was done for Cameroon, and no attempt has to be made to distinguish between main and contributory causes.

Based on the results of a few studies a recall period of 6–24 months has been recommended (Gray, 1990). The length of the recall period in DHS surveys is 0–4 years. In three of the surveys, there was a moderate increase in the proportion of don't know responses where the recall period was more than two years. However, there was no increase in four other surveys. This does not suggest that the length of the recall period is the major problem. However, information given for deaths more than two years ago may be less accurate as well, but this cannot be evaluated with the DHS data sets.

Further improvements can possibly be made when more emphasis is placed on traditional names and classifications of causes of death. Such an effort has been shown to be worthwhile in several studies, but may take at least six weeks of research. Since DHS surveys are often carried out in multiple languages, such anthropological studies may not be feasible within the short time-frame of a DHS survey.

Causes of neonatal mortality generally are more difficult to determine in verbal autopsy than causes of death among older children. Not much effort has been made to determine causes of neonatal mortality, except for tetanus mortality, in the DHS program, but efforts to determine these causes would certainly be worthwhile.

In summary, it remains to be seen whether it is possible to obtain reasonably accurate data on the leading causes of death in childhood in large-scale cross-sectional surveys. With a well-developed questionnaire (more validation studies are required) it is possible to obtain a general picture of the causes of death which can be used for advocacy purposes. If the objective is to assess cause-specific mortality trends (e.g., four of the World Summit for Children Goals are cause-specific mortality reductions) one has to be more cautious for two reasons: misclassification and sampling errors. The results of validation studies show that misclassification of causes of death is common, and such studies are assumed to give the best possible picture (since only hospital deaths are used).

## Acknowledgments

We are grateful to Ron Gray for comments on this paper.

## References

Gray, R.H., G. Smith, and P. Barss. 1990. The use of verbal autopsy methods to determine selected causes of death in children. Occasional Paper No. 10. Baltimore, Maryland: Institute for International Programs, the Johns Hopkins University.

Gray, R.H. 1991. Interview-based diagnosis of morbidity and causes of death. Paper presented at seminar on Measurement of Maternal and Child Mortality, Morbidity and Health Care: Interdisciplinary Approaches. IUSSP. Cairo, November 4–7, 1991.

Kalter, H.D., R.H. Gray, R.E. Black, and S.A. Gultiano. 1990. Validation of post-mortem interviews to ascertain selected causes of death in children. *International Journal of Epidemiology* 19(2): 380–386.

Koenig, M.A., B. Khan, J.D. Wojtyniak, J.D. Clemens, J. Chakraborty, V. Fauveau, J.F. Phillips, J. Akbar, and U.S. Barua. 1990. Impact of measles vaccination on childhood mortality in Matlab, Bangladesh. *Bulletin of the World Health Organization* 68(4): 441–447.

Moreno, L. and N. Goldman. 1990. An assessment of survey data on birth weight. *Social Science and Medicine* 31(4): 491–500.

Sommerfelt, A.E., J.T. Boerma, L.H. Ochoa, and S.O. Rutstein. 1991. Maternal and child health in Bolivia: Report on the in-depth DHS survey in Bolivia 1989. Columbia, Maryland: Institute for Resource Development/Macro Systems Inc.

8

# Using survey data to assess neonatal tetanus mortality levels and trends in developing countries

*J. Ties Boerma and George Stroh*

**Demography**, *vol. 30, no. 3, 1993, pp. 459–476.*

## Abstract

Demographic and health surveys are a useful source of information on the levels and trends of neonatal mortality in developing countries. Such surveys provide data on mortality occurring at 4–14 days of life, which is a sensitive indicator of neonatal tetanus mortality. We analyze birth history data from 37 national surveys in developing countries to assess the quality of neonatal mortality data and to estimate levels and trends in mortality occurring at 4–14 days. It is shown that mortality at 4–14 days has declined considerably during the last decade in most developing countries, concomitant with development and expansion of programs to reduce neonatal tetanus. These declines show that reductions in neonatal tetanus mortality probably have been an important contributor to the decline of neonatal and infant mortality during the 1980s.

## Introduction

Tetanus has been estimated to be responsible for 750,000 neonatal deaths annually and is considered one of the leading causes of neonatal mortality (Expanded Programme on Immunization, 1989). The organism causing tetanus *(Clostridium tetani)* is omnipresent in soil and dust. Newborn babies generally are infected through the umbilical stump because of unsterile methods of cutting the cord or dressing the stump. After a few days of life the baby becomes unable to suck and swallow because of muscle rigidity, which spreads quickly throughout the body. Tetanus deaths are rare during the first days of life, but rise rapidly to a peak at the end of the first week of life. Case fatality rates of untreated tetanus are estimated as high as 85% (Galazka and Stroh, 1986).

Tetanus has long been an overlooked disease (Stanfield and Galazka, 1984), but the elimination of neonatal tetanus mortality currently ranks high on the international health agenda. Elimination of neonatal tetanus is to be achieved by increasing passive immunity among newborns through immunization of women of childbearing ages with tetanus toxoid (TT) to prevent disease and by improving delivery care to prevent infection. Well before the use of tetanus toxoid, neonatal tetanus mortality declined in much of the Western world and Japan through changing delivery practices (Steinglass, Brenzel, and Percy, 1992).

The measurement of national levels of neonatal tetanus mortality is complicated and must be conducted carefully through surveillance or surveys, because reliable vital registration data are lacking. In this paper we first review sources of data on neonatal tetanus mortality, including surveillance and special tetanus surveys. Subsequently we explore the usefulness of demographic surveys for evaluating neonatal tetanus mortality by using age-specific neonatal mortality data collected in birth histories. After assessing the quality of such information, we present levels and trends of neonatal tetanus mortality for 32 developing countries with recent Demographic and Health Surveys (DHS).

## Measurement of neonatal tetanus mortality

The reporting of surveillance data on neonatal tetanus, by countries, to the Expanded Program on Immunization of the World Health Organization shows that the frequency of reporting of neonatal tetanus as a separate disease entity was poor in 1980 but has improved considerably during the last decade. The completeness of reporting of neonatal tetanus cases and deaths depends on the quality of reporting of neonatal tetanus by health facilities within each country. More emphasis on tetanus led to an increase in reported tetanus cases during the 1980s. For instance, Egypt began reporting neonatal tetanus in 1978, but the importance of the disease was not recognized until the mid 1980s. As a result, reported neonatal tetanus cases increased from about 4,000 in 1978 to 7,000 in 1981, and to almost 10,000 in 1986. Serious control efforts began in 1987–1988, when immunizations of pregnant women increased from 9% to 73%. The effect of these control efforts is reflected in a decline of neonatal tetanus cases to about 5,000 in 1990. These data indicate the recency of the emphasis given to neonatal tetanus and represent improvements of surveillance for that disease through routine reporting. Incomplete, irregular, and inaccurate reporting of tetanus, however, remains an obstacle in many countries.

During the last decade, population-based neonatal tetanus mortality surveys have been the method most commonly used to assess the magnitude of neonatal tetanus mortality and, to a lesser extent, to show the impact of health interventions on neonatal tetanus mortality, if multiple surveys are conducted. These surveys focus on births and deaths in a specified and relatively short period before the survey, usually 12 months, and pose questions about the classic symptoms of tetanus to ascertain whether tetanus was the cause of neonatal death (Galazka and Stroh, 1986). As of 1989, 42 countries had conducted more than 75 of these surveys (Gasse, 1990). Estimates of neonatal tetanus mortality range from 1 or 2 per 1,000 live births to more than 30 per 1,000 live births.

**Table 1** Sensitivity, specificity, and predictive values of mortality at 4–14 days as an indicator of neonatal tetanus mortality, Colombia 1961–66 and Senegal 1983–86

| | Colombia | | | Senegal | | |
|---|---|---|---|---|---|---|
| | Tetanus | | | Tetanus | | |
| Age at death | Yes | No | Total | Yes | No | Total |
| 4–14 days | 100 | 26 | 126 | 62 | 45 | 107[a] |
| Other neonatal | 9 | 76 | 85 | 4 | 100 | 104 |
| Total | 109 | 102 | 211 | 66 | 145 | 211 |
| Sensitivity (%) | | | 92 | | | 94 |
| Specificity (%) | | | 75 | | | 69 |
| Predictive value positive (%) | | | 79 | | | 58 |
| Predictive value negative (%) | | | 89 | | | 96 |

a. 4–13 days.
Note: The definitions are as follows:

| | | Tetanus present | |
|---|---|---|---|
| | | Yes | No |
| Classification | Yes | a | b |
| | No | c | d |

Sensitivity = a/(a+c)
Specificity = d/(b+d)
Predictive value positive = a/(a+b)
Predicitive value negative = d/(c+d)

Sources: Newell et al. (1966); Leroy and Garenne (1987).

Initially most neonatal tetanus mortality surveys were conducted to convince authorities that neonatal tetanus was an under-reported problem and to set a baseline for tetanus control programs. Now that the awareness of the neonatal tetanus problem has been raised in most countries, series of such surveys could now be used to monitor neonatal tetanus mortality trends, but the costs of repeated large surveys with a limited focus are prohibitive. In addition, the use of a short fixed recall period before the survey may lead to substantial under-reporting of neonatal deaths (Ewbank, 1984,1984; Tabutin, 1984). A comparison of neonatal mortality levels in neonatal tetanus surveys and in demographic surveys (which use a full birth history) showed that neonatal tetanus surveys may underestimate neonatal mortality by as much as 50% (Boerma and Van Ginneken, 1992). Therefore alternative ways of monitoring neonatal tetanus mortality should be explored, particularly when the incidence of neonatal tetanus declines (Stroh, 1990).

## An alternative: age-specific mortality data

Neonatal tetanus mortality has a very typical age-specific mortality pattern; the great majority of deaths occur 4 to 14 days after birth (Stanfield and Galazka, 1984, Stroh, 1990), whereas most neonatal deaths not due to tetanus occur during the first few days of life. Table 1 presents data from local studies in Colombia (Newell et al., 1966) and Senegal (Leroy and Garenne, 1987), which permit calculations of sensitivity and predictive value positive (pvp) of mortality at 4–14 days as an indicator of neonatal tetanus mortality. The sensitivity is high: almost all neonatal tetanus deaths occur between 4 and 14 days. Reviews of data from other studies in Indonesia, Mozambique, St. Kilda (Scotland) and India also indicate sensitivity of about 90% (Galazka and Stroh, 1986). The pvp – that is the proportion of all deaths occurring at 4–14 days that are neonatal tetanus – was 79% in Colombia and 58% in Senegal. Other age periods (e.g., 6–14 days or 4–16 days) did not result in more satisfactory combinations of sensitivity and pvp.

Mortality rates at 4–14 days also have been used to evaluate the mortality impact of health interventions, particularly tetanus toxoid immunization (Bhatia, 1989, Black, Huber and Curlin, 1980). In an intervention area in Matlab, Bangladesh, tetanus toxoid immunization of pregnant women was introduced in 1978; neonatal deaths at 4–14 days declined from 40% in 1977–1978 to 20% in 1982–1983 (Bhatia, 1989). In the comparison area, the proportion of neonatal deaths at 4–14 days remained at the same level during the study period. No significant changes in mortality occurred at 0–3 days or at 15–28 days in either area, which could have altered the proportion occurring at 4–14 days as well.

Because neonatal tetanus follows a very typical age pattern of mortality, mortality data from demographic surveys are a potential source of data for evaluating neonatal tetanus mortality. Demographic surveys, which focus on child mortality and fertility related issues, include a full birth (or maternity) history of the respondents (usually women of reproductive age) and data on the age at death of deceased children. The relevance of the demographic surveys for estimating neonatal tetanus mortality depends on two factors: the usefulness of mortality at 4–14 days as an indicator of neonatal tetanus mortality, and the quality of age-specific mortality data during the neonatal period.

In our analysis of age-specific mortality data from the demographic surveys, neonatal tetanus mortality is suspected to be high if the mortality rate at 4–14 days is high and if a relatively large proportion of neonatal deaths occur in the 4–14 day period. Mortality during the first days of life is higher than during any other period, but declines rapidly. To assess whether the mortality level at 4–14 days is high, it may be useful to compare 4–14 day mortality levels with mortality at 15–27 days in the same population. Analysis of data from Colombia (Newell et al., 1966), Bangladesh (Black et al., 1980), Indonesia and Colombia (Stanfield and Galazka, 1984), and Senegal (Leroy and Garenne, 1987) suggests that mortality levels, in the absence of neonatal tetanus, should be approximately the same for the two age periods. Excess mortality at 4–14 days then could point to the possibility of high neonatal tetanus mortality.

Only limited methods are available for assessing the quality of age-specific neonatal mortality data. Both under-reporting and misreporting are possible, and the biases may vary with the length of the recall period. Consistency of mortality estimates between subsequent surveys for the same population would support the accuracy of recall data on age at death in days. Some indication of the quality of neonatal mortality data is provided by the prevalence of missing values for age at death and by the extent of heaping of deaths at 7, 14, and 15 days, by the length of the recall period. Heaping of deaths at 14 and 15 days is particularly important, because it may cause misclassification of deaths into or out of the 4–14 day age period.

# Data

The data on age-specific mortality are derived from the surveys conducted as part of the Demographic and Health Surveys project (DHS), which is supported by the U.S. Agency for International Development. This project started in 1984 and has assisted more than 40 developing countries in conducting nationally representative surveys.[1] As of this writing, five countries have conducted two DHS surveys: Colombia, the Dominican Republic, Indonesia, Morocco, and Peru. The survey respondents are women of reproductive age. Our study includes all completed DHS surveys with data on age-specific neonatal mortality. Table 2 shows the year of the survey and the sample sizes for each survey.

The DHS surveys collect data on a full birth history from women age 15–49 at the time of the survey. The respondent is asked to provide information on all her children born alive, starting with the most recent birth. This information includes the child's sex, birth date, and survival status. If a child died, the age at death is recorded in months for children under two years, but in days for neonatal deaths.

One advantage of a full birth history is that time trends can be assessed. For the analysis of neonatal mortality trends during the last decade, we grouped births into two five-year intervals before the date of each survey: 0–4 years and 5–9 years. Shorter intervals make the numbers of births and deaths in each cohort too small to produce reliable estimates of mortality in surveys with smaller sample sizes. The most recent period does not include children born during the month of interview and children born one month before the survey month, because some of these children had not completed one month of life. Because the DHS surveys we are using are retrospective surveys with respondents age 15–49 years, births during the survey year are to women age 15–49, whereas births 10 years ago before the surveys were to (the same) women at ages 5–39 years. Therefore, we exclude births to women over age 40 to avoid possible biases in trend analysis created by the larger proportion of births to older women in the more recent birth cohorts.

The DHS surveys also collect information on child health-related topics for all births in the five years preceding the survey. This information includes whether the mother had received at least one tetanus toxoid infection during each pregnancy, and the kind of medical assistance rendered at each delivery.[2] From these questions it is possible to obtain a crude estimate of the proportion of newborns at lower risk of neonatal tetanus, even though neither a single dose of tetanus toxoid (even if recalled correctly by the respondent) nor the presence of a doctor, nurse, or midwife at the delivery eliminates the risk of this condition.

# Results

## Quality of the data
Missing values for age at death were rare for child deaths (data not shown). Less than 2% of data on the age at death in days were missing in all but two surveys. About 5%

**Table 2**  Characteristics of DHS surveys and heaping of neonatal deaths

| Survey | Year of survey | Number of | | Heaping % | | |
|---|---|---|---|---|---|---|
| | | Births | Deaths | 7 days | 14 days | 15 days |
| **West and Central Africa** | | | | | | |
| Cameroon | 1991 | 3,388 | 107 | 6.3 | 4.2 | 3.8 |
| Ghana | 1988 | 4,013 | 176 | 5.1 | 3.4 | 0.0 |
| Liberia | 1986 | 4,991 | 332 | 12.7 | 6.7 | 1.2 |
| Mali | 1987 | 3,313 | 166 | 11.2 | 0.5 | 1.4 |
| Nigeria | 1990 | 7,932 | 329 | 6.1 | 4.8 | 1.2 |
| Senegal | 1987 | 4,180 | 186 | 9.7 | 1.1 | 5.4 |
| Togo | 1988 | 3,047 | 119 | 7.6 | 3.4 | 5.0 |
| **East and Southern Africa** | | | | | | |
| Botswana | 1988 | 3,101 | 66 | 11.0 | 1.8 | 0.0 |
| Burundi | 1987 | 3,764 | 133 | 13.8 | 12.9 | 3.7 |
| Kenya | 1989 | 6,930 | 184 | 28.5 | 15.7 | 1.2 |
| Tanzania | 1991 | 7,876 | 287 | 14.7 | 10.4 | 0.2 |
| Uganda | 1988 | 4,886 | 201 | 17.0 | 6.3 | 1.5 |
| Zambia | 1992 | 6,085 | 254 | 11.7 | 9.3 | 0.0 |
| Zi mbabwe | 1989 | 3,278 | 87 | 8.0 | 6.9 | 1.1 |
| **North Africa and Middle East** | | | | | | |
| Egypt | 1989 | 8,470 | 323 | 22.9 | 0.7 | 4.5 |
| Jordan | 1990 | 8,032 | 177 | 8.2 | 2.8 | 3.5 |
| Morocco I | 1987 | 5,945 | 235 | 14.4 | 1.3 | 8.5 |
| Morocco II | 1992 | 5,091 | 159 | 10.6 | 1.9 | 6.9 |
| Sudan | 1989 | 6,375 | 274 | 12.4 | 1.1 | 2.2 |
| Tunisia | 1988 | 4,362 | 115 | 9.6 | 0.0 | 6.1 |
| **Asia** | | | | | | |
| Indonesia I | 1987 | 8,018 | 211 | 19.2 | 1.1 | 5.0 |
| Indonesia II | 1991 | 14,109 | 439 | 15.9 | 2.1 | 2.5 |
| Pakistan | 1991 | 6,245 | 296 | 6.7 | 1.1 | 5.2 |
| Sri Lanka | 1987 | 3,873 | 62 | 5.1 | 9.5 | 0.0 |
| Thailand | 1987 | 3,568 | 72 | 8.2 | 0.0 | 7.2 |
| **Latin America and Caribbean** | | | | | | |
| Bolivia | 1989 | 5,641 | 199 | 9.8 | 4.4 | 4.9 |
| Brazil | 1986 | 3,399 | 111 | 5.0 | 1.6 | 3.6 |
| Colombia I | 1986 | 2,620 | 51 | 0.0 | 0.0 | 0.0 |
| Colombia II | 1990 | 3,665 | 51 | 1.9 | 0.0 | 0.0 |
| Dominican Rep. I | 1986 | 4,306 | 165 | 1.3 | 2.6 | 2.8 |
| Dominican Rep. II | 1991 | 3,745 | 90 | 4.7 | 1.6 | 1.5 |
| Ecuador | 1987 | 2,977 | 100 | 7.0 | 0.0 | 9.0 |
| Guatemala | 1987 | 4,626 | 155 | 4.1 | 0.7 | 10.3 |
| Paraguay | 1990 | 3,882 | 74 | 4.5 | 0.0 | 5.1 |
| Peru I | 1986 | 3,052 | 105 | 11.4 | 1.9 | 6.7 |
| Peru II | 1992 | 8,409 | 212 | 5.5 | 1.8 | 4.6 |
| Trinidad and Tobago | 1987 | 1,903 | 45 | 4.4 | 0.0 | 0.0 |

Note: Live births and neonatal deaths refer to the five-year period before the survey, and exclude the month of survey and the preceding month.

were missing only in Kenya and Liberia, but these deaths are not necessarily neonatal. In addition, the comparison of the proportions with missing values for deaths 0–4 and 5–9 years before each survey generally shows no increase in the proportion of missing ages at death by the length of time elapsed before the survey.

The quality of data on the age at death is evaluated in Table 2 for births in the five years preceding each survey. Heaping of deaths at seven days is common. In 14 of the 36 surveys more than 10% of the neonatal deaths reportedly occurred at seven days; in Egypt and Indonesia I, about one-fifth of the neonatal deaths were recorded as deaths at seven days of life. There is no increase in heaping by the length of the recall period (not shown). We expect heaping at seven days to be somewhat more common in populations with high levels of neonatal tetanus mortality, because neonatal tetanus deaths are concentrated at 6–10 days (e.g., see Leroy and Garenne, 1987).

In eight countries more than 5% of the neonatal deaths were recorded at 14 days, including six surveys in eastern and southern Africa. The extent of heaping at 14 days is not affected by the length of the recall period (not shown). Heaping at 15 days is also common: in nine countries, at least 5% of the neonatal deaths were recorded as deaths at 15 days; Guatemala shows the strongest heaping (10%).

## Mortality levels

Table 3 presents the distribution of neonatal deaths by age at death in days in the DHS surveys for the five years before the survey. Four surveys had neonatal mortality rates below 20 per 1,000 live births; in nine surveys, neonatal mortality was more than 40 per 1,000 live births. Mortality levels at 4–14 days vary from 3 to 22 per 1,000 live births and are higher than 10 per 1,000 live births in more than half of the surveys. The proportion of neonatal deaths occurring at 4–14 days is more than 40% in five countries (Mali, Senegal, Burundi, Egypt, Indonesia) and less than 20% in three countries (Guatemala, Colombia, and Trinidad and Tobago).

Regionally, neonatal and 4–14 day mortality levels are highest in west and central Africa, followed by east and southern Africa, and by north Africa and the Middle East. The last-cited region has the highest proportion of neonatal deaths occurring at 4–14 days (39%). Mortality at 4–14 days is lower in Latin America and the Caribbean than in the other regions (25% of neonatal mortality). In Asia, 4–14 day mortality levels in Pakistan and Indonesia are relatively high, whereas Sri Lanka and Thailand have low levels.

## Mortality trends

The trends of neonatal mortality rates and mortality rates at 4–14 days are shown in Table 4 for two five-year periods before the survey. In virtually all countries neonatal mortality declined during the decade preceding the survey.[3] The strongest declines occurred in countries in west and central Africa (from 58 to 44 per 1,000 live births), but much of this decline is associated with a large decline in neonatal mortality in Mali. In eastern and southern Africa, neonatal mortality levels are lower and the decline is less pronounced. Neonatal mortality increased in Kenya and Zambia. In the case of Kenya this increase may be due partly to underestimation of mortality for the earlier periods. In Zambia the increase is consistent with a mortality increase in all age groups. In north

**Table 3** Neonatal mortality rates (per 1,000 live births) by age at death in days for the five years preceding DHS

| Survey | 0–3 days | 4–14 days | 15–27 days | Total | Percentage at 4–14 days |
|---|---|---|---|---|---|
| **West and Central Africa** | 25.8 | 16.3 | 3.2 | 45.3 | 36 |
| Cameroon | 18.7 | 10.9 | 2.0 | 31.6 | 34 |
| Ghana | 28.1 | 14.0 | 1.7 | 43.9 | 32 |
| Liberia | 40.9 | 21.8 | 3.9 | 66.6 | 33 |
| Mali | 25.5 | 20.6 | 3.9 | 50.0 | 41 |
| Nigeria | 24.8 | 12.7 | 4.0 | 41.5 | 31 |
| Senegal | 18.9 | 21.5 | 4.1 | 44.5 | 48 |
| Togo | 23.7 | 12.8 | 2.6 | 39.1 | 33 |
| **East and Southern Africa** | 19.5 | 11.3 | 3.1 | 33.9 | 33 |
| Botswana | 15.8 | 5.6 | 0.0 | 21.4 | 26 |
| Burundi | 17.5 | 15.0 | 2.8 | 35.2 | 43 |
| Kenya | 16.5 | 8.8 | 1.4 | 26.6 | 33 |
| Tanzania | 21.7 | 12.9 | 5.0 | 36.4 | 35 |
| Uganda | 23.0 | 14.5 | 3.6 | 41.1 | 35 |
| Zambia | 23.4 | 14.7 | 8.7 | 41.7 | 35 |
| Zimbabwe | 18.6 | 7.6 | 0.3 | 26.5 | 29 |
| **North Africa and Middle East** | 6.5 | 12.4 | 3.3 | 32.2 | 39 |
| Egypt | 17.1 | 17.4 | 3.7 | 38.2 | 46 |
| Jordan | 12.1 | 8.1 | 1.8 | 22.0 | 37 |
| Morocco I | 17.8 | 14.6 | 7.1 | 39.5 | 37 |
| Morocco II | 14.3 | 11.6 | 5.3 | 31.2 | 37 |
| Sudan | 25.0 | 15.5 | 2.5 | 43.0 | 36 |
| Tunisia | 13.8 | 9.2 | 3.4 | 26.4 | 35 |
| **Asia** | 15.2 | 10.2 | 3.3 | 28.7 | 35 |
| Indonesia I | 9.0 | 14.5 | 3.2 | 26.6 | 54 |
| Indonesia II | 15.5 | 12.6 | 3.0 | 31.1 | 40 |
| Pakistan | 23.9 | 16.4 | 7.1 | 47.4 | 35 |
| Sri Lanka | 9.2 | 5.7 | 1.2 | 16.1 | 36 |
| Thailand | 12.3 | 5.9 | 2.0 | 20.2 | 29 |
| **Latin America and Caribbean** | 16.5 | 6.5 | 3.5 | 26.5 | 25 |
| Bolivia | 19.9 | 11.4 | 4.0 | 35.2 | 35 |
| Brazil | 20.8 | 8.0 | 4.0 | 32.8 | 24 |
| Colombia I | 12.4 | 5.2 | 2.1 | 19.6 | 26 |
| Colombia II | 10.6 | 2.5 | 0.8 | 13.9 | 18 |
| Dominican Rep. I | 22.0 | 12.0 | 4.3 | 38.3 | 29 |
| Dominican Rep. II | 15.8 | 6.4 | 1.7 | 23.9 | 27 |
| Ecuador | 18.5 | 9.7 | 5.4 | 33.6 | 29 |
| Guatemala | 19.5 | 5.8 | 6.1 | 31.3 | 19 |
| Paraguay | 12.1 | 5.0 | 2.0 | 19.0 | 26 |
| Peru I | 18.7 | 11.8 | 3.9 | 34.4 | 34 |
| Peru II | 14.8 | 6.2 | 4.2 | 25.2 | 25 |
| Trinidad and Tobago | 16.8 | 3.7 | 3.2 | 23.6 | 16 |

Note: Regional means include only DHS 1I survey in countries where more than one survey was conducted.

**Table 4** Trends in neonatal mortality rates (per 1,000 live births) during decade preceding DHS

| Country | 0–4 Years before Survey | | | | | 5–9 Years before Survey | | | | |
|---|---|---|---|---|---|---|---|---|---|---|
| | 0–3 Days | 4–14 Days | 15–27 Days | Total | % at 4–14 | 0–3 Days | 4–14 Days | 15–27 Days | Total | % at Days |
| **West and Central Africa** | 25.5 | 15.5 | 3.0 | 44.1 | 35 | 30.7 | 22.6 | 4.3 | 57.7 | 39 |
| Cameroon | 18.4 | 10.8 | 2.0 | 31.3 | 35 | 29.6 | 18.7 | 3.8 | 52.2 | 36 |
| Ghana | 28.8 | 13.2 | 1.3 | 43.4 | 30 | 26.9 | 18.9 | 3.4 | 49.3 | 38 |
| Liberia | 39.5 | 21.3 | 3.2 | 64.0 | 33 | 41.2 | 26.5 | 3.2 | 70.9 | 37 |
| Nigeria | 24.9 | 17.6 | 3.6 | 46.1 | 38 | 43.8 | 33.0 | 6.2 | 83.1 | 40 |
| Mali | 24.5 | 12.2 | 4.2 | 40.9 | 30 | 22.0 | 22.4 | 3.0 | 47.4 | 47 |
| Senegal | 18.7 | 20.7 | 4.0 | 43.4 | 48 | 19.6 | 24.7 | 4.6 | 48.9 | 51 |
| Togo | 23.7 | 12.9 | 2.8 | 39.3 | 33 | 32.0 | 13.9 | 6.0 | 51.9 | 27 |
| **East and Southern Africa** | 19.0 | 11.0 | 2.0 | 32.0 | 34 | 20.4 | 13.6 | 1.6 | 35.7 | 38 |
| Botswana | 15.3 | 5.8 | 0.0 | 21.1 | 28 | 14.0 | 6.3 | 0.8 | 21.2 | 30 |
| Burundi | 17.5 | 14.6 | 3.0 | 35.1 | 42 | 20.6 | 19.2 | 1.7 | 41.5 | 46 |
| Kenya | 16.5 | 9.1 | 1.5 | 27.0 | 34 | 16.0 | 5.6 | 0.3 | 21.9 | 26 |
| Tanzania | 21.7 | 13.9 | 3.7 | 39.4 | 35 | 34.3 | 19.3 | 1.8 | 55.4 | 35 |
| Uganda | 22.0 | 11.3 | 1.9 | 35.2 | 32 | 24.8 | 13.8 | 2.4 | 41.0 | 34 |
| Zambia | 22.8 | 14.5 | 3.6 | 40.9 | 35 | 17.2 | 15.7 | 3.1 | 36.0 | 44 |
| Zimbabwe | 17.6 | 7.7 | 0.3 | 25.5 | 30 | 16.1 | 15.4 | 1.3 | 32.7 | 47 |
| **North Africa and Middle East** | 17.2 | 12.8 | 3.7 | 33.7 | 38 | 19.5 | 14.9 | 4.6 | 39.0 | 38 |
| Egypt | 17.3 | 17.5 | 3.7 | 38.4 | 45 | 19.3 | 30.2 | 5.3 | 54.8 | 55 |
| Jordan | 11.9 | 8.0 | 1.7 | 21.6 | 37 | 13.3 | 5.3 | 3.0 | 21.6 | 24 |
| Morocco I | 18.3 | 15.1 | 7.4 | 40.8 | 37 | 20.8 | 18.7 | 8.2 | 47.7 | 39 |
| Morocco II | 14.5 | 11.6 | 5.1 | 31.2 | 37 | 16.2 | 14.1 | 5.9 | 36.1 | 39 |
| Sudan | 13.6 | 8.4 | 3.1 | 25.1 | 33 | 18.1 | 7.6 | 3.8 | 29.5 | 26 |
| Tunisia | 24.9 | 15.3 | 2.6 | 42.9 | 36 | 25.8 | 12.7 | 2.7 | 41.2 | 31 |

*(continued)*

**Table 4** (continued)

| Country | 0–4 Years before Survey | | | | | 5–9 Years before Survey | | | | |
|---|---|---|---|---|---|---|---|---|---|---|
| | 0–3 Days | 4–14 Days | 15–27 Days | Total | % at 4–14 | 0–3 Days | 4–14 Days | 15–27 Days | Total | % at Days |
| Asia | 15.0 | 10.0 | 3.4 | 28.5 | 35 | 19.0 | 13.4 | 3.2 | 35.6 | 38 |
| Indonesia I | 8.7 | 15.0 | 3.2 | 26.9 | 56 | 15.0 | 20.8 | 4.6 | 40.4 | 52 |
| Indonesia II | 15.0 | 12.4 | 3.1 | 30.4 | 41 | 15.8 | 16.7 | 3.0 | 35.5 | 47 |
| Pakistan | 23.6 | 16.8 | 7.4 | 47.9 | 35 | 28.2 | 21.6 | 6.3 | 56.1 | 38 |
| Sri Lanka | 9.0 | 5.5 | 1.2 | 15.8 | 35 | 16.7 | 5.1 | 2.9 | 24.7 | 21 |
| Thailand | 12.5 | 5.5 | 2.0 | 19.9 | 27 | 15.5 | 10.2 | 0.5 | 26.2 | 39 |
| Latin America and Caribbean | 16.6 | 7.2 | 3.5 | 27.2 | 26 | 17.8 | 9.2 | 3.5 | 30.6 | 30 |
| Bolivia | 19.9 | 11.8 | 4.2 | 35.9 | 33 | 22.5 | 18.4 | 4.1 | 45.1 | 41 |
| Brazil | 20.4 | 7.5 | 4.0 | 31.9 | 23 | 20.8 | 9.9 | 5.0 | 35.6 | 28 |
| Colombia I | 12.4 | 5.3 | 2.2 | 19.9 | 27 | 14.8 | 3.8 | 1.9 | 20.5 | 19 |
| Colombia II | 10.0 | 2.5 | 0.6 | 13.1 | 19 | 10.3 | 4.2 | 1.9 | 16.4 | 25 |
| Ecuador | 21.7 | 12.1 | 4.3 | 38.1 | 32 | 25.3 | 11.0 | 3.4 | 39.7 | 28 |
| Dom. Rep. I | 16.0 | 5.7 | 1.5 | 23.3 | 25 | 12.3 | 8.9 | 3.8 | 25.0 | 35 |
| Dom. Rep. II | 18.5 | 9.1 | 5.6 | 33.2 | 27 | 18.9 | 11.4 | 6.5 | 36.9 | 31 |
| Guatemala | 19.1 | 6.1 | 6.1 | 31.4 | 20 | 26.7 | 10.3 | 2.3 | 39.3 | 26 |
| Paraguay | 11.6 | 4.7 | 2.1 | 18.4 | 26 | 11.4 | 5.7 | 2.5 | 19.6 | 29 |
| Peru I | 19.0 | 11.1 | 3.5 | 33.6 | 33 | 16.8 | 11.7 | 4.7 | 33.2 | 35 |
| Peru II | 14.0 | 6.2 | 4.2 | 24.4 | 25 | 18.3 | 10.6 | 5.4 | 34.3 | 31 |
| Trinidad and Tobago | 16.0 | 3.7 | 3.2 | 22.9 | 16 | 15.9 | 4.9 | 0.5 | 21.4 | 23 |

Notes: Includes only births to women age < 40 years. Excludes month of interview and month before. Regional means include only DHS II survey in countries where more than one survey was conducted.

**Figure I** Neonatal mortality trends

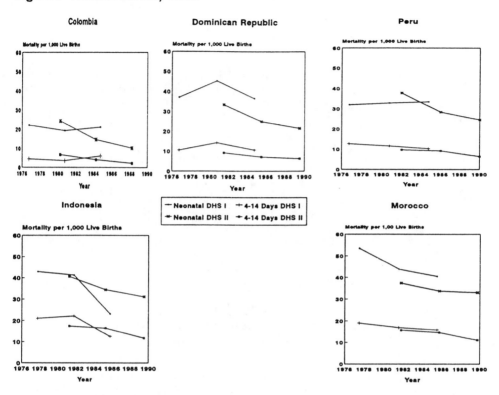

Africa and the Middle East, overall neonatal mortality levels and trends are similar to those in east and southern Africa, including a pronounced decline in Egypt, but no decline occurred in Jordan and Tunisia. In the four Asian countries, levels of mortality vary considerably, but all show a decline in neonatal mortality. A moderate decline can be observed in most countries in Latin America and the Caribbean, where neonatal mortality levels are lowest.

Mortality at 4–14 days also decreased in most countries and made a major contribution to the overall decline in neonatal mortality in many countries. In most countries, 4–14 day mortality declined faster than overall neonatal mortality, as evidenced by the decline in the proportion of neonatal deaths occurring at 4–14 days. In 19 of 32 countries, more than half of the neonatal mortality decline can be attributed to the decline in mortality at 4–14 days. Egypt is an example: neonatal mortality declined from 55 to 38 per 1,000 live births from 1980–1984 to 1985–1989 and the reduction in mortality at 4–14 days accounted for more than three-quarters of this decline. This change is consistent with the introduction of and major emphasis given to a neonatal tetanus control program in Egypt.[4]

**Figure 2**  Mortality rate at 4–14 days, by tetanus risk level

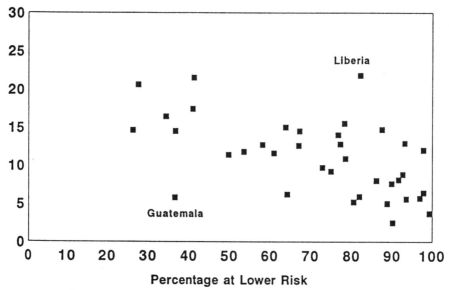

Percentage at Lower Risk

Each dot represents one survey. See text for definition of lower risk.

Figure 2. Mortality Rate at 4–14 Days, by Tetanus Risk Level

Figure 1 shows neonatal and 4–14 day mortality trends in countries with two DHS surveys.[5] For each survey, mortality has been estimated for three four-year intervals preceding the survey. The neonatal mortality trends are consistent between the two surveys in Peru, Morocco, and Colombia, but not in the other two countries. In Indonesia, the neonatal mortality estimate for the most recent four-year interval from the first survey appears to be about 10 per 1,000 too low, if the more consistent estimates of both surveys are assumed to be correct. Half of this deficit stems from the first two days. Under-reporting of very early deaths in the most recent period is a possibility, although this phenomenon does not repeat itself in the DHS II survey. In the Dominican Republic, considerable under-reporting of very early neonatal deaths seems to have occurred for the most distant periods in both surveys.

Trends in 4–14 day mortality, however, are much more consistent in all surveys and show a steady decline in Indonesia, Peru, Morocco, and the Dominican Republic. The rate does not decline in Colombia, where the level of 4–14 day mortality was already below 10 per 1,000 in 1980.

## Mortality differentials

Figure 2 presents a scatter diagram of 4–14 day mortality by the proportion of newborns at lower risk of neonatal tetanus among births in the five years before the surveys. We considered a birth lower-risk if the mother either had received at least one tetanus toxoid injection during pregnancy or had delivered in the presence of a medically trained person. A fairly strong correlation exists at the aggregate level: 50% of the variation in the 4–14 day mortality rate is explained by the 'tetanus risk' level (excluding the outliers Liberia and Guatemala; 30% if all are included). In countries with higher mortality at 4–14 days, the proportions of births at lower risk of neonatal tetanus are small, and mortality declines with increasing proportions of births at lower risk of tetanus. Liberia is an outlier with a much higher mortality level than expected; most likely this is due to errors made during data collection. Traditional birth attendants with some training were often misclassified as medically trained workers (doctors, nurses, midwives). Guatemala is also an outlier, but in the other direction: 4–14 day mortality is less common than expected on the basis of the proportion of children at lower risk of tetanus. In part this may be due to underestimation of the 4–14 day mortality level because of heaping at 15 days instead of 14 days, as shown in Table 1.

In Table 5 the relationship between mortality and being at lower risk of tetanus is examined at the individual level in each country. In almost all countries, 4–14 day mortality levels are markedly lower for births at lower risk of tetanus than for nonlower-risk births. We find little or no mortality-reducing effect of being at lower risk only in Liberia, Kenya, and Jordan. Kenya and Jordan both have low levels of 4–14 day mortality; also, neonatal tetanus is likely to be low in these countries, although problems in the data quality of survey data may have caused the lack of difference. The possibility of poor data cannot be excluded, especially in the case of Kenya.

The effect of being at lower risk of neonatal tetanus on 4–14 day mortality is not necessarily causal. In fact, receiving at least one dose of tetanus toxoid during pregnancy and delivering with medical assistance merely may be proxies for better overall maternity care or better socioeconomic conditions in the household. Even so, a comparison of the mortality levels among lower-risk and nonlower-risk births in Table 5 shows that the overall effect of being at lower risk is larger on 4–14 day mortality than on neonatal mortality in general for 26 of 30 surveys with sufficiently large numbers in both risk categories. In addition, we performed multivariate analysis (results not shown) with 4–14 days mortality as the dependent variable and with socioeconomic and biodemographic characteristics as control variables. The control variables did not significantly alter the effect of being at lower risk of tetanus on 4–14 day mortality.

## Discussion

Demographic data sources have been largely unexplored by epidemiologists and public health specialists working with neonatal tetanus. The usefulness of birth history data for the study of neonatal tetanus depends on a number of factors. First, are the birth history data on age at death in the neonatal period sufficiently accurate and complete to allow an estimate of 4–14 day mortality levels and trends? The analysis provided three arguments to demonstrate that recall of the day at death was fairly accurate: missing values were not a problem; heaping at 7, 14, and 15 days was within acceptable ranges; and data from five countries with two surveys were reasonably consistent. Complete-

**Table 5** Neonatal mortality and mortality per 1,000 live births at 4–14 days for lower risk of tetanus births (LR) and nonlower risk births (NLR) among births in the last five years

| Country | Number of Births | | Neonatal Mortality | | | 4–14 day Mortality | | |
|---|---|---|---|---|---|---|---|---|
| | LR | NLR | LR | NLR | LR/NLR | LR | NLR | LR/NLR |
| **West and Central Africa** | | | | | | | | |
| Cameroon | 2,725 | 747 | 25.4 | 52.2 | 0.49 | 7.6 | 23.5 | 0.32 |
| Ghana | 3,034 | 920 | 39.2 | 46.7 | 0.84 | 11.9 | 17.4 | 0.68 |
| Liberia | 2,433 | 529 | 43.5 | 47.9 | 0.91 | 17.4 | 18.7 | 0.93 |
| Mali | 824 | 2161 | 24.0 | 51.9 | 0.46 | 8.4 | 19.8 | 0.42 |
| Nigeria | 4,565 | 3276 | 36.1 | 47.3 | 0.73 | 9.1 | 17.9 | 0.51 |
| Senegal | 1,694 | 2409 | 30.7 | 49.4 | 0.62 | 12.4 | 27.4 | 0.45 |
| Togo | 2,310 | 681 | 36.8 | 35.2 | 1.04 | 8.7 | 22.0 | 0.39 |
| **East and Southern Africa** | | | | | | | | |
| Botswana | 2,865 | 198 | 19.2 | (21.8) | a | 5.1 | 14.7 | 0.34 |
| Burundi | 2,365 | 1,336 | 29.0 | 40.8 | 0.71 | 12.6 | 18.9 | 0.66 |
| Kenya | 6,346 | 505 | 24.4 | 37.6 | 0.65 | 8.4 | 7.9 | 1.06 |
| Tanzania | 8,130 | 597 | 35.3 | 52.1 | 0.68 | 11.2 | 19.6 | 0.59 |
| Uganda | 3,272 | 1,591 | 35.7 | 50.4 | 0.71 | 10.8 | 21.8 | 0.50 |
| Zambia | 5,288 | 760 | 34.1 | 67.1 | 0.51 | 13.0 | 18.0 | 0.72 |
| Zimbabwe | 2,865 | 324 | 18.8 | 30.9 | 0.61 | 5.9 | 9.3 | 0.64 |
| **North Africa and Middle East** | | | | | | | | |
| Egypt | 3,414 | 4,914 | 37.5 | 37.4 | 1.00 | 9.7 | 22.0 | 0.44 |
| Jordan | 6,896 | 634 | 23.4 | 20.4 | 1.15 | 9.3 | 8.7 | 1.07 |
| Morocco I | 1,545 | 4,345 | 33.7 | 39.6 | 0.85 | 7.1 | 17.0 | 0.42 |
| Morocco II | 3,103 | 1,979 | 21.3 | 46.5 | 0.46 | 6.8 | 19.2 | 0.35 |
| Sudan | 4,950 | 1,376 | 36.2 | 63.2 | 0.57 | 10.9 | 30.5 | 0.36 |
| Tunisia | 3,245 | 1,081 | 24.3 | 30.5 | 0.80 | 7.4 | 13.0 | 0.57 |

*(continued)*

**Table 5** (continued)

| Country | Number of Births | | Neonatal Mortality | | | 4–14 day Mortality | | |
|---|---|---|---|---|---|---|---|---|
| | LR | NLR | LR | NLR | LR/NLR | LR | NLR | LR/NLR |
| Asia | | | | | | | | |
| Indonesia I | 2,917 | 5,050 | 16.3 | 29.4 | 0.55 | 7.2 | 17.6 | 0.41 |
| Indonesia II | 9,726 | 4,768 | 22.8 | 48.2 | 0.47 | 7.3 | 22.6 | 0.32 |
| Pakistan | 2,098 | 4,019 | 41.4 | 44.0 | 0.94 | 12.6 | 17.0 | 0.74 [a] |
| Sri Lanka | 3,709 | 116 | 13.8 | (4.3) | [a] | 5.5 | (0.0) | [a] |
| Thailand | 2,859 | 631 | 12.3 | 40.1 | 0.31 | 3.7 | 10.8 | 0.34 |
| Latin America and Caribbean | | | | | | | | |
| Bolivia | 2,759 | 2,782 | 21.3 | 45.7 | 0.47 | 5.9 | 16.6 | 0.35 |
| Brazil | 2,855 | 461 | 30.9 | 42.5 | 0.73 | 7.4 | 11.3 | 0.65 |
| Colombia I | 2,079 | 503 | 16.1 | 25.7 | 0.63 | 4.7 | (5.6) | [a] |
| Colombia II | 3,302 | 363 | 10.9 | 34.4 | 0.32 | 2.3 | 10.5 | 0.21 |
| Dom.Rep. I | 4,176 | 91 | 36.8 | (90.2) | [a] | 11.9 | (20.9) | [a] |
| Dom.Rep. II | 3,642 | 79 | 22.6 | (77.0) | [a] | 5.4 | (41.7) | [a] |
| Ecuador | 2,093 | 777 | 27.7 | 37.3 | 0.74 | 8.1 | 11.6 | 0.70 |
| Guatemala | 1,606 | 2,800 | 31.1 | 31.4 | 0.99 | 4.4 | 6.4 | 0.68 |
| Paraguay | 3,437 | 436 | 17.6 | 28.2 | 0.62 | 3.5 | 14.7 | 0.24 |
| Peru I | 1,605 | 1,392 | 22.4 | 40.9 | 0.55 | 4.4 | 17.2 | 0.25 |
| Peru II | 5,355 | 2,976 | 15.8 | 41.3 | 0.38 | 2.3 | 12.6 | 0.19 |
| Trinidad & Tob. | 1,739 | 12 | 20.1 | b | | 3.5 | b | |

[a] Mortality rate is based on less than 250 births, and no LR/NLR ratio is given.
[b] Fewer than 50 births.
Note: Excludes month of interview and month before.

ness of death reporting is difficult to evaluate. In general, mortality rates showed fairly consistent trends and did not suggest serious under-reporting of neonatal deaths for the more distant periods in comparison with the most recent.

Second, how accurate is 4–14 day mortality as an indicator of tetanus mortality? There is sufficient evidence to show that mortality at 4–14 days is a sensitive indicator of neonatal tetanus mortality: about 90% of the neonatal tetanus deaths occur in that age period, when the predominant route of infection is the umbilical stump. The proportion of deaths at 4–14 days that is actually due to tetanus, however, may vary according to the level of mortality and the incidence of neonatal tetanus. Other important causes of death during the neonatal period include birth trauma, sepsis due to perinatal infections, pneumonia, diarrhoea, and mortality associated with low birth weight. If diarrhoea and pneumonia are common, mortality at 15–27 days also should be high. If low birth weight (prematurity and small size for gestational age) and birth trauma are important, mortality during the first three days of life should be elevated even more. Neonatal sepsis can be associated with unsterile delivery conditions, and has a mortality peak similar to that for neonatal tetanus. Both tetanus and sepsis can be prevented by 'clean' delivery, but tetanus toxoid vaccinations affects only tetanus. Clearly some of the 4–14 day mortality trends may be associated with reductions in neonatal sepsis.

Comparisons with data from other sources could support the validity of the DHS data as an indicator of the magnitude of neonatal tetanus mortality. Data from Senegal (Leroy and Garenne, 1987), Indonesia (Arnold, Soewarso and Karyadi, 1986, Budiarso, 1984, Yusuf et al,. 1986), and Thailand (Swaddiwudhipong et al., 1989) show similar levels or trends in neonatal tetanus mortality, as indicated by the results of the DHS surveys, but a thorough external comparison is not possible because very little information has been available on national levels and trends. Reasons for the lack of reliable data have been described (Stanfield and Galazka, 1984). Much of the effort to initiate or improve surveillance for neonatal tetanus is current and (with few exceptions) follows the introduction of intensified immunization programs with tetanus toxoid and emphasis on clean delivery. Therefore, declines in neonatal tetanus must be demonstrated retrospectively, on the basis of existing data sets. Maputo, Mozambique, provides an example of the use of health facility data to retrospectively demonstrate a decline in the incidence of neonatal tetanus (Cutts et al., 1990). Such data, however, cannot be extrapolated to the national level. In countries with relatively reliable vital registration data during the period of implementation of a tetanus control program, changes in the patterns of ages at death should be a means of indirectly measuring the decline of neonatal tetanus on a national scale. For example, a review of vital event data for Egypt beginning in 1986 should demonstrate the decline in 4–14 day mortality, concomitant with and inversely related to recent efforts at neonatal tetanus: control.

Data on 4–14 day mortality levels and trends are not an accurate indicator of the level of neonatal tetanus mortality if tetanus is not common. For example, surveillance data from government hospitals in Sri Lanka suggest a decline of neonatal tetanus mortality from about 2 per 1,000 live births during 1970–1978 to less than 0.5 per 1,000 after 1980 (WHO, 1984). Such a decline cannot be assessed by examining at 4–14 day mortality trends (mortality at 4–14 days remained at about 5 per 1,000 live births during 1976–1987).

What are the implications of the findings on 4–14 day mortality levels for the global efforts to eliminate tetanus? Generally, neonatal tetanus is not likely to be a major public health problem in countries with 4–14 day mortality levels below 7 per 1,000 live births; tetanus mortality is then probably less than 2 per 1,000. In such countries, monitoring the impact of tetanus elimination programs can be monitored most effectively through increased national surveillance, especially in high-risk subpopulations. Among the DHS countries, this description applies to six of the nine countries in Latin America and the Caribbean, two countries in Asia, and one country in Africa (Botswana).

A second group includes countries with 4–14 day mortality levels of 7–10 per 1,000 live births: three countries in Sub-Saharan Africa, Jordan and Tunisia, and Brazil and Ecuador. All of the countries in this group have fairly high proportions of persons at lower risk of tetanus (at least 70%). In these countries neonatal tetanus probably is still associated with 1–5 deaths per 1,000 live births, but considerable variation within this group is likely. Surveys may contribute to the assessment of mortality trend for neonatal tetanus, but surveillance is increasingly important.

The third group includes countries with 4–14 day mortality rates of 11 per 1,000 or more: 10 countries in Sub-Saharan Africa, three in North Africa, two in Asia, and one in mortality associated with low birth weight. If diarrhoea and pneumonia are common, mortality at 15–27 days also should be high. If low birth weight (prematurity and small size for gestational age) and birth trauma are important, mortality during the first three days of life should be elevated even more. Neonatal sepsis can be associated with unsterile delivery conditions, and has a mortality peak similar to that for neonatal tetanus. Both tetanus and sepsis can be prevented by "clean" delivery, but tetanus toxoid vaccinations affects only tetanus. Clearly some of the 4–14 day mortality trends may be associated with reductions in neonatal sepsis.

Comparisons with data from other sources could support the validity of the DHS data as an indicator of the magnitude of neonatal tetanus mortality. Data from Senegal (Leroy and Garenne, 1987), Indonesia (Arnold, Soewarso and Karyadi, 1986; Budiarso, 1984; Yusuf et al., 1986), and Thailand (Swaddiwudhipong et al., 1989) show similar levels or trends in neonatal tetanus mortality, as indicated by the results of the DHS surveys, but a thorough external comparison is not possible because very little information has been available on national levels and trends. Reasons for the lack of reliable data have been described (Stanfield and Galazka, 1984). Much of the effort to initiate or improve surveillance for neonatal tetanus is current and (with few exceptions) follows the introduction of intensified immunization programs with tetanus toxoid and emphasis on clean delivery. Therefore, declines in neonatal tetanus must be demonstrated retrospectively, on the basis of existing data sets. Maputo, Mozambique, provides an example of the use of health facility data to retrospectively demonstrate a decline in the incidence of neonatal tetanus (Cutts et al., 1990). Such data, however, cannot be extrapolated to the national level. In countries with relatively reliable vital registration data during the period of implementation of a tetanus control program, changes in the patterns of ages at death should be a means of indirectly measuring the decline of neonatal tetanus on a national scale. For example, a review of vital~ event data for Egypt beginning in 1986 should demonstrate the decline in 4–14 day mortality, concomitant with and inversely related to recent efforts at neonatal tetanus control.

Data on 4–14 day mortality levels and trends are not an accurate indicator of the level of neonatal tetanus mortality if tetanus is not common. For example, surveillance data from government hospitals in Sri Lanka suggest a decline of neonatal tetanus mortality from about 2 per 1,000 live births during 1970–1978 to less than 0.5 per 1,000 after 1980 (WHO, 1984). Such a decline cannot be assessed by examining at 4–14 day mortality trends (mortality at 4–14 days remained at about 5 per 1,000 live births during 1976–1987).

What are the implications of the findings on 4–14 day mortality levels for the global efforts to eliminate tetanus? Generally, neonatal tetanus is not likely to be a major public health problem in countries with 4–14 day mortality levels below 7 per 1,000 live births; tetanus mortality is then probably less than 2 per 1,000. In such countries, monitoring the impact of tetanus elimination programs can be monitored most effectively through increased national surveillance, especially in high-risk subpopulations. Among the DHS countries, this description applies to six of the nine countries in Latin America and the Caribbean, two countries in Asia, and one country in Africa (Botswana).

A second group includes countries with 4–14 day mortality levels of 7–10 per 1,000 live births: three countries in Sub-Saharan Africa, Jordan and Tunisia, and Brazil and Ecuador. All of the countries in this group have fairly high proportions of persons at lower risk of tetanus (at least 70%). In these countries neonatal tetanus probably is still associated with 1–5 deaths per 1,000 live births, but considerable variation within this group is likely. Surveys may contribute to the assessment of mortality trend for neonatal tetanus, but surveillance is increasingly important.

The third group includes countries with 4–14 day mortality rates of 11 per 1,000 or more: 10 countries in Sub-Saharan Africa, three in North Africa, two in Asia, and one in Latin America. Mortality rates at 4–14 days range from 11 to 22 per 1,000 in this group, and neonatal tetanus mortality levels may range correspondingly from 4 to 15 per 1,000 live births. In these countries, demographic surveys can provide useful information on the national trend in neonatal tetanus mortality.

The overall picture leaves no doubt that neonatal mortality has declined in developing countries. The consistent and pronounced decline of mortality at 4–14 days, observed in most developing countries during the past decade, indicates the importance of the decline in neonatal tetanus mortality to the overall decline in neonatal mortality. In some cases the decline can be linked to programmatic efforts; in other cases it appears to have started well before the program achieved nationwide coverage. Changes in traditional practices (e.g., reductions in the application of contaminated cord dressings) and the training of traditional birth attendants in sterile delivery practices may account for such changes before the beginning of an immunization program.

In summary, demographic surveys with birth histories have been, and in several countries should continue to be, an important source of data for assessing the magnitude of neonatal tetanus mortality and evaluating trends in neonatal tetanus mortality.

## Acknowledgements

We are grateful to George Bicego, Michel Garenne, and Robert Steinglass for their comments, and to Virginia Sturwold for editorial assistance.

## Notes

1   A number of DHS surveys are not based on nationally representative samples, especially in politically unstable countries, such as Uganda in 1988 and Sudan in 1989. In Indonesia the first DHS survey included 20 of the 27 provinces; the second survey comprised all provinces.

2   Two doses of tetanus toxoid (TT), with at least four weeks between, are recommended to prevent tetanus in the newborn. Five doses of TT are considered to provide lifetime protection. During the first five years of DHS the women were asked only if they had received a TT injection. In the DHS II questionnaire the respondent also is asked to recall the number of injections.

3   Sampling errors must be taken into consideration in interpreting the mortality rates. For a mortality rate of 20 per 1,000 live births with a sample size of 4,000, for example, the 95 per cent confidence interval is 15.9–24.8. In addition, a design effect must be taken into account. On the other hand, comparative analysis can be a powerful tool for drawing conclusions in spite of large sampling errors in individual countries. If the results of most of 37 surveys show a decline in 4–14 days mortality, this finding may be highly significant.

4   The major impact of the control program on 4–14 day mortality should become evident in the next DHS survey in Egypt, scheduled for 1992–1993.

5   The DHS I survey in Indonesia included 20 provinces. Therefore the data from the second survey are limited to the same 20 of Indonesia's 27 provinces.

## References

Arnold, Richard B., Titi Indijati Soewarso, and Albertus Karyadi. 1986. 'Mortality from neonatal tetanus in indonesia: results from two surveys.' *Bulletin of the World Health Organization* 64:259–62.

Bhatia, Shushum. 1989. "Patterns and causes of neonatal and postneonatal mortality in rural Bangladesh." *Studies in Family Planning* 20:136–46.

Black, Robert E., D.H. Huber, and George T. Curlin. 1980. 'Reduction of neonatal tetanus by mass immunization of non-pregnant women: duration of protection provided by one or two doses of aluminium-absorbed tetanus toxoid.' *Bulletin of the World Health Organization* 58:927–30.

Boerma, J. Ties and Jeroen K. Van Ginneken. 1992. 'Comparison of substantive results from demographic and epidemiological surveys.' Pp. 27–60 in *Measurement of maternal and child mortality, morbidity and health care: interdisciplinary approaches,* edited by J. Ties Boerma. Liege: Derouaux-Ordina Editions for IUSSP.

Budiarso, L.R. 1984. 'Prospective study on infant and childhood mortality in Sukabumi 1982–83.' Jakarta: Government of Indonesia, Department of Health.

Cutts, Felicity T., A. Soares, A.V. Jecque, J. Cliff, S. Kortbeek, and S. Colombo. 1990. 'The use of evaluation to improve the expanded programme on immunization in Mozambique.' *Bulletin of the World Health Organization* 68:199–208.

Expanded Programme on Immunization. 1989. 'A vision for the world: global elimination of neonatal tetanus by the year 1995: plan of action.' EPI/GAG/89/WP9. Geneva: World Health Organization.

Ewbank, Douglas C. 1984. 'Uses of mortality data for evaluating the success of specific health and development programmes' Pp. 18–30 in *Data bases for mortality measurement,* United Nations, New York: Department of International Economic and Social Affairs. Population Studies #84, ST/ESA/SER.A/84.

Galazka, Arthur and George Stroh. 1986. 'Neonatal Tetanus: guidelines on the community-based survey on neonatal tetanus mortality.' EPI/GEN/86.8. Geneva: World Health Organization.

Gasse, Francois. 1990. 'Neonatal tetanus elimination initiative: progress report and recommendation.' EPI/MCH/NNT/GEN/90.1. Geneva: World Health Organization.

Leroy, Odile and Michel Garenne. 1987. 'La mortalité par tétanos néonatal: la situation a Niakhar.' Proceedings of the IUSSP seminar on Comparative Studies of Mortality and Society in Africa South of the Sahara, Yaoundé, October.

Newell, K.W., D. Lehrnann, D.R. Leblanc and N.G. Osorio. 1986. 'The use of toxoid for the prevention of tetanus: final report of a double blind controlled field trial.' *Bulletin of the World Health Organization* 35:863–71.

Stanfield, J. Paget and Arthur Galazka. 1984. 'Neonatal tetanus in the world today.' *Bulletin of the World Health Organization* 62:647–69.

Steinglass, Robert, Logan Brenzel and Allison Percy. 1992. 'Tetanus.' In *Disease control priorities in developing countries* edited by Dean T. Jamison and W. Henry Mosley. New York: Oxford University Press.

Stroh, George. 1990. 'Suggested tools for surveillance of neonatal tetanus elimination.' EPI/NNT/90/WP.2. Geneva: World Health Organization.

Swaddiwudhipong, Witaya, Sirisak Warintrawat, Prayura Kunasol and Orapun Sangwanloy. 1989. "Surveillance of neonatal tetanus in Thailand, 1977–86." *Journal of the Medical Association of Thailand* 72:638–41.

Tabutin, Dominique. 1984. "'Comparison of single and multi-round surveys for measuring mortality in developing countries.' Pp. 11–25 in *Methodologies for the Collection and Analysis of Mortality Data* edited by Jacques Vallin, John H. Pollard and Larry Heligman. Liege: Ordina Editions.

Yusuf, B., S. Solter, Z. Bakri, A.A. Hasiban, T.I. Soewarso, E.R. Aiyub and R.B. Arnold. 1986. 'Neonatal tetanus mortality in Aceh Province, Indonesia.' *Annales de la Societé Belge de Médicine Tropicale* 66:349–54.

World Health Organization (WHO). 1984. 'Expanded programme on immunization: tetanus surveillance.' *Weekly Epidemiological Record* 41:319.

9

# Data on birth weight in developing countries: can surveys help?

*J. Ties Boerma, Kia Reinis, Shea O. Rutstein and A. Elisabeth Sommerfelt*

## Abstract

The main source of birth weight data in developing countries are health facility statistics, although most developing countries do not produce annual estimates of the incidence of low birth weight from these data. Even so, such estimates would be subject to a selection bias: data are usually limited to babies born within health facilities, and therefore pertain to babies who are markedly different from the overall population. Since 1990 the Demographic and Health Surveys programme (DHS) has included questions on recalled birth weight and relative size at birth in 15 national surveys.

In this paper, we show that cross-sectional surveys can provide a useful source for making national estimates of mean birth weight and the incidence of low birth weight. The level of misclassification is, however, too large to use reported data on subjective size at the individual level as an indicator of low birth weight.

## Introduction

Data on birth weight are important for several reasons. First, national and regional estimates of the incidence of low birth weight are internationally recognized indicators of the well-being of neonates and women of reproductive ages. Recently, the incidence of low birth weight was selected as one of the indicators to monitor the health goals of the World Summit for Children. The goal is to reduce the incidence of low birth weight (less than 2500 grams) to 10 percent of births. Second, birth weight has been shown to be a leading determinant of the survival chances of a new born.[1]

The main source of birth weight data in developing countries are health facility statistics, although most developing countries do not produce annual estimates of the incidence of low birth weight from these data. In many countries, the majority of babies are born outside health facilities; for example over three-quarters of recent births in Niger, Morocco, Indonesia, Pakistan and Yemen were delivered at home.[2] Estimates limited to babies born within health facilities would be subject to selection bias, as there are good reasons to assume that these babies are markedly different from the overall population. It is likely that the incidence of low birth weight would be underestimated, and the findings on factors affecting the risk of low birth weight could be misleading as well.

Retrospective data collected in surveys are an alternative source of information on birth weight. DaVanzo et al. showed how retrospective data from the 1976 Malaysia Family Life Survey[3] could be used to investigate correlates of birth weight, but that inferences derived solely from reported numerical weights would be biased. In an analysis of the Peru Demographic and Health Survey[4] Moreno and Goldman showed how retrospective data could be used to estimate the incidence of low birth weight, concluding that estimates restricted to babies with reported birth weights were substantially underestimated. These analyses spurred the Demographic and Health Surveys programme (DHS) to include questions on recalled birth weight and relative size at birth in national surveys. In this paper, we use these data to assess whether data collected in cross-sectional surveys can be used to improve national estimates of mean birth weight and of the incidence of low birth weight. In addition, we examine whether size at birth data can be used in individual level analyses, such as studies of the determinants of infant mortality, child anthropometry, and effects of maternity care.

## Data and methods

DHS, funded by the US Agency for International Development (USAID), assists developing countries in the organization of nationally representative surveys, aiming to provide information for policy and program decision making and for scientific research. Survey information include a full birth history, which is used for fertility and child mortality estimation, and various maternal and child health indicators. Survey respondents are women of childbearing ages.

Since 1990, DHS surveys have included the following questions for all children born in the five years preceding the survey:

- When (NAME) was born was he/she: very large, larger than average, average, smaller than average or very small?
- Was (NAME) weighed at birth?
- IF YES: How much did (NAME) weigh?

We analyze data from fifteen surveys which included these questions. In 12 of the 15 surveys, the question on size at birth was exactly as phrased above. In Cameroon and Yemen, the categories 'very large' and 'larger than average' were combined into one category. In Paraguay, only three size categories were used: small, average and large.

In all surveys, size at birth were asked for all children, including children whose mothers reported a numerical birth weight.

The usefulness of survey data on birth weight depends on the ability of mothers to accurately recall the birth weight of children weighed at birth, and on the quality of the data on subjective size at birth. Because the United States maintains an accurate vital registration system that includes recording of birth weights from birth certificates, Ekouevi and Morgan[5] were able to assess the validity of retrospective reporting of birth weights in the USA National Surveys of Family Growth by comparing reports to vital registration data. They were also able to assess the reliability of retrospective birth weight reporting by comparing reports across repeated surveys. They found that levels and trends of low birth weight estimates from the retrospective data 'generally matched' the data from vital registration, confirming the validity of such reports; and that levels and trends estimated across repeated surveys were found to be 'similar', thus confirming reliability of retrospective reporting of birth weight. In DHS surveys, the quality of numerical data on birth weight can only be assessed by comparing these results to other national studies in the same country. Such studies are based on hospital data, and are generally not available for similar time periods in most countries.

The quality of subjective size at birth data can only be assessed for births with numerical birth weights. Mean birth weight and the incidence of low birth weight should correspond with reported size at birth. If so, survey data on birth weight can be used to obtain better estimates of the national incidence of low birth weight.

Low birth weight is defined by the World Health Organization as less than 2500 grams. Heaping of birth weight data on multiples of 500 grams is common, and this affects the estimates of the incidence of low birth weight. Therefore, the amount of heaping at 2500 grams will be examined in DHS surveys. For aggregate analyses, half of the responses at 2500 grams will be classified as low birth weight.

In addition, the analysis focuses on the usefulness of using very small size at birth (or very small and small size) as an indicator of low birth weight. The magnitude of the misclassification bias is assessed through analysis of the sensitivity and predictive value positive (PVP) of size at birth as an indicator of low birth weight. If misclassification bias is found to be low, the proportion classified as very small or small could be used as an indicator of the incidence of low birth weight (or another cutoff point). More importantly, size at birth data could be used in individual level analysis of the determinants and consequences of low birth weight.

## Results

Table 1 presents the DHS surveys included in this study, the year of survey and the number of births in the five years preceding the survey. The proportion of children

**Table 1**  Survey characteristics and distribution of births according to availability of birth weight data (percents)

| Survey | Year | Number of births | Weighed at birth | Births with weight / size | | | |
|--------|------|------------------|------------------|-------------------|-----------|-----------------|-------|
| | | | | Weight recalled | Size only | Missing both | Total |
| **Sub-Saharan Africa** | | | | | | | |
| Cameroon | 1991 | 3350 | 61.1 | 50.7 | 49.2 | 0.1 | 100.0 |
| Namibia | 1992 | 3966 | 71.6 | 44.3 | 54.0 | 1.8 | 100.0 |
| Nigeria | 1990 | 7899 | 26.2 | 9.5 | 88.9 | 1.6 | 100.0 |
| Niger | 1992 | 6962 | 16.8 | 12.6 | 86.3 | 1.1 | 100.0 |
| Tanzania | 1991–92 | 8138 | 51.9 | 49.3 | 49.9 | 0.8 | 100.0 |
| Zambia | 1992 | 6479 | 50.5 | 41.9 | 57.8 | 0.3 | 100.0 |
| **North Africa & Middle East** | | | | | | | |
| Jordan | 1991 | 8364 | na | 85.7 | 13.9 | 0.4 | 100.0 |
| Morocco | 1992 | 5245 | 29.5 | 21.6 | 78.3 | 0.1 | 100.0 |
| Yemen | 1991–92 | 7230 | 8.8 | 5.8 | 73.3 | 20.9 | 100.0 |
| **Asia** | | | | | | | |
| Indonesia | 1990–91 | 15708 | 37.1 | 36.8 | 62.0 | 1.2 | 100.0 |
| Pakistan | 1991 | 6424 | 9.3 | 7.4 | 91.1 | 1.5 | 100.0 |
| **Latin America & Caribbean** | | | | | | | |
| Colombia | 1990 | 3751 | 80.7 | 62.2 | 37.5 | 0.3 | 100.0 |
| Dominican Rep. | 1991 | 4164 | 90.7 | 90.3 | 9.5 | 0.2 | 100.0 |
| Paraguay | 1991–92 | 4246 | 72.5 | 71.7 | 27.7 | 0.6 | 100.0 |
| Peru | 1991 | 9461 | 64.2 | 62.0 | 37.6 | 0.4 | 100.0 |

weighed at birth varies greatly between surveys: from 9 percent in Pakistan and Yemen to 91 percent in the Dominican Republic. The proportion of children with reported birth weight varies from 6 percent in Yemen to 90 percent in the Dominican Republic. Most, but not all women who said their child had been weighed could recall the birth weight. In 10 of 14 surveys more than three-quarters of the mothers who said their children had been weighed could actually recall the weight. In Nigeria, however, only 36 percent of the mothers who said their child had been weighed reported the birth weight to the interviewer. (In Jordan only the reported weight was recorded without first asking whether the child had been weighed).

Table 2 shows the unit of measurement used to record birth weight and the extent to which responses are heaped at multiples of 500 grams. Weights were recorded in grams in 7 surveys, in kilograms with one decimal in 5 surveys, and in kilograms with 2 decimals in one survey. In the Dominican Republic, weights were recorded in (avoirdupois) pounds and ounces, and in Pakistan, recording in either pounds or kilograms was possible.

There is considerable heaping in all surveys where the metric system is used, with a third to half of the responses occurring at multiples of 500 grams. Heaping is particu-

**Table 2**  Method of recording birth weight, and heaping at multiples of 500 gr and at 2500 gr, DHS surveys

| Survey | Method of recording weight[1] | Heaping at multiples of 500 gr[2] | Heaping at 2500 gr[3] |
|---|---|---|---|
| Cameroon | gr | 33.6 | 4.9 |
| Namibia | gr | 22.2 | 2.9 |
| Nigeria | kg1 | 44.1 | 6.7 |
| Niger | kg1 | 29.6 | 8.6 |
| Tanzania | kg2 | 46.6 | 9.1 |
| Zambia | kg1 | 31.8 | 6.5 |
| Jordan | gr | 31.6 | 6.8 |
| Morocco | kg1 | 49.2 | 5.7 |
| Yemen | gr | 54.7 | 23.5 |
| Indonesia | gr | 37.7 | 6.2 |
| Pakistan | p/gr | 0.6 | 0.2 |
| Colombia | gr | 51.3 | 5.7 |
| Dominican Rep. | p | 0 | 0 |
| Paraguay | gr | 30.5 | 2.7 |
| Peru | kg1 | 29.2 | 3.7 |

1. gr = grams; kgn = kilograms with n decimals; p = pounds and ounces
2. Proportion of all reported weights which are multiples of five
3. Proportion of all reported weights which are 2500 grams.

larly problematic at 2500 grams, just above the cut off point for low birth weight. Among the surveys using the metric system, only five countries have less than 5 percent heaping, and eight countries have 5–9 percent heaping at 2500 grams. In Yemen, almost one-fourth of responses are 2500 grams. In Dominican Republic and Pakistan, responses are heaped on whole pounds: 42 percent in the Dominican Republic and 85 percent in Pakistan. Generally, there does not appear to be a relationship between the level of heaping and the unit of measurement used to record weights.

The distributions of reported relative size of new borns are presented in Table 3 by whether the numerical birth weight was reported or not. The distributions of relative size vary considerably across surveys; for example, the proportion reported as 'average' varies from 29 percent in the Dominican Republic to 81 percent in Tanzania. The distribution of sizes in Yemen differs from all other surveys in that virtually all responses are in two categories: 'average' and 'very small'.

Within countries, the distributions of reported relative size differ by whether the numerical birth weight was recalled or not. In all countries, the distributions are tilted towards smaller sizes if no birth weight was reported. The difference between the two distributions is significant in all surveys (Kolmogorov-Smirnov test, P<.05), except Zambia.
The quality of the size at birth data can only be assessed among children with numerical birth weights. Therefore, Tables 4 and 5 include only children whose mothers reported a numerical birth weight. Table 4 and Figure 1 show the mean birth weight

**Table 3** Percent distribution of size at birth according to recall of numerical birth weight, DHS surveys

| Survey | Weight known | Very large | Large | Average | Small | Very small | Missing | Total | N |
|---|---|---|---|---|---|---|---|---|---|
| Cameroon | Yes | na | 38.7 | 49.7 | 9.0 | 2.5 | 0.2 | 100.0 | 1699 |
| | No | na | 26.6 | 54.4 | 16.0 | 2.9 | 0.1 | 100.0 | 1649 |
| Namibia | Yes | 6.3 | 5.5 | 72.3 | 10.5 | 5.3 | 0.2 | 100.0 | 1755 |
| | No | 6.4 | 4.7 | 66.3 | 9.8 | 9.6 | 3.2 | 100.0 | 2140 |
| Nigeria | Yes | 16.0 | 18.5 | 54.3 | 7.4 | 3.6 | 0.3 | 100.0 | 752 |
| | No | 16.7 | 12.5 | 52.1 | 10.3 | 6.7 | 1.8 | 100.0 | 7020 |
| Niger | Yes | 8.2 | 26.8 | 40.2 | 17.4 | 5.9 | 1.6 | 100.0 | 875 |
| | No | 5.3 | 14.4 | 40.6 | 22.5 | 16.0 | 1.3 | 100.0 | 4357 |
| Tanzania | Yes | 1.8 | 10.2 | 78.7 | 7.0 | 2.1 | 0.3 | 100.0 | 4015 |
| | No | 1.3 | 6.7 | 80.8 | 7.1 | 2.6 | 1.5 | 100.0 | 4060 |
| Zambia | Yes | 4.5 | 15.3 | 68.0 | 9.4 | 2.6 | 0.3 | 100.0 | 2792 |
| | No | 2.3 | 17.5 | 68.3 | 9.4 | 2.0 | 0.5 | 100.0 | 3666 |
| Jordan | Yes | 2.5 | 12.4 | 68.4 | 10.2 | 6.4 | 0.2 | 100.0 | 7169 |
| | No | 0.8 | 6.7 | 73.4 | 8.7 | 7.6 | 2.7 | 100.0 | 1163 |
| Morocco | Yes | 3.0 | 24.1 | 53.8 | 14.8 | 4.3 | 0.0 | 100.0 | 1133 |
| | No | 1.3 | 18.0 | 52.8 | 23.6 | 4.2 | 0.1 | 100.0 | 4108 |
| Yemen | Yes | na | 2.9 | 87.0 | 0.4 | 8.8 | 0.9 | 100.0 | 421 |
| | No | na | 1.6 | 63.1 | 0.3 | 12.9 | 22.2 | 100.0 | 3894 |
| Indonesia | Yes | 8.5 | 29.8 | 49.4 | 10.3 | 1.9 | 0.1 | 100.0 | 5787 |
| | No | 4.2 | 21.2 | 59.8 | 11.7 | 1.4 | 1.8 | 100.0 | 9739 |
| Pakistan | Yes | 2.0 | 16.6 | 64.3 | 11.6 | 5.4 | 0.0 | 100.0 | 477 |
| | No | 1.9 | 9.1 | 64.6 | 16.4 | 6.4 | 1.6 | 100.0 | 5850 |
| Colombia | Yes | 8.9 | 23.6 | 49.3 | 10.9 | 7.2 | 0.2 | 100.0 | 2334 |
| | No | 4.1 | 24.9 | 47.5 | 13.7 | 8.9 | 1.0 | 100.0 | 1405 |
| Dominican Rep. | Yes | 4.7 | 47.0 | 29.1 | 16.0 | 3.2 | 0.1 | 100.0 | 3761 |
| | No | 3.1 | 39.6 | 26.9 | 22.1 | 6.3 | 2.1 | 100.0 | 394 |
| Paraguay | Yes | na | 35.0 | 47.3 | 17.3 | na | 0.3 | 100.0 | 3045 |
| | No | na | 34.6 | 37.1 | 26.2 | na | 2.1 | 100.0 | 1364 |
| Peru | Yes | 1.8 | 22.4 | 57.9 | 14.1 | 3.5 | 0.3 | 100.0 | 5867 |
| | No | 0.7 | 15.7 | 57.9 | 20.5 | 4.2 | 1.0 | 100.0 | 3558 |

within each size category, the standard deviation, the coefficient of variation (SD/mean), and the number of standard deviations units the mean in each category is from the overall mean in that survey. The mean birth weight varies considerably by size at birth category and has the expected pattern with 'very small' having the lowest mean, 'small' the next-to lowest etc. in all countries.

With the exceptions of Colombia and Niger, the mean birth weights for 'very small' babies are well below the cut-off for low birth weight, and are in the range of 1800 to 2300 grams. The mean for 'very small' babies falls 1.4 to 2 SD units below the overall mean in 11 of the 14 surveys. The coefficient of variation is largest in the 'very small' category in all surveys but Colombia, indicating considerable individual variability in what is meant by 'very small'.

**Table 4** Mean birth weight according to size at birth, with standard deviation (SD), coefficient of variation (CV) and standard deviations from the mean, DHS surveys

| Survey | Size | N | Mean | SD | CV | SD from mean |
|---|---|---|---|---|---|---|
| Cameroon | All | 1967 | 3306 | 640 | 0.19 | 0.00 |
| | Very large | na | na | na | na | na |
| | Large | 767 | 3709 | 604 | 0.16 | 0.63 |
| | Average | 967 | 3162 | 443 | 0.14 | −0.23 |
| | Small | 181 | 2640 | 414 | 0.16 | −1.04 |
| | Very small | 49 | 2059 | 476 | 0.23 | −1.95 |
| Namibia | All | 1659 | 3098 | 687 | 0.22 | 0.00 |
| | Very large | 120 | 3647 | 817 | 0.22 | 0.80 |
| | Large | 95 | 3491 | 596 | 0.17 | 0.57 |
| | Average | 1171 | 3170 | 603 | 0.19 | 0.10 |
| | Small | 172 | 2572 | 405 | 0.16 | −0.77 |
| | Very small | 98 | 2110 | 610 | 0.29 | −1.44 |
| Nigeria | All | 993 | 3308 | 752 | 0.23 | 0.00 |
| | Very large | 163 | 3970 | 897 | 0.23 | 0.88 |
| | Large | 207 | 3608 | 650 | 0.18 | 0.40 |
| | Average | 507 | 3165 | 536 | 0.17 | −0.19 |
| | Small | 72 | 2810 | 499 | 0.18 | −0.66 |
| | Very small | 40 | 2060 | 547 | 0.27 | −1.66 |
| Niger | All | 1821 | 3062 | 533 | 0.17 | 0.00 |
| | Very large | 146 | 3596 | 558 | 0.16 | 1.00 |
| | Large | 509 | 3230 | 479 | 0.15 | 0.32 |
| | Average | 711 | 3058 | 423 | 0.14 | −0.01 |
| | Small | 316 | 2744 | 440 | 0.16 | −0.60 |
| | Very small | 121 | 2554 | 606 | 0.24 | −0.95 |
| Tanzania | All | 3756 | 3026 | 613 | 0.20 | 0.00 |
| | Very large | 89 | 3735 | 653 | 0.17 | 1.16 |
| | Large | 370 | 3703 | 532 | 0.14 | 1.10 |
| | Average | 2953 | 3024 | 477 | 0.16 | −0.00 |
| | Small | 254 | 2250 | 560 | 0.25 | −1.27 |
| | Very small | 76 | 1791 | 611 | 0.34 | −2.01 |
| Zambia | All | 2627 | 3128 | 616 | 0.20 | 0.00 |
| | Very large | 118 | 4048 | 660 | 0.16 | 1.49 |
| | Large | 421 | 3665 | 456 | 0.12 | 0.87 |
| | Average | 1763 | 3098 | 436 | 0.14 | −0.05 |
| | Small | 250 | 2348 | 477 | 0.20 | −1.27 |
| | Very small | 67 | 1950 | 539 | 0.28 | −1.91 |
| Jordan | All | 7083 | 3227 | 717 | 0.22 | 0.00 |
| | Very large | 173 | 4566 | 737 | 0.16 | 1.87 |
| | Large | 862 | 4012 | 535 | 0.13 | 1.09 |
| | Average | 4858 | 3249 | 464 | 0.14 | 0.03 |
| | Small | 744 | 2562 | 485 | 0.19 | −0.93 |
| | Very small | 434 | 2014 | 603 | 0.30 | −1.69 |
| Morocco | All | 1134 | 3335 | 697 | 0.21 | 0.00 |
| | Very large | 34 | 4382 | 647 | 0.15 | 1.50 |
| | Large | 274 | 3855 | 681 | 0.18 | 0.75 |
| | Average | 609 | 3343 | 379 | 0.11 | 0.01 |
| | Small | 168 | 2609 | 456 | 0.17 | −1.04 |
| | Very small | 49 | 2096 | 505 | 0.24 | −1.78 |

## Table 4 (continued)

| Survey | Size | N | Mean | SD | CV | SD from mean |
|--------|------|-----|------|------|------|------|
| Yemen | All | 571 | 2750 | 592 | 0.22 | 0.00 |
| | Very large | na | na | na | na | na |
| | Large | 34 | 3578 | 469 | 0.13 | 1.40 |
| | Average | 451 | 2809 | 511 | 0.18 | 0.10 |
| | Small | 4 | 2651 | 522 | 0.20 | −0.17 |
| | Very small | 76 | 1915 | 591 | 0.31 | −1.41 |
| Indonesia | All | 5896 | 3188 | 581 | 0.18 | 0.00 |
| | Very large | 533 | 3852 | 612 | 0.16 | 1.14 |
| | Large | 1919 | 3467 | 441 | 0.13 | 0.48 |
| | Average | 2757 | 3096 | 395 | 0.13 | −0.16 |
| | Small | 589 | 2528 | 448 | 0.18 | −1.14 |
| | Very small | 90 | 1808 | 482 | 0.27 | −2.38 |
| Pakistan | All | 607 | 3169 | 804 | 0.25 | 0.00 |
| | Very large | 14 | 4157 | 987 | 0.24 | 1.23 |
| | Large | 101 | 3683 | 758 | 0.21 | 0.64 |
| | Average | 392 | 3230 | 758 | 0.23 | 0.08 |
| | Small | 73 | 2427 | 758 | 0.31 | −0.92 |
| | Very small | 27 | 2074 | 1068 | 0.51 | −1.36 |
| Colombia | All | 2419 | 3436 | 778 | 0.23 | 0.00 |
| | Very large | 215 | 4339 | 782 | 0.18 | 1.16 |
| | Large | 570 | 3790 | 637 | 0.17 | 0.46 |
| | Average | 1193 | 3353 | 587 | 0.18 | −0.11 |
| | Small | 263 | 2997 | 793 | 0.26 | −0.56 |
| | Very small | 173 | 2564 | 600 | 0.23 | −1.12 |
| Dominican Rep. | All | 4033 | 3316 | 705 | 0.21 | 0.00 |
| | Very large | 186 | 4261 | 690 | 0.16 | 1.34 |
| | Large | 1837 | 3648 | 480 | 0.13 | 0.47 |
| | Average | 1133 | 3132 | 426 | 0.14 | −0.26 |
| | Small | 727 | 2714 | 634 | 0.24 | −0.85 |
| | Very small | 143 | 1944 | 818 | 0.42 | −1.95 |
| Paraguay | All | 2857 | 3446 | 758 | 0.22 | 0.00 |
| | Very large | na | na | na | na | na |
| | Large | 1029 | 4067 | 605 | 0.15 | 0.82 |
| | Average | 1300 | 3343 | 395 | 0.12 | −0.14 |
| | Small | 519 | 2476 | 633 | 0.26 | −1.28 |
| | Very small | na | na | na | na | na |
| Peru | All | 5728 | 3294 | 639 | 0.19 | 0.00 |
| | Very large | 92 | 4160 | 750 | 0.18 | 1.36 |
| | Large | 1212 | 3701 | 576 | 0.16 | 0.64 |
| | Average | 3417 | 3318 | 464 | 0.14 | 0.04 |
| | Small | 797 | 2704 | 563 | 0.21 | −0.92 |
| | Very small | 196 | 2247 | 666 | 0.30 | −1.64 |

**Figure 1** Mean birth weight by size at birth

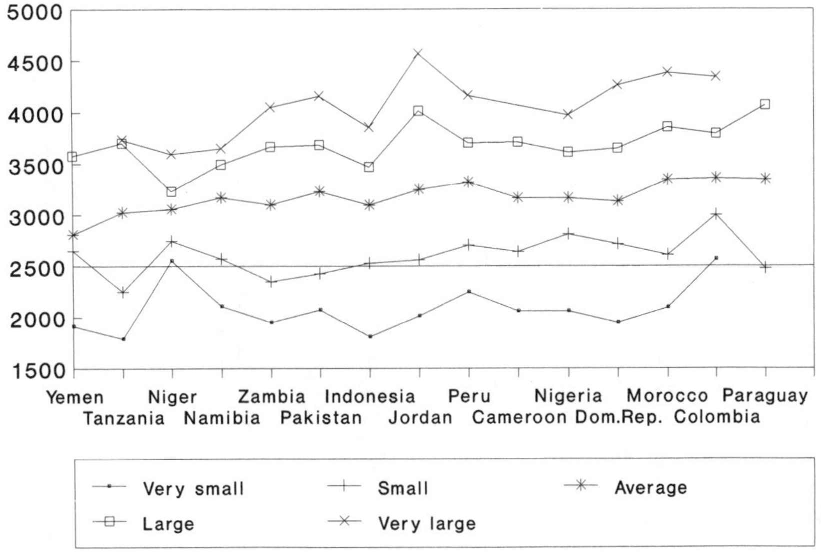

Countries ranked according to mean
birth weight

Babies reported to be 'very large' at birth have mean birth weights above 3500 grams in all surveys and over 4000 grams in 7 of 12 surveys, while the mean is on the order of 1 to 1.5 SD units above the overall mean birth weight in most surveys.

Can the proportion reported as 'very small' or 'small' be used as an indicator of the proportion of children with low birth weights? Table 5 shows the sensitivity, predictive value positive (PVP) and specificity of size at birth as an indicator of low birth weight. Sensitivity is here defined as the ability of the indicator to detect true positives, i.e. the proportion of low birth weight children identified by the size indicator; PVP as the proportion of true positives among those identified by the indicator (size at birth) and; specificity as the proportion of true negatives among children who are not low birth weight.

The first panel of Table 5 focuses on children born at less than 2500 grams and identified as 'very small'. Sensitivity is very low in all surveys (mean 29 percent), even though the PVP is 70 percent or more in most surveys. Thus, we can be confident that most babies reported as 'very small' are indeed of low birth weight (high PVP), but we are only capturing on the order of one-quarter of all low birth weight babies (low sensitivity).

The sensitivity of the indicator improves markedly when we use both 'very small' and 'small' as indicators of low birth weight (indicated as small in second panel of Table 5). However, while 'small' size captures two-thirds of low birth weight babies (mean sensitivity 66 percent), we are now less confident that the babies reported to be 'very

**Table 5** Sensitivity, predictive value positive (PVP), specificity and predictive value negative (PVN) of size at birth as indicator of low birth weight

| Survey | Very Small | | | | Small[1] | | | |
|---|---|---|---|---|---|---|---|---|
| | Sens[2] | PVP | Spec[3] | PVN | Sens[2] | PVP | Spec[3] | PVN |
| Cameroon | 29 | 72 | 99 | 95 | 62 | 33 | 97 | 97 |
| Namibia | 30 | 70 | 98 | 91 | 60 | 47 | 91 | 94 |
| Nigeria | 31 | 63 | 99 | 95 | 46 | 31 | 92 | 96 |
| Niger | 24 | 35 | 96 | 93 | 61 | 23 | 80 | 96 |
| Tanzania | 13 | 86 | 100 | 88 | 46 | 69 | 97 | 92 |
| Zambia | 20 | 89 | 100 | 91 | 68 | 65 | 95 | 96 |
| Jordan | 45 | 71 | 98 | 94 | 75 | 46 | 90 | 97 |
| Morocco | 36 | 63 | 98 | 95 | 90 | 35 | 87 | 99 |
| Yemen | 31 | 73 | 97 | 84 | 32 | 71 | 97 | 84 |
| Indonesia | 23 | 88 | 100 | 94 | 71 | 42 | 92 | 98 |
| Pakistan | 29 | 85 | 99 | 88 | 68 | 64 | 93 | 94 |
| Colombia | 55 | 37 | 95 | 97 | 83 | 23 | 85 | 99 |
| Dom. Rep | 24 | 81 | 99 | 91 | 78 | 46 | 88 | 97 |
| Paraguay | | | | | 87 | 41 | 89 | 99 |
| Peru | 23 | 66 | 99 | 96 | 41 | 70 | 88 | 97 |
| Average | 29 | 70 | 98 | 92 | 66 | 45 | 91 | 96 |

1. Includes very small
2. Proportion of low-birth-weight children identified by the size-at-birth indicator.
3. Proportion of non low-birth-weight children included in the very small or small categories.

small' or 'small' are indeed low birth weight: in 11 of 15 surveys fewer than 50 percent of the 'very small' and 'small' babies are in fact low birth weight (mean PVP 45 percent).

Table 6 presents estimates of mean birth weight and low birth weight incidence for births with reported weights, for births with size data only and for all births. Weights for births with size only were calculated using the mean birth weight of each size category among births with known weights and the distribution of sizes among births with no weights. All births present the weighted average of both birth weight estimates.

As expected on the basis of the size distributions presented in Table 3, the incidence of low birth weight is higher if all births are taken into account. In eight countries the increase in the incidence of low birth weight is more than 1 percent, and in Niger, Nigeria, Pakistan and Morocco the increase is well over 2 percent. Yemen data are very different from all other surveys, which is most likely due to data quality problems, as will be discussed below.

**Table 6**  Mean birth weight and incidence of low birth weight among children with reported birth weight, children with size data only, and all children

| | Numeric | | Size only | | All | |
|---|---|---|---|---|---|---|
| | Mean | % LBW | Mean | % LBW | Mean | % LBW |
| Cameroon | 3302 | 8.6 | 3193 | 11.6 | 3248 | 10.1 |
| Namibia | 3098 | 13.9 | 3042 | 17.3 | 3067 | 15.8 |
| Niger | 3062 | 13.3 | 2958 | 17.9 | 2971 | 17.3 |
| Nigeria | 3308 | 10.9 | 3232 | 14.1 | 3240 | 13.8 |
| Tanzania | 3024 | 18.4 | 2992 | 19.2 | 3008 | 18.8 |
| Zambia | 3128 | 14.6 | 3126 | 14.2 | 3127 | 14.4 |
| Jordan | 3228 | 13.6 | 3154 | 14.9 | 3218 | 13.8 |
| Morocco | 3335 | 10.4 | 3219 | 13.7 | 3244 | 13.0 |
| Yemen | 2751 | 32.8 | 2253 | 29.7 | −[1] | |
| Indonesia | 3188 | 10.3 | 3118 | 11 | 3144 | 10.8 |
| Pakistan | 3169 | 16.1 | 3030 | 19.3 | 3041 | 19 |
| Colombia | 3436 | 8.3 | 3374 | 9.5 | 3413 | 8.7 |
| Dom. Rep | 3316 | 11.7 | 3210 | 16.9 | 3313 | 11.8 |
| Paraguay | 3446 | 9.5 | 3366 | 13.4 | 3424 | 10.6 |
| Peru | 3294 | 10.2 | 3211 | 12.7 | 3263 | 11.2 |

1. No estimate was made.

## Discussion

Surveys can improve estimates of the incidence of low birth weight in developing countries, where a substantial proportion of children are not weighed at birth. The assessment of the quality of birth weight data has shown that data on the subjective size at birth are reasonably good indicators of birth weight at the aggregate level. However, two caveats need to be made. First, the assessment of the quality of the data on size can only be done for children with numerical birth weights. We have assumed that the quality of data on size among children with no numerical weight is the same as that for children with numerical weights. However, if mothers can attach meaning to the numerical weights, it is possible that the mothers who know the birth weights may be able to provide more accurate assessments of relative size than mothers of children who were not weighed at birth. We have no reason to suspect that the quality of data on size among children with no numerical weights would be better than for children with numerical weights. Second, the quality of the numerical data cannot be evaluated in detail. There is considerable heaping, which may be the result of recall error. However, data from health facilities are also strongly heaped on multiples of 500 grams, indicating the measurer often rounds the weight off.

There are no national estimates of the incidence of low birth for most countries included in this study, based on health facility data. Only Tanzania had a sufficiently large number of birth weight studies in the WHO data bank to be able to compare our estimates with health facility data.[6] Data on more than 100,000 births in 16 different locations during 1975–86 show a mean birth weight slightly under 3000 grams, and an incidence of low birth weight of 14 percent. The mean is very close to our survey-based estimate (3024 grams), while the lower incidence of low birth weight in the hospital data may partly be due to excluding all children with weights recorded as 2500 grams in health facilities (while we considered half of these births of low birth weight).

Because we assign birth weights to children with only size data, the overall estimates of birth weight generally become more uncertain as the proportion of children with recalled birth weights declines. In the case of Yemen, we refrained from estimating the incidence of low birth weight not only because weight was recalled for only 6 percent of births, but because the overall data were poor. One-fourth of numerical responses were heaped on 2500 grams, one-fifth of children had no data on either weight or size, and subjective sizes at birth were heaped on only two choices. We recommend that size not be used for estimating the incidence of low birth weight in surveys where the small and very small categories contain fewer than 25 children for whom there is also a measure of birth weight. Estimates for countries like Nigeria and Pakistan, with recalled weights for less than 50 births, are less accurate than estimates for countries in which a birth weight was recalled for at least 40 percent of births (9 of the 15 countries). Ideally, we would be able to say at what point are there too few births with a recalled weight to produce a reliable overall estimate. In addition, if the reporting of numerical birth weights is largely limited to a highly selective group – e.g. better-off urban women – national estimates of the incidence of low birth weight cannot be made. At the individual level, there is considerable misclassification of birth weights into the various size categories. Therefore, it does not appear useful to use 'very small' as an indicator of less than 2500 grams in analyses of the determinants of low birth weight and the effects of low birth weight on infant mortality.

In sum, cross-sectional surveys can provide a useful source of data for making national estimates of mean birth weight and the incidence of low birth weight, and, if sample sizes are sufficiently large, regional estimates can also be made within a country.


## References

1  McCormick, M.C. The contribution of low birth weight to infant mortality and childhood mortality. *New England Journal of Medicine*, 1985;312: 82–90.

2  Govindasamy P, Stewart MK, Rutstein SO et al. High-risk births and maternity care. *DHS Comparative Studies* No.8, Macro International Inc., Columbia, Maryland, 1994.

3  DaVanzo J, Habicht JP and Butz WP. Assessing socioeconomic correlates of birthweight in Peninsular Malaysia: ethnic differences and changes over time. *Social Science and Medicine* 1984;18: 387–404.

4  Moreno L and Goldman N. An assessment of survey data on birthweight. *Social Science and Medicine* 1990;31: 491–500.

5  Ekouevi K and Morgan SP. Note on the reliability and validity of mother's retrospective reports of their children's birthweights. *Social Biology* 1991;38: 140–145.

6  World Health Organization. Low birth weight: a tabulation of available information. WHO/MCH/92.2. Geneva, 1992.

10

# Child anthropometry in cross-sectional surveys in developing countries: an assessment of the survivor bias

*J. Ties Boerma, A. Elisabeth Sommerfelt, and George T. Bicego*

**American Journal of Epidemiology**, *vol. 135, no. 4, 1992, pp. 438—449.*

## Abstract

In cross-sectional surveys, the sample of children with anthropometric measurements is not representative of all children in a birth cohort, since only children surviving to the survey date are measured. This survivor bias may have implications for studies of trends and differentials in anthropometric indicators. In this paper, the effects of the survivor bias on the estimates of child anthropometric indicators are assessed by 1) reviewing evidence from longitudinal studies on the prevalence of malnutrition among deceased children and among surviving children and by 2) analyzing retrospective data on child mortality and cross-sectional data on child anthropometry in 17 national surveys that are part of the Demographic and Health Surveys Program. It is concluded that comparisons of anthropometric data across geographic units, population subgroups, and calendar time are marginally affected by the survivor bias, unless mortality differences between the birth cohorts are very large (e.g., well over 50 per 1,000 births).

anthropometry; bias (epidemiology); developing countries; mortality

## Introduction

There is considerable evidence of the relation between malnutrition and mortality in childhood. For example, in a large study in Latin America, malnutrition was considered an important contributing cause to as much as half of the deaths among children under 5 years of age.[1] Several longitudinal studies have also shown that anthropometric measures are significant indicators of subsequent mortality risks.[2] The risk of mortality is increased many times for the severely malnourished, and moderately malnourished children are also at greater risk of dying in most studies. At the population level, the association between malnutrition and child mortality is less pronounced than at the individual level. An international comparison of prevalence of underweight and mortality showed that there are substantial differences among countries. For example, countries in southern Asia have relatively high levels of malnutrition in relation to their child mortality levels, while countries in Sub-Saharan Africa appear to have relatively low levels of malnutrition for their mortality levels.[3]

In cross-sectional surveys, the nutritional status of preschool children is usually assessed by measurement of weight and height of living children under 5 years of age. The sample of children with anthropometric measurements is, however, not representative of a birth cohort of children, since only children surviving to the survey date are measured. The level of mortality and the extent to which anthropometric status is related to subsequent mortality will determine the level of bias in cross-sectional estimates of nutritional status in a population. If this bias is not uniform across populations or across subgroups of a population, comparative analysis and analysis of differentials in nutritional status are affected. Similarly, in a population experiencing a decline in childhood mortality, the survivor bias within subgroups of a trend analysis (i.e., real or synthetic birth cohorts) will change, and the trend in measures of nutritional status will be distorted. For example, it has been suggested that the child mortality decline in Panama and Guatemala between 1965 and 1975 contributed to the increase in the proportion of children under 5 years with moderate to severe malnutrition during the same period, since more children with malnutrition survived.[4]

In this paper, an attempt is made to assess the effects of this survivor bias on the estimates of the anthropometric indicators in cross-sectional surveys. This includes a review of data from longitudinal studies that provide data on anthropometry of children who subsequently died. In addition, data from the Demographic and Health Surveys Program (DHS) will be analyzed. Retrospective data on child mortality and cross sectional data on child anthropometry in DHS surveys enable an evaluation of the potential magnitude of the survivor bias.

## Materials and methods

DHS, funded by the US Agency for International Development (USAID), assists developing countries in the organization of nationally representative surveys, aiming to provide information for policy and program decision making and for scientific research. Survey information includes a full birth history, which is used for child mortality estimation, and various maternal and child health indicators. Survey respondents are women of childbearing ages. DHS is the only large international data base that includes data on both child mortality and anthropometry.

In 17 DHS surveys in the period 1986–1989, anthropometric data were collected from national samples. Children aged 3–36 months of the respondents were weighed and measured after the completion of the interview. The validity of the anthropometric indicators calculated from these data depends on the accuracy of the height, weight, and age data collected. Therefore, thorough training of measurers was ensured. The procedures used were those recommended by the United Nations.[5] The children were weighed using hanging spring scales and measured with portable measuring boards.

The anthropometric measurements were evaluated using the reference population of the US National Center for Health Statistics/Centers for Disease Control, as recommended by the World Health Organization (referred to as the NCHS reference). The indicators used here are height for age, weight for age, and weight for height, with minus two standard deviations (–2 SD) and minus three standard deviations (–3 SD) from the median of the reference population chosen as cutoff points to determine the degree of malnutrition. Children with missing data on date of birth (which have been imputed for other analyses of DHS data) have been excluded from the analysis. DHS samples are weighted to obtain national estimates. In the present study, the weighted data are used.

The magnitude of the effect of the survivor bias on anthropometric indicators depends on three factors: 1) child mortality level, the proportion deceased in a cohort of children between birth and the survey date; 2) prevalence of malnutrition among living children that varies by population, indicators, and cutoff point used; and 3) prevalence of malnutrition among deceased children.

The odds ratio of the prevalence of malnutrition among deceased children and among living children will be referred to as $K$. If $K = 1$, malnutrition among deceased children and living children is the same, and there is no survivor bias. If all deceased children would have been malnourished at the time of the survey, the proportion malnourished is simply the sum of malnourished living children and all the dead children, divided by all children in the birth cohort. This scenario would be similar to the propositions made by Mosley and Chen.[6] They suggested that an index of health status could be created from the nutritional status of living children in a cross-sectional survey and that child deaths would be incorporated into the index by assigning deaths to the worst grade of malnutrition. In the Gomez classification of weight for age, where grade III is below 60 percent of standard weight for age, this would be grade IV.

The prevalence of malnutrition among all children ($P_{MN,all}$) is thus:

$$P_{MN,all} = P_{MN,S}*P_S + P_{MN,D}*P_D \qquad (1)$$
$$= P_{MN,S}*(1 - P_D) + P_{MN,D}*P_D$$

where $P_{MN,S}$ and $P_{MN,D}$ are the prevalences of malnutrition among survivors and deceased children, respectively, and $P_S$ and $P_D$ are the proportions of children surviving and deceased, respectively (where $P_S + P_D = 1$).

The relative increase in malnutrition by including deceased children is then:

$$P_{MN,all}/P_{MN,S} = (P_{MN,S}*(1 - P_D)$$
$$+ P_{MN,D}*P_D)/P_{MN,S} \qquad (2)$$
$$= (1 - P_D) + P_D*K$$

where $K$ = the ratio $P_{MN,D}/P_{MN,S}$.

Table 1 shows the relative increase in the prevalence of malnutrition by different levels of mortality (2.5, 7.5, and 12.5 percent of the birth cohort died before the survey), different levels of $K$, and different levels of malnutrition. For example, consider a population where 7.5 percent of the children in a birth cohort died before the survey, and 25

**Table I**   Relative increase in prevalence of malnutrition by different levels of mortality and different levels of K (see text) at three levels of malnutrition among survivors

| % dead of cohort | % malnourished among survivors | K 1.0 | 1.5 | 2.0 | 3.0 | 5.0 | Max [a] |
|---|---|---|---|---|---|---|---|
| 2.5 | 5 | 1.00 | 1.01 | 1.03 | 1.05 | 1.10 | 1.48 |
|  | 25 | 1.00 | 1.01 | 1.03 | 1.05 |  | 1.08 |
|  | 50 | 1.00 | 1.01 | 1.03 |  |  | 1.03 |
| 7.5 | 5 | 1.00 | 1.04 | 1.08 | 1.15 | 1.30 | 2.43 |
|  | 25 | 1.00 | 1.04 | 1.08 | 1.15 |  | 1.23 |
|  | 50 | 1.00 | 1.04 | 1.08 |  |  | 1.08 |
| 12.5 | 5 | 1.00 | 1.06 | 1.13 | 1.25 | 1.50 | 3.38 |
|  | 25 | 1.00 | 1.06 | 1.13 | 1.25 |  | 1.38 |
|  | 50 | 1.00 | 1.06 | 1.13 |  |  | 1.13 |

a. $K$ = max implies that all deceased children would have been malnourished.

percent of the living children were malnourished at the time of the survey. In this population, the assumption of $K = 3$ (malnutrition three times more common among dead children than among living children) leads to a relative increase of 15 percent in the prevalence of malnutrition (i.e., from 25 to almost 29 percent).

Although the prevalence of malnutrition is not included in equation 2, it does have an effect on the potential magnitude of the survivor bias, since it determines the maximum value of $K$ that is possible. For example, if malnutrition is found among 50 percent of the surviving children, the maximum value of $K$ is 2. The relative increase will therefore be relatively small. However, the absolute increase may still be considerable.

To assess the magnitude of the effect of omitting dead children in cross-sectional surveys, it has to be estimated how much worse the nutritional status of deceased children is compared with that of surviving children. Such data can only be derived from longitudinal surveys. It will be assumed that children who were poorly nourished at some point in time before death would have been malnourished at the time of the measurement had they survived to the survey date. Using the data from longitudinal studies, an estimate will be made of how much more common malnutrition is among children who subsequently died.

To evaluate the effect of the survivor bias on the differentials in anthropometric indicators, five countries will be used with differing levels of mortality and malnutrition. Two of the most important variables affecting child survival are used: mother's level of education and preceding birth interval.

The mother's level of education is one of the most important determinants of both mortality and malnutrition in childhood. Different assumptions can be made to enable an assessment of the magnitude of the survivor bias. As in the case of the analysis of the effects of the survivor bias on levels of malnutrition, one can assume that all children who died would have been malnourished at the time of the survey *(K is maximal)* and that malnutrition would be somewhat higher among deceased children, both regardless of mother's educational level *(K greater than 1 and less than maximum)*. An addi-

**Table 2** Comparison of anthropometric indicators between children who died after the measurement and children who survived a specified time period in longitudinal studies

| Study | Dead children | | Survivors | | Indicator | Cutoff point[a] | Reference population | Age group |
|---|---|---|---|---|---|---|---|---|
| | $n$ | % MN[b] | $n$ | % MN | | | | |
| India, Punjab [7] | 148 | 73.0 | 8,009 | 54.8 | wt[b]/age | 80% | Harvard | 1–35 months |
| | | 34.5 | | 20.1 | wt/age | 70% | | |
| | | 17.6 | | 3.8 | wt/age | 60% | | |
| Bangladesh, Matlab [8] | 112 | 82.1 | 1,907 | 72.4 | wt/age | 75% | Harvard | 13–23 months at |
| | | 42.9 | | 19.9 | wt/age | 60% | | first measurement |
| | | 71.4 | | 56.1 | ht[b]/age | 90% | | and then followed |
| | | 47.3 | | 21.8 | ht/age | 85% | | for 2 years |
| | | 34.8 | | 31.6 | wt/ht | 80% | | |
| | | 9.8 | | 3.4 | wt/ht | 70% | | |
| Senegal, Niakhar [9] | 363 | 42.7 | 13,894[c] | 20.4 | wt/age | −2SD | NCHS[b] | 0–59 months |
| | | 16.8 | | 5.0 | wt/age | −3SD | | |
| | | 29.5 | | 19.3 | ht/age | −2SD | | |
| | | 14.6 | | 6.9 | ht/age | −3SD | | |
| | | 11.8 | | 5.1 | wt/ht | −2SD | | |
| | | 3.9 | | 0.7 | wt/ht | −3SD | | |
| Guinea-Bissau, Bandim [10] | 109 | 15.6 | 17,092[c] | 12.4 | wt/age | 75% | NCHS | 6–59 months at |
| | | 9.2 | | 12.3 | ht/age | 90% | | first measurement |
| | | 15.6 | | 10.7 | wt/ht | 85% | | and then followed |
| | | | | | | | | for 8–12 months |
| Malawi, Chingale [11] | 84 | 44.0 | 18,151[c] | 29.0 | wt/age | −2SD | NCHS | 0–59 months |
| | | 21.4 | | 6.2 | wt/age | −3SD | | |
| | | 47.6 | | 48.1 | ht/age | −2SD | | |
| | | 25.0 | | 20.6 | ht/age | −3SD | | |
| | | 13.1 | | 4.2 | wt/ht | −2SD | | |
| Yemen, South[12] | 32 | 25.0 | 2,123 | 39.5 | ht/age | −2SD | NCHS | 0–6 years |
| | | 21.9 | | 12.9 | ht/age | −3SD | | |
| | | 18.8 | | 7.5 | wt/ht | −2SD | | |
| | | 6.2 | | 0.8 | wt/ht | −3SD | | |
| India, Tamil Nadu 13 | 110 | 60.0 | 14,950 | 50.2 | ht/age | −2SD | NCHS | 0–71 months, |
| | | 54.5 | | 42.2 | wt/ht | −2SD | | followed for 1 year |
| Papua New Guinea, Southern Highlands [14] | 47 | 66.0 | 1,100 | 35.8 | wt/age | 80% | Harvard | 6–30 months, |
| | | 19.2 | | 7.1 | wt/age | 70% | | followed for 18 |
| | | 8.5 | | 1.3 | wt/age | 60% | | months |
| | | 44.7 | | 30.6 | ht/age | 90% | | |
| | | 12.8 | | 4.5 | ht/age | 85% | | |
| | | 8.5 | | 1.3 | wt/ht | 80% | | |

a   Refers to the percentage of median or standard deviation (SD) units below median of the reference population: −2 SD refers to approximately 77% from the median for weight/age, 90% for height/age, and 80% for weight/height; − 3 SD refers to approximately 65%, 85%, and 70%, respectively.

b   % MN, percentage malnourished; wt, weight; ht, height; NCHS, US National Center for Health Statistics/Centers for Disease Control, as recommended by the World Health Organization.

c   Refers to number of measurements.

tional scenario is possible. The combination of death and malnutrition may be much more common among children of less educated mothers than among children of more educated mothers. The factor $K$ will thus be greater for estimating the prevalence of malnutrition among deceased children in the lower education groups than in the higher education groups.

The length of the preceding birth interval is also often reported as one of the leading determinants of child survival, but much less evidence exists of its influence on child growth. To assess the effects of the survivor bias, it will be assumed that all children who died would have been malnourished at the time of the survey $(K$ is maximal) and that malnutrition would be somewhat higher among deceased children $(K$ greater than 1 and less than maximal). A fourth scenario, as for mother's education, with different values of $K$ by birth interval length, does not appear plausible for birth interval analysis and was not used.

## Results

### Anthropometry of deceased children: review of longitudinal studies

Table 2 presents a comparison of anthropometric indicators between children who died after the initial measurements and children who survived the specified time period. Most studies used different standards, different observation periods, and different age groups, but the general picture is clear; the nutritional status among children who died was poorer than among the surviving children. Unfortunately, samples in most surveys were too small to focus on differentials by age of the child. Only data from the Narangwal study in India allowed for a separate analysis of infants (1-11 months) and children (12–35 months).[7]

Among children who died, the proportion of children underweight was higher in both age groups compared with survivors, and the relative difference was slightly larger among infants than among children 12–35 months. It is also obvious that to assume that all deceased children are malnourished is not justified. Only in the studies of Bangladesh and India, where the prevalence of malnutrition is very high among surviving children, are the proportions of children who are underweight and stunted well above 50 percent. However, in most studies, less than half of the children who subsequently died were considered malnourished.

Based on the data summarized in Table 2, a summary of the ratio of the proportions malnourished among children who subsequently died and children who survived is presented in Table 3. The ratios are higher if the malnutrition is more severe, implying that such conditions are indeed much more commonly found among deceased children. The differences are more pronounced for weight for age and weight for height than for height for age. In fact, there is little evidence showing that stunting (below –2 SD from the median height for age) is much more common among dead children. For severe stunting (below –3 SD from the median height for age or similar cutoff points), there are differences between living children and deceased children. Regarding weight for age, the proportion underweight is 1.5–2.0 times higher among deceased children than

**Table 3** Prevalence of malnutrion among surviving children and ratio of proportion malnourished among dead and surviving children in longitudinal studies (K) (data from Table 2)

| Study area | Weight for age | | | |
| | % underweight | K | % severely underweight | K |
| --- | --- | --- | --- | --- |
| Matlab | 72.4 | 1.13 | 19.9 | 2.16 |
| Punjab | 54.8 | 1.33 | 20.1 | 1.72 |
| Papua New Guinea | 35.8 | 1.84 | 6.3 | 3.05 |
| Chingale | 29.0 | 1.52 | 6.2 | 3.45 |
| Niakhar | 20.4 | 2.09 | 5.0 | 3.36 |
| Bandim | 12.4 | 1.26 | | |

| | Height for age | | | |
| | % stunted | K | % severely stunted | K |
| --- | --- | --- | --- | --- |
| Matlab | 56.1 | 1.27 | 21.8 | 2.17 |
| Tamil Nadu | 50.3 | 1.19 | | |
| Chingale | 48.1 | 0.99 | 20.6 | 1.21 |
| Yemen | 39.5 | 0.63 | 12.9 | 1.70 |
| Papua New Guinea | 30.6 | 1.46 | 4.5 | 2.84 |
| Bandim | 12.3 | 0.75 | | |

| | Weight for height | | | |
| | % wasted | K | % severely wasted | K |
| --- | --- | --- | --- | --- |
| Tamil Nadu | 42.2 | 1.29 | | |
| Matlab | 31.6 | 1.10 | 3.4 | 2.88 |
| Bandim | 10.7 | 1.46 | | |
| Yemen | 7.5 | 2.51 | 0.8 | 7.75 |
| Niakhar | 5.1 | 2.31 | 0.7 | 5.57 |
| Chingale | 4.2 | 3.12 | | |
| Papua New Guinea | 1.3 | 6.54 | | |

among surviving children, although the difference is smaller in populations with a very high prevalence of underweight. The differences in the proportion who are severely underweight are larger with $K$ values of 2–3. The largest differences are observed for wasting. The range of the values of $K$ is also larger, partly due to the very low prevalence of wasting among surviving children in some studies.

## Nutritional status and mortality

Table 4 presents the prevalence of malnutrition using three anthropometric indicators and two different cutoff points among children aged 3–35 months. There is considerable variation among countries, indicators, and cutoff points, which implies that the effects of the survivor bias may also be different. Table 4 also includes the proportion of children deceased in this birth cohort as well as the proportions of children dead in the cohorts born 3–11 and 12–35 months before the survey. The proportion dead among children 3–35 months at the time of the survey varies from 2.5 percent in Sri

**Table 4**  Percentage of children 3–35 months who fall below –2 standard deviations (SD) and –3 SD from the median of the NCHS[1] reference population for height (ht)/age, weight (wt)/age, and weight/height (wt/ht), and proportion dead by birth cohort: 3–11 months, 12–35 months, and 3–35 months

| Country | No. of children | ht/age | | wt/age | | wt/ht | | Proportion dead | | |
|---|---|---|---|---|---|---|---|---|---|---|
| | | <–3SD | <–2SD | <–3SD | <–2SD | <–3SD | <–2SD | 3–35 months | 3–11 months | 12–35 months |
| **Sub-Saharan Africa** | | | | | | | | | | |
| Burundi | 1,889 | 18.8 | 47.4 | 10.0 | 37.5 | 0.8 | 5.7 | 7.9 | 5.8 | 8.8 |
| Ghana | 1,795 | 9.7 | 29.4 | 7.1 | 30.3 | 0.4 | 8.0 | 9.8 | 5.9 | 11.2 |
| Mali | 909 | 8.2 | 23.8 | 9.2 | 30.6 | 1.3 | 11.5 | 14.9 | 8.5 | 18.1 |
| Senegal | 618 | 7.6 | 23.0 | 5.3 | 22.0 | 0.3 | 5.8 | 11.3 | 8.4 | 12.4 |
| Togo | 1,281 | 10.2 | 31.0 | 6.3 | 26.1 | 0.5 | 5.7 | 9.8 | 8.1 | 10.5 |
| Uganda | 2,326 | 17.3 | 43.8 | 6.1 | 25.1 | 0.2 | 2.2 | 12.3 | 8.6 | 13.8 |
| Zimbabwe | 1,496 | 8.0 | 29.8 | 1.5 | 12.6 | 0.3 | 1.2 | 5.7 | 5.1 | 5.9 |
| **North Africa** | | | | | | | | | | |
| Egypt | 1,885 | 12.0 | 30.9 | 2.5 | 13.4 | 0.1 | 1.1 | 7.9 | 5.4 | 7.9 |
| Morocco | 2,523 | 7.6 | 23.7 | 3.2 | 14.0 | 0.7 | 3.7 | 7.9 | 6.5 | 8.4 |
| Tunisia | 1,970 | 5.4 | 17.9 | 1.7 | 10.3 | 0.6 | 3.0 | 4.5 | 3.2 | 4.9 |
| **Asia** | | | | | | | | | | |
| Sri Lanka | 1,962 | 7.9 | 27.2 | 8.3 | 37.3 | 0.6 | 11.6 | 2.5 | 1.9 | 2.8 |
| Thailand | 1,808 | 4.1 | 21.5 | 4.0 | 25.3 | 0.4 | 5.3 | 3.5 | 2.4 | 3.8 |
| **Latin America and Caribbean** | | | | | | | | | | |
| Bolivia | 2,511 | 14.5 | 37.7 | 2.6 | 13.2 | 0.3 | 1.6 | 9.5 | 6.3 | 10.7 |
| Colombia | 1,301 | 8.2 | 25.3 | 1.9 | 12.0 | 0.2 | 1.3 | 3.2 | 2.6 | 3.5 |
| Dominican Rep. | 1,767 | 7.6 | 20.6 | 2.8 | 12.4 | 0.2 | 2.3 | 7.0 | 5.5 | 7.6 |
| Guatemala | 2,207 | 30.1 | 57.7 | 8.5 | 33.2 | 0.1 | 1.3 | 7.9 | 5.0 | 9.1 |
| Trinidad and Tobago | 817 | 0.4 | 4.8 | 0.4 | 6.5 | 0.7 | 3.8 | 2.6 | 2.5 | 2.7 |

1. NCHS, US National Center for Health Statistics/Centers for Disease Control, as recommended by the World Health Organization.

Lanka to almost 15 percent in Mali. As expected, the proportion deceased is higher in the birth cohort 12–35 months than in the cohort born 3–11 months before the survey, suggesting that the survivor bias is potentially larger in the 12- to 35-month birth cohort.

There is a relation between the levels of mortality and malnutrition in the same birth cohort, even without taking the survivor bias into account. There is, however, considerable variation among countries. Figure 1 displays the relation between the proportion deceased in the cohort of children born 3–35 months before the survey and the proportion of children severely underweight (weight for age below –3 SD) among children 3–35 months in 17 DHS surveys (23 percent of the variation in the proportion severely underweight is explained by the mortality level). In line with previous reports, the only DHS country in southern Asia, Sri Lanka, has a very high prevalence of underweight in

**Figure I** Mortality 3–35 months by proportion severly underweight. Regression line excludes Sri Lanka. m., months; SD, standard deviation

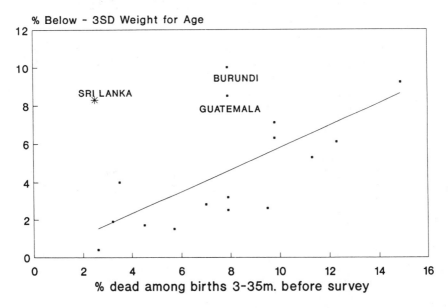

relation to its mortality level. If Sri Lanka is excluded from the linear regression analysis, a stronger relation exists between nutritional status and mortality (44 percent of the variation in proportion severely underweight is explained by variation in mortality). In addition to Sri Lanka, Guatemala and Burundi also have levels of underweight that are much higher than expected on the basis of their mortality levels.

The other five anthropometric indicators showed similar but weaker associations between nutritional status and mortality. The strongest relations occurred between mortality and weight/age below –2 SD ($R^2 = 0.29$, excluding Sri Lanka), weight/height below –2 SD ($R^2 = 0.26$, excluding Sri Lanka), and height/age below –3 SD ($R^2 = 0.27$, excluding Guatemala).

## Prevalence of malnutrition

Table 5 illustrates the possible effects of the survivor bias in four countries with different levels of malnutrition and mortality: Mali (14.9 percent deceased), Bolivia (9.5 percent), Egypt (7.2 percent), and Sri Lanka (2.5 percent). For each indicator, the prevalence of malnutrition is shown for surviving children (or for all children assuming that malnutrition prevalence among surviving and deceased children would have been the same, i.e., $K = 1$), for all children assuming that all deceased children would have been malnourished ($K = $ max), and for all children using the most probable value for K, i.e., the odds ratio of malnutrition among deceased children and among surviving children. The results from Table 2 were used to select the most probable values of $K$, which are shown in Table 5.

**Table 5**  Changes in the percentage malnourished (% MN) when adjusting for the survivor bias: for K is maximal (K = max) and for K with the most probable value (K = probable), with absolute and relative changes compared with survivors only

| Country | % MN (survivors) | K - max % MN | K - probable % MN | Increase of K - probable | |
|---|---|---|---|---|---|
| | | | | Absolute | Relative |
| *Weight for age below −2 SD[a] (K - 2.0)* | | | | | |
| Mali | 30.6 | 39.6 | 35.2 | 4.6 | 1.15 |
| Bolivia | 13.2 | 20.7 | 14.5 | 1.3 | 1.10 |
| Egypt | 13.4 | 19.2 | 14.4 | 1.0 | 1.07 |
| Sri Lanka | 37.3 | 38.8 | 38.2 | 0.9 | 1.03 |
| *Weight for age below −3 SD (K - 3.0)* | | | | | |
| Mali | 9.2 | 21.0 | 11.9 | 2.7 | 1.30 |
| Bolivia | 2.6 | 11.1 | 3.1 | 0.5 | 1.19 |
| Egypt | 2.5 | 9.0 | 2.9 | 0.4 | 1.14 |
| Sri Lanka | 8.3 | 10.5 | 8.7 | 0.4 | 1.05 |
| *Height for age below −2 SD (K - 1.2)* | | | | | |
| Mali | 23.8 | 33.7 | 24.5 | 0.7 | 1.03 |
| Bolivia | 37.7 | 43.1 | 38.4 | 0.7 | 1.02 |
| Egypt | 30.9 | 35.5 | 31.3 | 0.4 | 1.01 |
| Sri Lanka | 27.2 | 29.0 | 27.3 | 0.1 | 1.01 |
| *Height for age below −3 SD (K - 2.0)* | | | | | |
| Mali | 8.2 | 20.1 | 9.4 | 1.2 | 1.15 |
| Bolivia | 14.5 | 21.9 | 15.9 | 1.4 | 1.10 |
| Egypt | 12.0 | 17.9 | 12.9 | 0.9 | 1.07 |
| Sri Lanka | 7.9 | 10.1 | 8.1 | 0.2 | 1.03 |
| *Weight for height below −2 SD (K - 2.0)* | | | | | |
| Mali | 11.5 | 23.0 | 13.2 | 1.7 | 1.15 |
| Bolivia | 1.6 | 10.1 | 1.8 | 0.2 | 1.10 |
| Egypt | 1.1 | 7.7 | 1.2 | 0.1 | 1.07 |
| Sri Lanka | 11.6 | 13.8 | 11.9 | 0.3 | 1.03 |
| *Weight for height below −3 SD (K - 4.0)* | | | | | |
| Mali | 1.3 | 14.1 | 1.9 | 0.6 | 1.45 |
| Bolivia | 0.3 | 8.9 | 0.4 | 0.1 | 1.29 |
| Egypt | 0.1 | 6.8 | 0.1 | 0.0 | 1.22 |
| Sri Lanka | 0.6 | 3.0 | 0.6 | 0.0 | 1.08 |

a. SD, standard deviation.

It is obvious that the effects of the survivor bias are very large if all deceased children would have been malnourished. These estimates of the prevalence of malnutrition are much higher than the estimates based on a 'probable' value of K. Regarding height for age, the effects of the survivor bias appear to be negligible if −2 SD is used as a cut-off point and small for severe stunting (below −3 SD). The effects of the survivor bias are large on the prevalence of severe wasting if the relative increases are considered (more than 20 percent increase in three of the four countries). However, the absolute increase is very small (less than 1 percent), since severe wasting is rare.

**Table 6** Differentials in the percentage of children 3–35 months underweight by mother's level of education and odds of being underweight for different values of K, with children of mothers with secondary education as reference category

| Mother's education | % below −2 SD[a,b] | Relative odds | | | |
|---|---|---|---|---|---|
| | | (A) [b] | (B) [b] | (C) [b] | (D) [b] |
| **Uganda** | | | | | |
| None | 28.9 | 1.8 | 1.8 | 2.2 | 1.4 |
| Primary | 23.8 | 1.5 | 1.5 | 1.6 | 1.2 |
| Secondary [c] | 15.8 | 1.0 | 1.0 | 1.0 | 1.0 |
| **Zimbabwe** | | | | | |
| None | 21.5 | 3.3 | 3.5 | 3.7 | 2.8 |
| Primary | 12.5 | 2.0 | 2.0 | 2.2 | 1.8 |
| Secondary [c] | 6.3 | 1.0 | 1.0 | 1.0 | 1.0 |
| **Sri Lanka** | | | | | |
| None | 52.4 | 1.6 | 1.6 | 1.6 | 1.6 |
| Primary | 44.4 | 1.4 | 1.3 | 1.3 | 1.3 |
| Secondary [c] | 32.8 | 1.0 | 1.0 | 1.0 | 1.0 |
| **Egypt** | | | | | |
| None | 16.4 | 2.6 | 2.8 | 3.0 | 2.5 |
| Primary | 13.9 | 2.2 | 2.2 | 2.3 | 2.0 |
| Secondary [c] | 6.2 | 1.0 | 1.0 | 1.0 | 1.0 |
| **Bolivia** | | | | | |
| None | 22.9 | 3.2 | 3.4 | 3.8 | 2.6 |
| Primary | 13.7 | 1.9 | 2.0 | 2.0 | 1.9 |
| Secondary [c] | 7.1 | 1.0 | 1.0 | 1.0 | 1.0 |

a. For living children measured during the survey.
b. SD, standard deviation; (A), $K = 1$; (B), $K = 2$; (C), $K$ differs between education groups (none, $K = 2.5$; primary, $K = 1.5$; and secondary and over, $K = 1.0$); (D), $K =$ maximal.
c. Reference category.

The largest effect of the survivor bias can be observed for weight for age. In Mali, where mortality is highest, the proportion underweight increased by 4.6 percent and severely underweight by 2.7 percent. The increases in Bolivia and Egypt were substantial in relative terms, but still small in absolute terms, while the increase in Sri Lanka was smallest.

### Differentials by education and birth interval

Five DHS surveys were selected to illustrate the potential impact of the survivor bias on differentials in child anthropometric indicators. Regarding the effect of the mother's education, four different assumptions were tested, with different values of $K$: 1 (A), 2 (B), and maximal (D). In addition, $K$ was assumed to vary among the education groups: $K = 1$ for children of mothers with at least secondary education, 1.5 among children of mothers with primary education, and 2.5 among children of mothers with no education (C).

Table 6 presents the results for the four assumptions in five surveys and compares the results with the differentials among surviving children. Even though mortality levels and levels of malnutrition vary considerably among the countries, the results are fairly consistent. There is an increase in the differentials by education if dead children are included with a higher prevalence of malnutrition. The increase is moderate. The largest increase can be observed in Uganda, where the odds ratio increases from 1.8 to 2.2 if the prevalence of underweight is assumed to be 2.5 times higher for deceased children of uneducated mothers. If all deceased children are considered malnourished, differentials tend to decrease, because the absolute increase in the percentage underweight is lower in the no education category.

The effect of the length of the preceding birth interval on the anthropometric indicators is less pronounced than the impact of the mother's education (Table 7). The proportion underweight among children 3–35 months is only 1.1–1.3 times higher among children with short preceding birth intervals (less than 24 months) compared with children with longer birth intervals (at least 24 months). One may argue, however, that differentials would be much larger if deceased children are taken into consideration. Table 7 shows that the effect of including deceased children on the relative proportion underweight by birth interval is negligible in four countries. Only in Bolivia can a moderate increase be observed if deceased children are included.

## Discussion

A review of longitudinal studies showed that malnutrition is indeed much more common among deceased children. There is considerable variation among studies, which were carried out in very different settings, but still a fairly consistent pattern emerges. Wasting and underweight are about twice as common among deceased children. This, however, does not pertain to stunting (defined as height for age below –2 SD). For severe stunting (height for age below –3 SD), there are again marked differences between children who subsequently died and survivors. The review of the literature on anthropometric data of deceased children, however, also shows that it is not appropriate to assign all child deaths to the worst grade of malnutrition.

In the DHS surveys, there is a relation between the level of malnutrition and child mortality at the country level. This relation turned out to be strongest between weight for age and mortality. There is, however, considerable variation among countries, and there are a few major outliers. For example, in some countries the level of malnutrition is much higher than expected on the basis of their mortality levels. The most notable exceptions are Sri Lanka and, to a lesser extent, Guatemala.

It has been suggested that differences in child mortality need to be taken into account in trends assessments and comparative studies using anthropometric indicators.

However, if the assumptions made in this study concerning the increased prevalence of malnutrition among deceased children compared with surviving children are correct, the effects of the survivor bias are generally small. Only if large mortality differences

**Table 7** Differentials in the percentage of children 3–35 months underweight by length of preceding birth interval and odds of being underweight for different values of $K$, with children with birth intervals of at least 24 months as reference category

| Birth interval | % below −2 SD[a,b] | Relative odds (A)[b] | Relative odds (B)[b] | Relative odds (C)[b] |
|---|---|---|---|---|
| Uganda | | | | |
| < 24 months | 28.6 | 1.2 | 1.2 | 1.2 |
| ≥ 24 months | 23.9 | 1.0 | 1.0 | 1.0 |
| Zimbabwe | | | | |
| < 24 months | 14.5 | 1.2 | 1.2 | 1.0 |
| ≥ 24 months | 12.3 | 1.0 | 1.0 | 1.0 |
| Sri Lanka | | | | |
| < 24 months | 40.8 | 1.1 | 1.1 | 1.1 |
| ≥ 24 months | 37.6 | 1.0 | 1.0 | 1.0 |
| Egypt | | | | |
| < 24 months | 15.8 | 1.1 | 1.2 | 1.4 |
| ≥ 24 months | 14.0 | 1.0 | 1.0 | 1.0 |
| Bolivia | | | | |
| < 24 months | 16.7 | 1.3 | 1.5 | 1.7 |
| ≥ 24 months | 12.5 | 1.0 | 1.0 | 1.0 |

a.  For living children measured during the survey.
b.  SD, standard deviation; (A), $K = 1$; (B), $K = 2$; (C), $K =$ maximal.

exist between two cohorts does the survivor bias need to be taken into account. Among the four surveys analyzed in Table 5, the mortality difference between Sri Lanka and Egypt and between Mali and Bolivia was about 5 percent, or 50 per 1,000 births in more conventional terms. Under the most probable assumptions concerning the nutritional status of deceased children, the effect of the survivor bias is still fairly small. Only if Mali and Sri Lanka are compared, i.e., a mortality difference of more than 100 per 1,000 births between the birth cohorts, does the effect of the survivor bias become important. In this case, the cross-sectional prevalences of underweight are 30.6 and 37.3 percent in Mali and Sri Lanka, respectively. If deceased children are included under the most probable assumption, the corresponding prevalences are 35.2 and 38.2 percent. The difference is narrowed.

The effects of the survivor bias are more important for the indicators weight for age and weight for height than for height for age. In addition, the older the children in the age group under study, the larger the potential effect of the survivor bias, since greater cumulative mortality is related to a greater fraction of the birth cohort being selected out of the cross-sectional sample.

Regarding the effect of selectivity on the study of differentials in anthropometric indicators, it is concluded that the effects of selectivity are small and in most cases would not have a substantial effect on the study of differentials by socioeconomic or family formation variables. This was also shown in a multivariate analysis of anthropometric data from the Bolivia DHS survey, where all deceased children were considered malnourished.[15] These findings indicate that it is sound to study differentials in anthropometric indicators by socioeconomic and other variables without taking mortality differentials into account. Studies that attempt to link the determinants of growth faltering with those of childhood mortality appear unencumbered by the issue of survivor bias.

## References

1  Puffer R.R., Serrano C.V., Pattern of mortality in childhood. Washington, DC: Pan American Health Organization, 1973. (PAHO scientific publication no. 262).

2  Martorell R., Ho T.J., Malnutrition, morbidity, and mortality. Popul Dev Rev 1984;10 (suppl): 49–68.

3  Haaga J., Kenrick C., Test K., et al., An estimate of the prevalence of child malnutrition in developing countries. World Health Stat Q 1985;38:331–47.

4  Teller C., Sibrian R., Talavera C., et al., Population and nutrition: impiications of sociodemographic trends and differentials for food and nutrition policy in Central America and Panama. Ecol Food Nutr 1979;8:95–109.

5  United Nations, How to weigh and measure children: assessing the nutritional status of young children in household surveys. New York: Department of Technical Cooperation for Development and Statistical Office, 1986.

6  Mosley W.H., Chen L.C., An analytical framework for the study of child survival in developing countries. Popul Dev Rev 1984;10(suppl):25–48.

7  Kielmann A.A., McCord C., Weight–for-age as an index of risk of death in children. Lancet 1978;1:1247–50.

8  Chen L.C., Chowdhury A.K.M.A., Huffman S.L., Anthropometric assessment of energy-protein malnutrition and subsequent risk of mortality among preschool aged children. Am J Clin Nutr 1980;33:1836–45.

9  Garenne M., Maire B., Fontaine O., et al., Risques de déces associés a différents états nutritionnels chez l'enfant d'age préscolaire. (In French). Dakar, Senegal: ORSTOM, 1987.

10  Smedman L., Sterky G., Mellander L., et al., Anthropometry and subsequent mortality in groups of children aged 6–59 months in Guinea-Bissau. Am J Clin Nutr 1987;46:369–73.

11  Lindskog U., Lindskog P., Carstensen J., et al., Childhood mortality in relation to nutritional status and water supply – a prospective study from rural Malawi. Acta Paediatr Scand 1988,77;260–8.

12  Bagelholm G.C., Nasher A.A.A., Mortality among children in rural areas of the People's Democratic Republic of Yemen. Ann Trop Paediatr 1989;9: 75–81.

13  Rahmathullah L., Underwood B.A., Thulasiraj R.D., et al. Reduced mortality among children in southern India receiving a small weekly dose of vitamin A. N Engl J Med 1990;323:929–35.

14  Heywood P., The functional significance of malnutrition – growth and prospective risk of death in the highlands of Papua New Guinea. J Food Nutr 1982;39:13–19.

15  Bicego G.T., Boerma J.T., Maternal education, use of health services, and child survival: an analysis of data from the Bolivia DHS survey. Columbia, MD: Institute for Resource Development, 1990. (DHS working paper no. 1).

# Preceding birth intervals and child survival: searching for pathways of influence

*J. Ties Boerma and George T. Bicego*

**Studies in Family Planning**, *vol. 23, no. 4, 1992, pp. 243–256.*

## Abstract

The importance of the length of preceding birth intervals for the survival chances of young children has been established, but the debate concerning the causal biomedical or behavioral mechanisms continues. This article uses data from 17 Demographic and Health Surveys to investigate the effect of birth intervals on child mortality: anthropometry of children, recent morbidity of children, and use of health services are examined in addition to child survival data for children born in the five years before the survey. Various methodological approaches are used to investigate the relative importance of the postulated mechanisms linking birth intervals and child survival. Short preceding birth intervals are associated with increased mortality risks in the neonatal period and at 1–6 months of age, and, to a much lesser extent, at 7–23 months of age. The effects of short birth intervals on nutritional status are rather moderate, and there is a weak relationship with lower attendance at prenatal care services. No consistent relationship exists between the length of birth intervals and other health status or health-service utilization variables. The results indicate that prenatal mechanisms are more important than postnatal factors, such as sibling competition, in explaining the causal nature of the birth interval effect. (*Studies in Family Planning*, 1992; 23, 4:)

## Introduction

Many studies have demonstrated the importance of the length of preceding birth intervals for the survival chances of young children. In particular, analyses of data from the World Fertility Survey have made a strong case for increased mortality risks among children born after short birth intervals (Hobcraft et al., 1985). Little is known, however, about the actual biological and behavioral mechanisms responsible for the child spacing–child survival relationship. The current evidence for the most frequently suggested mechanisms of maternal depletion, sibling competition, and increased infectious-disease transmission is fragmentary and sometimes contradictory.

In this article, data from the Demographic and Health Surveys (DHS) Project are used to investigate the pathways through which preceding birth intervals may affect early childhood mortality. Following a review of the possible causal mechanisms, we discuss the methodological approach taken here to evaluate the relative importance of prenatal vs. postnatal, and behavioural vs. biological effects. The approach includes analysis of differential age patterns of mortality, the effects of controlling for the survival status of the previous child and for breastfeeding practices, and analysis of the effects of birth intervals on the current health status of surviving children and on utilization of maternal and child health services. The study aims to discern the common patterns among diverse populations in the relative importance of various factors and the pathways through which the relationship between preceding birth intervals and child survival is affected.

## Possible pathways of influence

Figure 1 summarizes the possible prenatal and postnatal mechanisms that link the length of preceding birth intervals and child survival.

### Prenatal mechanisms

Maternal depletion is often cited as the primary mechanism responsible for the adverse effects of short birth intervals.[1] Women with short intervals between two pregnancies have insufficient time to restore their nutritional reserves, which is thought to affect fetal growth. Several studies have documented an increased risk of intrauterine growth retardation for interpregnancy intervals of fewer than nine months (that is, birth intervals of fewer than 18 months) (Lieberman et al., 1989, Brody and Bracken, 1987, Ferraz et al., 1988). Intrauterine growth could also be retarded by a short recuperative interval between the end of lactation and the beginning of a new pregnancy, or, even stronger, by the existence of an overlap between lactation and gestation. In Guatemala, Merchant et al. (1990) observed that the absence of an overlap between lactation and gestation and a longer recuperative interval were less stressful for mothers and somewhat favoured better intrauterine growth. The birth-weight differentials, however, were small, and it was suggested that fetal growth was protected at the cost of maternal nutritional status.

Short interpregnancy intervals may be a cause of premature delivery (Miller, 1989, Fedrick and Adelstein, 1973); however, the evidence for such an effect is mixed. Although no relationship was observed in studies in the US (Lang et al., 1990, Lieberman et al., 1989, Brody and Bracken, 1987), Brazil (Ferraz et al., 1988), and the Philippines (Miller et al., 1992), studies in India (Mavalankar and Gray, 1991), Great Britain (Fedrick and Adelstein, 1973), and Bangladesh and the Philippines (Miller et al., 1992) reported increased risks of preterm birth among infants conceived within six months after the previous birth.[2]

**Figure I** Possible mechanisms linking short preceding birth intervals and child survival, and the outcomes used to study the importance of these mechanisms

| Mechanisms | Study outcomes |
|---|---|
| **Prenatal and biological** | |
| Prematurity | Mortality (by age) |
| Intrauterine growth retardation (maternal depletion due to pregnancies and lactation) | Overlap gestation-lactation Breastfeeding initiation |
| **Prenatal and behavioural** | |
| Poor pregnancy care | Mortality (by age) Health-service utilization (prenatal and delivery care) |
| **Postnatal and biological** | |
| Impaired lactation Increased disease transmission | Mortality (by age) Diarrhoea prevalence Poor nutritional status Breastfeeding initiation |
| **Postnatal and behavioural** | |
| Poor care and nutrition (sibling competition) | Mortality (by age) Poor nutritional status Diarrhoea prevalence Health-services utilization |
| Confounding variables affecting birth interval length and child survival | |
| Socioeconomic and biodemographic variables | Control for mother's education; residence; economic status of the household; birth order; maternal age; sex of the child; and twin |
| Prematurity | – |
| Breastfeeding | Control for breastfeeding duration of index child in mortality analysis |
| Intrafamilial mortality risks | Control for survival status of preceding sibling |

Both intrauterine growth retardation and prematurity lead to low birth-weight babies. Since low birth weight is a strong determinant of early infant mortality, controlling for small size at birth is expected to attenuate the effect of short birth intervals on mortality during the first months of life. However, data from Malaysia on the child's size at birth, as recalled by the mother, did not explain much of the relationship between child spacing and child survival in Malaysia (Millman and Cooksey, 1987).

Apart from the biological mechanisms operating in the prenatal period, behavioural factors may also affect the outcome of pregnancy. Because pregnant mothers with short spacing of births still have very young children, they may not attend prenatal care services at all or they may attend much later in pregnancy than might otherwise be the case. Illnesses during pregnancy, such as malaria, may then last longer and have an adverse effect on the outcome of pregnancy. On the other hand, women with longer birth intervals may be better disposed toward self-monitoring their pregnancy and toward having higher levels of attendance at prenatal care services; they may also be more likely to deliver in institutions.

### Postnatal mechanisms

A mother's poor health and poor nutritional status may also have postnatal consequences, such as impaired lactation (Pebley and Millman, 1986, Retherford et al., 1989) and an inability to give adequate care to her children. Evidence from studies of the adequacy of breastmilk suggests, however, that mild to moderate malnutrition does not have a strong effect on lactation or the composition and quantity of breastmilk, at least during the first months of life (Van Steenbergen et al., 1989).[3]

Sibling competition is considered a plausible mechanism in the birth interval-child survival association during the postnatal period. The newborn child has to compete with another young sibling for household resources and the mother's care. This situation may have a bearing on the nutrition of the youngest child (the child with a short preceding birth interval), although reliance on breastfeeding during the first months of life may ensure adequate nutrition at least very early on. Lack of adequate care for the child may result in a higher incidence of illnesses (due to an unclean environment or to higher exposure to infectious agents, a lack of immunizations, and so on), and accidents, and higher case-fatality rates from illnesses, because the symptoms are recognized too late or curative health services are not used at all.

An additional biomedical mechanism that has been proposed is the increased risk of infectious-disease transmission. A short preceding birth interval implies that the index child has an older sibling aged under 24 months, or perhaps two siblings under the age of five. The older child is more likely to bring infections into the household, and the youngest sibling is put at risk of becoming ill more frequently. Furthermore, the youngest child, as a secondary case, may suffer more severe infection with higher mortality risks, such as has been shown with measles (Aaby, 1988). Increased disease transmission is primarily a consequence of crowding and thus is not strictly an effect of short birth intervals per se, but it is possible that short birth intervals put the youngest child in a dangerous position. Consequently, short intervals may indirectly heighten the risk of morbidity and mortality through crowding and may increase the probability of child-to-child transmission of disease.

## Searching for evidence with DHS data

Retrospective birth-history information does not present the ideal data base for studying possible pathways through which short preceding birth intervals influence child survival. Yet, it is worthwhile to use data from DHS surveys to obtain some insight into the mechanisms that link birth intervals and child survival. The analysis of a large number of surveys that use comparable methodology can be a powerful tool in discerning common patterns, as was shown with World Fertility Survey (WFS) data. In addition, DHS surveys include data on child anthropometry, child morbidity, and health-service utilization, which have rarely been used in birth-interval analysis.[4]

Various methodological approaches are used to investigate the relative importance of the postulated mechanisms linking birth intervals and child survival. These approaches include analysis of age-specific mortality patterns, assessment of the effects of controlling for the survival status of the preceding birth and for breastfeeding duration, and, perhaps most interestingly, a multivariate analysis of the effects of birth intervals on child-health indicators, health-service utilization, and breastfeeding practices.

## Age-specific mortality patterns

Analysis of mortality risks for short birth intervals by the age of the child can provide information on the relative importance of the factors that mediate the birth interval-child survival relationship. If prenatal influences are the predominant mechanisms, then the effect of a short preceding birth interval should be greatest early in life, primarily due to low birth weight. If maternal depletion has a major effect on impaired lactational performance, the effect on mortality should become weaker as the child ages (Palloni, 1989). The consequences of sibling competition and infectious-disease transmission are expected to be observed primarily in the postneonatal and toddler-age periods.

For 39 countries included in the WFS, the median relative risk of dying was higher, at all periods, among children with preceding birth intervals of fewer than two years than among children born after longer intervals: it was 58 percent higher in the neonatal period, 96 percent greater in the postneonatal period, 45 percent greater during the second year of life, and 30 percent greater during the 2–5 year-old age period (Pebley and Millman, 1986). In a longitudinal study in Bangladesh, the effects of short preceding birth intervals were limited to the neonatal period (Koenig et al., 1990), although it cannot be excluded that postneonatal mortality differentials by birth intervals may have been erased by a concurrent famine. On the other hand, Winikoff (1983) reviewed a number of cross-sectional and longitudinal surveys and concluded that the effects of short preceding birth intervals were most striking in the postneonatal period. Differential under-reporting of neonatal deaths, however, may have led to this pattern. Palloni and Millman (1986) analyzed the effects of short preceding birth intervals (< 18 months) on age-specific mortality rates during infancy (1–2, 3–5 and 6–11 months) in nine Latin American countries; they found no consistent differences between the effects in the three age segments.

## Control for survival status of previous child

The effect of short birth intervals on mortality may be spurious, if intrafamilial mortality risks are correlated, as was shown in Nepal (Gubhaju, 1985) and Bangladesh (Majumder, 1990). In this case, the short birth interval is associated with the death of the previous child and the increased mortality risk of the index child is due to factors other than short birth intervals. Hobcraft et al. (1985) showed that controlling for the survival status of the previous child in a family results in a small reduction of the deleterious effects of short birth intervals in WFS surveys. Longitudinal studies in Bangladesh (Koenig et al., 1990) and India (De Sweemer, 1984) reported a weaker relationship between interval length and neonatal mortality when the previous child survived, but a significant birth interval effect remains.

Interpreting the results of controlling for previous child death can be difficult, because two counteractive mechanisms can be operating: (1) If mortality risks between successive children are correlated because of common familial characteristics, the effect of birth intervals on child mortality would be reduced by controlling for previous child death;[5] and (2) If sibling competition is important, then the death of the previous child removes the potential effects of sibling competition and disease transmission; therefore, controlling for the survival status of the previous child would be expected to increase the effect of birth intervals on child survival. If the net effect of controlling for the survival status of the previous child is a reduction of the birth-interval effect on child mortality (as found by Hobcraft et al., 1985, for example), the implication is that (1) is apparently stronger than (2), but it does not suggest that sibling competition is not operating.

## Control for breastfeeding

Breastfeeding could potentially be a confounding factor, since it affects both child survival and the length of the birth interval. For example, in Malaysia, it was observed that children with short preceding birth intervals were less likely than others to have ever been breastfed, even after controlling for neonatal health status (Millman and Cooksey, 1987). Studies in Latin America (Palloni and Millman, 1986), Nepal (Retherford et al., 1989), and Malaysia (Millman and Cooksey, 1987), however, report only minor changes in the effects of preceding birth intervals on postneonatal mortality, and no changes after the first birthday, when breastfeeding is controlled.

## Child health and health-service utilization

Children born after a short birth interval may have poorer growth than children born after a longer birth interval, due to postnatal influences such as inadequate breastmilk, inadequate care, and increased disease transmission. The risk of being undernourished – with a low score on anthropometric indicators – is also higher among children of low birth weight, since they usually do not catch up in growth with normal birth-weight children during the first two years of life (Jansen et al., 1984). Only a few studies have looked at the relationship between growth retardation and birth intervals. In Senegal, the risk of stunting – height-for-age below –2 standard deviations from the NCHS/WHO reference population – was more than two times greater among children whose preceding birth interval was shorter than two years, compared with other children (Goldberg and M'Bodji, 1985). Studies in Kenya (Boerma and Van Vianen, 1984) and Nigeria (Doyle et al., 1978) did not find a significant relationship between preceding birth interval and growth of the child.

Very little research exists on the effects of short birth intervals on the use of health services. It has only been suggested that longer intervals are associated with higher levels of health-service utilization, which leads to higher use of contraceptives, longer birth intervals, and lower child mortality (Potter, 1988).

## Data and methods

This analysis uses data from 17 DHS surveys, which were carried out during the period 1986–89. The 17 countries were selected because they included anthropometric data on children.[6] Although DHS surveys include a full birth history, our analysis will be limited to births that occurred in the five years preceding the survey. The decision to limit analysis to this subset of births was largely based on the consideration that births that occurred more than five years before the survey cannot be linked with important information on breastfeeding patterns, health-service utilization, anthropometry, and morbidity, which was collected only for children born in the last five years. Moreover, the short recall period may have the advantage of providing better data quality. Last, using the last five years also reduces the magnitude of the bias created by including multiple observations in the same family, compared with a 15-year recall period, for example.

For the purposes of analysis, the length of the preceding birth interval is classified as (1) fewer than 24 months, (2) 24–35 months (used as the reference category), or (3) 36 months and over.[7] First births were excluded from the analysis. The following dependent variables are used in the analysis:

1 Mortality: neonatal (0 months), 1–6 months, and 7–23 months. The more conventional cut-off point of 12 months of age was not chosen, because there is considerable heaping of deaths at this month (Sullivan et al., 1990). In addition, the number of deaths at ages 12–23 months was prohibitively small in many surveys. Children born in the month of interview were excluded from the analysis.
2 Anthropometry: stunting was coded as a dichotomous variable, and 1 indicates a height-for-age z-score below –2 standard deviations from the median of the NCHS reference population, and zero otherwise. Underweight was coded the same way using weight-for-age data. Anthropometric data in most surveys were collected for children aged 3–36 months, but for this analysis only children under 24 months of age were included.
3 Morbidity: diarrhoea prevalence in the two weeks preceding the interview was the only morbidity variable available for all surveys.
4 Prenatal and delivery care: coded 1 if the woman did not make a visit to a prenatal clinic during pregnancy, and zero if otherwise; and for delivery care, coded 1 if the delivery was not attended by a modern health worker.
5 Breastfeeding: coded 1 if the child had never been breastfed, and 0 if otherwise.
6 Immunization: coded 1 if the child was never immunized, and 0 if it was immunized. Most surveys only collected information on specific vaccinations if the mother could present a health card; therefore, information on specific vaccinations could not be used.
7 Medical treatment: coded 1 if the child with diarrhoea in the two weeks before the survey was not taken to a medical person for assistance, and zero if otherwise.

The following independent control variables are used in the analysis:

1 Socioeconomic status: mother's level of education (none, some primary, at least some secondary); mother's current residence (urban or rural); and economic status of the

household based on household assets and floor material of the house (see Bicego and Boerma, 1991).

2 Biodemographic variables: sex of the child; multiple-birth status; maternal age (under age 20, 20–34, and 35 years and over); birth order (second through fifth, and sixth and over); and breastfeeding duration (whether the child was breastfed or not at the beginning of each month).

3 Survival status of the preceding birth at the time of the index birth. For neonatal mortality, the survival status at the time of conception of the index child is used (thereby excluding prenatal competition associated with an overlap of gestation and lactation in case the previous child died before conception). Gestation is assumed to be uniformly nine months long.

4 Use of maternity services: no use; either prenatal care or delivery care; and both prenatal and delivery care (the reference category). This variable will be used in mortality-risk analysis.

With the exception of postneonatal mortality, all dependent variables were analyzed as dichotomous outcomes, using a logistic regression model.[8] In the case of postneonatal mortality, a Cox hazards regression model[9] is used, obviating the exclusion of a large number of children born within two years of survey.[10] Independent measures are reference parameterized, with the theoretically low-risk category serving as reference.[11]

Breastfeeding was included as a time-varying covariate in the postneonatal mortality models.[12] From the information on breastfeeding duration (collected for each child born in the five years before the survey), a dichotomous variable was constructed to indicate whether the child is still breastfeeding at the beginning of the age segment (month) of risk.[13]

There are three data quality problems that necessitate caution when interpreting the impact of breastfeeding controls on the birth interval-child survival relationship (see Appendix Table A1). First, there are many missing values for breastfeeding duration, especially for deceased children. In many countries, more than 10 percent of the post-neonatal deaths have no data on breastfeeding duration. Second, a large proportion of deceased children were reportedly breastfed until they died. In some countries, virtually all deceased children are breastfed until death, and an estimate of the effect of breast-feeding is neither possible nor relevant. In other cases, reverse causality is possible: a sick child is taken off the breast or is unable to suckle well, and dies within a few weeks or months due to the primary disease. Third, the recalled durations of breastfeeding are rather imprecise, as evidenced by the massive heaping on multiples of six and by the unlikely high level of overlap between gestation and breastfeeding.[14]

In the analyses of anthropometric status, morbidity, and use of health services (as outcome measures), the relative odds are converted to relative risks.[15] The relative odds will overstate the relative risk to different degrees when the outcome is common (occurring in more than 10 percent of cases) (Gray, 1990), as in these analyses; this will be a misleading base for comparison of different outcomes, such as mortality and stunting, within a country, and for comparisons among countries.

**Table 1** Number of births in the past five years, number of deaths by age group (in months), percentage of births in each birth-interval category, and level of mortality for the five years before the survey, DHS

| Country | No. of births | Number of deaths by age group (months) | | | Preceding birth interval (%) (months) | | | Mortality levels (per 1,000 live births) | | + |
|---|---|---|---|---|---|---|---|---|---|---|
| | | 0 | 1–6 | 7–23 | <18 | <24 | >35 | Neo-natal | Infant | <5 years |
| **Sub-Saharan Africa** | | | | | | | | | | |
| Burundi | 3,114 | 91 | 67 | 81 | 8.8 | 22.9 | 33.8 | 34.9 | 74.5 | 151.8 |
| Ghana | 3,255 | 137 | 63 | 99 | 7.2 | 18.1 | 42.5 | 43.8 | 77.2 | 154.7 |
| Mali | 2,740 | 107 | 72 | 101 | 9.6 | 25.3 | 37.5 | 53.6 | 108.4 | 249.6 |
| Senegal | 3,465 | 140 | 86 | 137 | 6.1 | 20.0 | 33.0 | 44.2 | 85.8 | 191.2 |
| Togo | 2,507 | 90 | 57 | 72 | 5.2 | 16.4 | 44.1 | 43.3 | 80.5 | 158.2 |
| Uganda | 3,951 | 154 | 108 | 154 | 11.7 | 30.1 | 28.7 | 45.5 | 100.7 | 178.7 |
| Zimbabwe | 2,647 | 73 | 38 | 37 | 6.2 | 18.5 | 39.1 | 27.4 | 52.7 | 75.0 |
| **North Africa** | | | | | | | | | | |
| Egypt | 6,743 | 246 | 142 | 137 | 17.8 | 34.3 | 34.3 | 30.0 | 70.2 | 102.0 |
| Morocco | 4,973 | 190 | 111 | 79 | 12.2 | 29.3 | 33.1 | 16.3 | 25.3 | 102.2 |
| Tunisia | 3,511 | 89 | 48 | 27 | 19.0 | 36.7 | 29.7 | 20.1 | 35.6 | 65.2 |
| **Asia** | | | | | | | | | | |
| Sri Lanka | 2,775 | 42 | 13 | 13 | 11.9 | 28.8 | 40.3 | 16.3 | 25.3 | 34.6 |
| Thailand | 2,257 | 52 | 22 | 11 | 11.5 | 24.4 | 52.3 | 20.1 | 35.6 | 45.1 |
| **Latin America and Caribbean** | | | | | | | | | | |
| Bolivia | 4,615 | 154 | 143 | 143 | 12.7 | 29.3 | 36.0 | 34.6 | 85.7 | 132.0 |
| Brazil | 2,559 | 82 | 85 | 39 | 23.8 | 41.4 | 34.2 | 33.0 | 74.7 | 84.9 |
| Colombia | 1,896 | 39 | 19 | 13 | 18.0 | 35.6 | 38.7 | 19.4 | 33.4 | 42.6 |
| Domin. Rep. | 3,426 | 107 | 70 | 64 | 22.4 | 41.0 | 30.6 | 38.7 | 67.4 | 88.4 |
| Guatemala | 3,728 | 116 | 87 | 97 | 12.6 | 30.4 | 31.3 | 32.9 | 73.3 | 110.1 |

The statistical significance of the estimated birth-interval effects was assessed using the Wald statistic (the square of the ratio of the estimated coefficient to its standard error), compared with a Chi-square distribution with one degree of freedom.[16]

## Results

### Pace of childbearing

Table 1 presents the sample sizes, number of deaths by age group, age-specific mortality levels, and proportion of births with short and long preceding birth intervals for 17 DHS surveys (all data are unweighted, except mortality rates). Very short birth intervals (< 18 months) are much less common in the Sub-Saharan African and Asian countries than in the North African and Latin American ones. The same applies to the frequency of birth intervals lasting fewer than 24 months, although the differences are less pronounced. Birth intervals shorter than 24 months are common, accounting for more than 20 percent of all births in 14 countries, and more than 30 percent in seven countries. About one-third of the birth intervals are three years or longer in most countries, but in Thailand, more than half of the birth intervals are long.

## Overlap of gestation and lactation

A high prevalence of overlap of gestation and lactation indicates that many women are exposed to the risks of becoming malnourished (maternal depletion), which may affect the birth weight and breastfeeding of the newborn. The proportion of women who are still breastfeeding during the three trimesters of pregnancy is shown in Table 2, based on current status data. The figures include women who had at least one living child and who were pregnant at the time of the survey. During the first trimester, more than 10 percent of the pregnant women in 11 countries are still breastfeeding: The trimean[17] for 17 countries is 16 percent. Most women have ceased breastfeeding by the second and third trimesters: The trimean for all countries drops to 4 percent in the second trimester and 2 percent in the third trimester. Continuation of breastfeeding into the second trimester is relatively common in Egypt (13 percent) and Guatemala (25 percent), but even in these countries fewer than 5 percent continue into the third trimester.

Table 2 also shows the extent of overlap between gestation and lactation by birth interval, from current status data. If early termination of breastfeeding were the sole cause of short birth intervals, then the proportions of women still lactating during the current pregnancy would be relatively low for short intervals. In most countries, however, overlap is more common for short intervals than for intervals of 24–35 months, and it is rare for long birth intervals. The proportion of pregnant women still breastfeeding with short intervals is particularly high in Egypt, Thailand, and Guatemala. The large variation between populations suggests that maternal depletion due to overlap of lactation and gestation (or short recuperative intervals) is of varying importance in different populations.

## Mortality

### Age-specific patterns

Table 3 presents the relative risks of mortality for short and long birth intervals, compared with the reference category of birth intervals lasting 24–35 months, during three age segments. The relative risks are estimated net of twin status, sex, mother's age, birth order, mother's education, economic status of the household, and residence. The effect of controlling for the survival status of the previous birth is shown separately. For three countries (Colombia, Sri Lanka, and Thailand) with small numbers of deaths (see Table 1), the age periods 1–6 months and 7–23 months were combined.

The adverse effects of short birth intervals are greatest in the neonatal and 1–6 months periods, and are relatively small in the age group 7–23 months. During the neonatal period, the relative risks of dying associated with short preceding intervals are substantially higher in the African and Asian countries surveyed and in the two high mortality countries in Latin America (Bolivia and Guatemala). In Senegal, there is no

**Table 2** Percentage of pregnant women reported to be still breastfeeding, by trimester of pregnancy and by length of preceding birth interval, taken from current status data, DHS

| Survey | N | Pregnancy trimester | | | Birth interval (months) | | | |
|---|---|---|---|---|---|---|---|---|
| | | First | Second | Third | < 24 | 24–35 | > 35 | All |
| **Sub-Saharan Africa** | | | | | | | | |
| Burundi | 313 | 18.8 | 3.5 | 0.0 | (0.7) | 8.0 | 1.9 | 4.9 |
| Ghana | 295 | 8.6 | 2.9 | 3.3 | (10.7) | 5.6 | 2.1 | 4.4 |
| Mali | 301 | 16.3 | 2.3 | 1.5 | 7.2 | 5.5 | 3.4 | 5.2 |
| Senegal | 393 | 5.4 | 1.7 | 1.6 | 9.7 | 2.0 | 0.0 | 2.5 |
| Togo | 251 | 14.1 | 7.8 | 2.4 | (15.4) | 11.5 | 1.9 | 8.0 |
| Uganda | 443 | 20.3 | 4.4 | 0.8 | 17.1 | 6.3 | 2.8 | 8.0 |
| Zimbabwe | 255 | 0.0 | 0.0 | 1.1 | (0.0) | 0.8 | 0.0 | 0.4 |
| **North Africa** | | | | | | | | |
| Egypt | 680 | 30.9 | 13.2 | 4.0 | 25.7 | 8.7 | 2.7 | 12.7 |
| Morocco | 472 | 9.9 | 2.4 | 2.3 | 12.6 | 1.6 | 0.7 | 4.4 |
| Tunisia | 300 | 17.3 | 7.2 | 3.0 | 17.4 | 5.6 | 0.0 | 8.3 |
| **Asia** | | | | | | | | |
| Sri Lanka | 210 | (33.3) | 1.5 | 3.9 | (6.0) | 19.1 | 4.7 | 9.9 |
| Thailand | 154 | (26.7) | 8.5 | (8.0) | 29.9 | (10.6) | 0.0 | 12.9 |
| **Latin America and Caribbean** | | | | | | | | |
| Bolivia | 432 | 17.5 | 1.5 | 0.3 | 7.6 | 4.6 | 0.0 | 4.2 |
| Brazil | 228 | 11.5 | 3.0 | 2.1 | 8.5 | 4.4 | 1.2 | 5.0 |
| Colombia | 181 | (8.5) | 5.1 | 1.5 | 8.5 | 4.0 | 0.0 | 4.7 |
| Dominican Rep. | 315 | 2.8 | 1.1 | 1.8 | 1.2 | 2.2 | 2.3 | 1.8 |
| Guatemala | 386 | 31.0 | 25.3 | 4.5 | 29.0 | 15.3 | 10.8 | 17.9 |
| Trimean | – | 16.2 | 3.8 | 2.3 | 10.8 | 6.0 | 1.6 | 5.9 |

Note: Includes only women pregnant at the time of the survey and with at least one living child born in the five years before the survey. Parentheses ( ) indicate 25 < N < 50.

effect of intervals lasting fewer than 24 months, but if intervals of under 18 months are considered, the relative risk is 2.41. During the postneonatal period, from 1–6 months of age, the relative risks of mortality in the Sub-Saharan African countries are considerably lower than in the neonatal period, while three of the five Latin American countries show more than a doubling of the relative mortality risks for short intervals. The North African countries continue to have high relative risks, while the relative risks in the two Asian countries decline after the neonatal period. During the late postneonatal and toddler periods (age 7–23 months), the adverse effects of short birth intervals are smaller. In seven countries, however, there is still a significant increase of the relative risks of mortality for short birth intervals. There is no consistent relationship between the country levels of mortality and the magnitude of the effect of short intervals on mortality.

Children born after long birth intervals (lasting three years or more) appear to have better survival chances in all three age periods than do children with shorter preceding birth intervals, even though the relative risks are not significantly lower in most coun-

**Table 3** Relative risks of neonatal mortality at 1–6 months and at 7–23 months associated with short and long birth intervals, compared with birth intervals of 24–35 months

| Country | Neonatal mortality | | | | Mortality at 1–6 months | | | | Mortality at 7–23 months | | | |
|---|---|---|---|---|---|---|---|---|---|---|---|---|
| | <18 months[b] | <24 months | | >35 months | <18 months[b] | <24 months | | >35 months | <18 months[b] | <24 months | | >35 months |
| | | No PREMO[c] | With PREMO[c] | | | No PREMO[c] | With PREMO[c] | | | No PREMO[c] | With PREMO[c] | |
| **Sub-Saharan Africa** | | | | | | | | | | | | |
| Burundi | 2.27** | 1.93** | 1.76* | 0.69 | 1.95* | 1.90* | 1.79* | 0.61 | 0.87 | 1.15 | 1.14 | 1.17 |
| Ghana | 2.31** | 2.34*** | 2.17** | 1.35 | 2.26* | 2.68** | 2.38** | 0.96 | 0.85 | 1.45 | 1.40 | 1.30 |
| Mali | 4.85** | 3.71*** | 3.54*** | 0.84 | 1.59 | 1.35 | 1.36 | 0.52* | 1.30 | 1.58* | 1.60* | 0.42** |
| Senegal | 2.41** | 1.32 | 1.21 | 0.63 | 0.75 | 0.81 | 0.84 | 0.66 | 0.97 | 1.11 | 1.03 | 0.84 |
| Togo | 2.37† | 2.78** | 2.52** | 2.21** | 1.86 | 1.56 | 1.65 | 0.61 | 0.87 | 1.18 | 1.21 | 0.94 |
| Uganda | 2.41*** | 1.66† | 1.52* | 0.98 | 1.68† | 1.53† | 1.45† | 0.97 | 2.41** | 1.91** | 1.89** | 1.04 |
| Zimbabwe | 1.11 | 1.74† | 1.57 | 1.00 | 2.41† | 2.07 | 1.95 | 0.78 | 0.91 | 1.54 | 1.36 | 0.96 |
| **North Africa** | | | | | | | | | | | | |
| Egypt | 2.65*** | 2.37*** | 2.34*** | 0.79 | 2.59*** | 2.41*** | 2.42*** | 0.76 | 2.21*** | 2.03** | 2.04* | 0.76 |
| Morocco | 2.32*** | 2.12*** | 2.01*** | 0.70 | 2.83*** | 2.62*** | 2.57*** | 0.89 | 0.96 | 0.86 | 0.81* | 0.62 |
| Tunisia | 2.53*** | 2.00** | 1.91* | 0.85 | 2.64*** | 2.16* | 2.16* | 0.45 | 1.51 | 4.86** | 4.70** | 1.18 |
| **Asia** | | | | | | | | | | | | |
| Sri Lanka | 2.63* | 2.35† | 1.94 | 0.53 | 1.95 | 1.25 | 1.25 | 1.02 | na | na | na | na |
| Thailand | 1.41 | 2.70* | 2.50* | 1.04 | 1.87 | 1.82 | 1.75 | 1.41 | na | na | na | na |
| **Latin America and Caribbean** | | | | | | | | | | | | |
| Bolivia | 2.13*** | 1.88** | 1.85** | 0.72 | 3.15*** | 2.70*** | 2.43*** | 0.61† | 0.88 | 1.60* | 1.59* | 0.64* |
| Brazil | 1.48 | 1.18 | 1.21 | 0.73 | 2.48*** | 2.79*** | 2.79** | 0.92 | 1.87† | 1.60 | 1.60 | 0.60 |
| Colombia | 1.40 | 1.04 | 1.04 | 0.89 | 1.79 | 1.12 | 1.09 | 0.70 | | | | |
| Dominican Republic | 2.10** | 1.40 | 1.44 | 0.81 | 2.25** | 2.65*** | 2.66** | 2.93*** | 1.66† | 1.96* | 1.97* | 0.92 |
| Guatemala | 2.35*** | 1.95** | 1.92** | 0.74 | 2.21** | 2.14** | 2.03** | 0.76 | 1.60† | 1.86** | 1.79* | 0.91 |
| Trimean | 2.29 | 1.98 | 1.88 | 0.83 | 2.24 | 2.13 | 2.06 | 0.76 | 1.20 | 1.57 | 1.57 | 0.88 |

† significant at p<.10; * significant at p<.05; ** significant at p<.01; *** significant at p<.001.

a Controlled for twin, sex of child, mother's age, birth order, mother's education, economic status of the household, and residence.     b RR compared with an interval of 18–35 months.     c PREMO is the survival status of preceding birth at time of conception of the index birth for neonatal mortality, and at the time of the index child's birth for postneonatal mortality.     na = not applicable.

**Note:** RRs of mortality at 1–6 and 7–23 months are combined into 1–23 months.

tries. The long interval effect is not age specific: The trimean relative risks of the 14 countries with estimates for the three age periods are 0.83 for the neonatal period, 0.76 for 1–6 months of age, and 0.88 for 7–23 months of age. In two cases, Togo in the neonatal period and the Dominican Republic in the postneonatal period, long intervals are associated with significantly increased mortality risks.

In sum, these age-specific mortality patterns indicate that the adverse effects of short intervals are strongest in the neonatal and early postneonatal periods, but appear to weaken thereafter. This pattern is very similar to the one observed in the WFS. The pattern suggests that prenatal mechanisms are more important, but not exclusively so, since the effect at ages 1–6 months is not smaller than the effect for neonatal mortality. For children born after a long birth interval, no age-specific effects can be observed, suggesting that other mechanisms are responsible for the advantageous position of such children.

### Control for previous child survivorship

In the analysis of neonatal mortality, controlling for the survival status of the preceding child at the time of the conception of the index child reduces the relative risk associated with short intervals in all countries with significant effects, but the reductions are generally modest. In seven countries (five in Sub-Saharan Africa and the two in Asia), the reduction in the relative risks is greater than 10 percent. In Sri Lanka, Zimbabwe, and Uganda, the reduction is greater than 20 percent.

The effects of controlling for the survival status of the previous child at the time of the index child's birth in the analysis of mortality after the neonatal period are smaller. At ages 1–6 months, a relative reduction in the relative risk of about 10 percent or more occurs in six of the 11 countries with significantly increased relative risks of mortality. At ages 7–23 months, the only reduction of relative risk greater than 5 percent is observed in Guatemala.

In sum, the control for the survival status of the previous child suggests that part of the association between short birth intervals and neonatal mortality is due to increased intrafamilial mortality risks. It cannot, however, be excluded that both deaths of an interval pair are a consequence of a rapid succession of pregnancies (that is, that the increased intrafamilial mortality risks are due to short birth intervals).[18]

### Control for breastfeeding duration

Birth interval effects on mortality with and without breastfeeding controls are shown in Table 4.[19] There is a small attenuation (less than a 5 percent reduction of the excess risk) of the effect of short birth intervals on mortality in Burundi, Ghana, Tunisia, and Brazil. Bolivia, Morocco, and the Dominican Republic have reductions of 7–9 percent, whereas in Guatemala, a reduction of 22 percent is observed when the breastfeeding control is introduced. At 7–23 months of age, the effects of controlling for breastfeeding duration are negligible, except in Egypt and Guatemala, where a small reduction in the birth interval effect was observed. Generally, it can be concluded that breastfeeding duration does not appear to be a major confounding variable in the birth spacing-child survival relationship.

**Table 4** Relative risks of mortality at 1–6 months and at 7–23 months associated with short preceding birth intervals, without and with controls for breastfeeding, DHS

| Country | 1–6 months | | | 7–23 months | | |
|---|---|---|---|---|---|---|
| | No breast-feeding | With breast-feeding | Breast-feeding effect significant [1] | No breast-feeding | With breast-feeding | Breast-feeding effect significant [1] |
| **Sub-Saharan Africa** | | | | | | |
| Burundi | 1.61 | 1.58 | Yes | 0.79 | 0.81 | No |
| Ghana | 2.81 [4] | 2.77 [4] | Yes | 1.52 | 1.52 | No |
| Mali | 1.60 | 1.59 | No | 1.60 | 1.63 | No |
| Senegal | 0.82 | 0.82 | No | 1.06 | 1.07 | No |
| Togo | 1.63 | 1.63 | No | 1.43 | 1.40 | No |
| Uganda | 1.54 [2] | 1.54 [2] | No | 1.71 [4] | 1.75 [4] | No |
| Zimbabwe | 2.07 [2] | 2.09 [2] | No | 1.15 | 1.15 | No |
| **North Africa** | | | | | | |
| Egypt | 2.37 [5] | 2.18 [5] | Yes | 1.91 [4] | 1.86 [4] | Yes |
| Morocco | 3.47 [5] | 3.26 [5] | Yes | 0.89 | 0.69 | No |
| Tunisia | 2.19 [3] | 2.13 [3] | No | 4.83 [4] | 4.81 [4] | No |
| **Latin America and Caribbean** | | | | | | |
| Bolivia | 2.61 [5] | 2.49 [5] | Yes | 1.58 [4] | 1.58 [4] | No |
| Brazil | 3.31 [5] | 3.24 [5] | Yes | 1.34 | 1.26 | Yes |
| Dominican Rep. | 2.53 [4] | 2.39 [4] | Yes | 2.28 [4] | 2.29 [4] | No |
| Guatemala | 2.09 [4] | 1.85 [3] | Yes | 1.76 [4] | 1.72 [3] | No |
| Trimean | 2.10 | 2.08 | | 1.50 | 1.49 | |

1. Breastfeeding effect is significant at $p < .05$. 2. Significant at $p < .10$;  3. Significant at $p < .05$;
4. Significant at $p < .01$;  5. Significant at $p < .001$.
Note: All effects are controlled for twin, sex, maternal age, birth order, mother's education, residence, and economic status.

*Control for use of health services*
The effects of controlling for health-service utilization (prenatal and delivery care) on the relative mortality risks for short birth intervals are negligible (not shown). Furthermore, the relative advantage in survival enjoyed by children born after a long interval is not related to greater use of maternity services, since introducing this variable did not substantially alter the long interval effect in any of the 13 countries for which the control could be done.

## Child health status

*Anthropometry*
Table 5 presents the relative risks of poor growth associated with short and long intervals. Poor nutritional status is slightly more common among children with short preceding birth intervals than among those with longer ones. In most countries, however, the

**Table 5** Relative risks of stunting and underweight among children under 24 months of age associated with short and long birth intervals, compared with 24–35-month birth intervals[1]

| Country | N | Stunting | | | Underweight | | |
|---|---|---|---|---|---|---|---|
| | | P(ref) | Short | Long | P(ref) | Short | Long |
| **Sub-Saharan Africa** | | | | | | | |
| Burundi | 991 | 0.388 | 1.02 | 0.93 | 0.321 | 1.12 | 0.94 |
| Ghana | 949 | 0.226 | 1.31 | 0.86 | 0.245 | 1.54[4] | 1.11 |
| Mali | 593 | 0.215 | 1.24 | 0.67[2] | 0.311 | 0.97 | 0.85 |
| Senegal | 348 | 0.196 | 0.86 | 1.20 | 0.182 | 0.96 | 1.00 |
| Togo | 740 | 0.282 | 0.76 | 0.88 | 0.247 | 1.06 | 0.87 |
| Uganda | 1,451 | 0.373 | 1.13 | 0.82 | 0.213 | 1.21 | 0.88 |
| Zimbabwe | 724 | 0.278 | 1.47[3] | 1.00 | 0.116 | 1.58 | 0.90 |
| **North Africa** | | | | | | | |
| Egypt | 959 | 0.315 | 1.03 | 0.99 | 0.148 | 1.27 | 1.16 |
| Morocco | 1,748 | 0.238 | 1.02 | 0.70[4] | 0.164 | 1.17 | 0.79 |
| Tunisia | 1,040 | 0.183 | 1.25 | 0.56[5] | 0.109 | 1.40 | 0.70 |
| **Asia** | | | | | | | |
| Sri Lanka | 891 | 0.306 | 1.03 | 0.68[3] | 0.349 | 1.09 | 0.90 |
| Thailand | 693 | 0.178 | 1.32 | 0.98 | 0.189 | 1.60[3] | 1.02 |
| **Latin America and Caribbean** | | | | | | | |
| Bolivia | 1,362 | 0.329 | 1.16 | 0.82[2] | 0.142 | 1.10 | 0.77 |
| Brazil | 347 | 0.301 | 1.21 | 0.64 | 0.161 | 1.21 | 0.49 |
| Colombia | 588 | 0.295 | 1.02 | 0.50[4] | 0.122 | 1.40 | 0.85 |
| Dominican Rep. | 841 | 0.320 | 0.72[3] | 0.46[5] | 0.193 | 0.91 | 0.38[5] |
| Guatemala | 1,173 | 0.539 | 1.04 | 1.03 | 0.293 | 1.21 | 1.11 |
| Trimean | | | 1.09 | 0.82 | | 1.22 | 0.89 |

1. Controlled for age, twin, sex, maternal age, birth order, mother's education, residence, and economic status. Significance levels refer to relative odds: 2. $p < .10$; 3. $p < .05$; 4. $p < .01$; 5. $p < .001$.
Note: P(ref) is the prevalence of the outcome in the reference group.

increased risks are small. The trimean relative risk for short intervals is 1.09. The relative risk of stunting associated with short intervals is increased by more than 20 percent in six of the 17 countries surveyed, and by more than 40 percent in Zimbabwe. The effects of short birth intervals on low weight-for-age are slightly larger than for stunting – five countries have an increase in relative risk of 40 percent or more (trimean 1.22). Controlling for the survival status of the previous birth has only minor effects or no effects on the relative risk estimates.

More remarkable is the better growth of children born after long birth intervals. The relative risks of stunting are more than 25 percent lower in seven countries, and the trimean of the 17 countries is 0.82. Data on the relative risks of being underweight show the same pattern, but the differences are less pronounced compared with the reference group.

**Table 6**  Trimean relative risks for different outcomes associated with short and long birth intervals, compared with an interval of 24–35 months, 17 DHS countries

| Outcome | P(ref) | Short | Long |
|---|---|---|---|
| Diarrhoea in the last two weeks among children < 24 months at survey | 0.34 | 1.05 | 1.01 |
| Child NOT taken for medical assistance during diarrhoea in the last two weeks | 0.69 | 1.03 | 0.96 |
| Mother NOT attending prenatal care for births during five years prior to survey | 0.34 | 1.15 | 0.95 |
| Mother NOT delivering with medical assistance for births during five years prior to survey | 0.57 | 1.00 | 0.92 |
| Child < 24 months NOT receiving any vaccination | 0.24 | 0.98 | 0.96 |

Note: P(ref) = prevalence or frequency in the reference group.

*Diarrhoea*

The estimated relative risks of having diarrhoea in the two weeks before the survey among children under 24 months of age are summarized in Table 6. There is generally little or no effect of either short or long birth intervals on diarrhoea prevalence. Regarding short intervals, in three countries (Burundi, Ghana, and Colombia), the relative risks are increased by more than 20 percent, while in two countries (Togo and Sri Lanka), the risks are decreased by more than 20 percent (not shown). For long intervals, significantly lower risks can be observed for Togo and the Dominican Republic, but no other countries exhibit substantial differences from the reference category. The control for survival status of the preceding birth at the time of the survey does not result in substantial changes.

## Health-service utilization

Table 6 also shows that there are only minor differences associated with the length of birth intervals in the relative risk of not being taken for medical assistance during diarrhoea in the past two weeks. It must be taken into consideration that the numbers of children sampled are small. Only in Thailand was nonuse of medical assistance during diarrhoea significantly lower for short intervals (not shown). For long intervals, there does not appear to be either a higher or lower use of curative services than existed in the reference interval group.

The relative risks of not attending prenatal care and not delivering with medical assistance are also summarized in the table. The risk of not attending prenatal care is higher among women with short preceding birth intervals and somewhat lower among women with long intervals. The effect of short intervals is significant (at p<.05) in Burundi, Ghana, Togo, Uganda, Zimbabwe, Tunisia, and the Dominican Republic (not shown). Effects of short birth intervals are minor for delivery care (except in Togo and Mali), and only children born after a long preceding birth interval are somewhat less likely to be delivered without the assistance of a modern health worker. The latter effect was significant (at p<.05) in Zimbabwe, Egypt, Morocco, Sri Lanka, Thailand, Bo-

**Table 7** Relative risks among children born in the five years preceding the survey of never being breastfed associated with short and long birth intervals, compared with an interval of 24–35 months, [1] DHS

| Country | N | P(ref) | No neonatal mortality | | Control for neonatal mortality | |
|---|---|---|---|---|---|---|
| | | | Short | Long | Short | Long |
| **Sub-Saharan Africa** | | | | | | |
| Burundi | 3,114 | 0.014 | 1.58 | 0.88 | 1.14 | 0.97 |
| Ghana | 3,255 | 0.017 | 2.66 [4] | 2.08 [4] | 2.09 [2] | 2.19 [3] |
| Mali | 2,740 | 0.009 | 2.66 [3] | 1.32 | 1.06 | 1.81 |
| Senegal | 3,465 | 0.017 | 1.62 | 1.50 | 1.41 | 1.84 [3] |
| Togo | 2,507 | 0.020 | 1.77 | 1.42 | 1.26 | 0.92 |
| Uganda | 3,951 | 0.018 | 1.29 | 0.95 | 0.92 | 0.94 |
| Zimbabwe | 2,647 | 0.007 | 3.22 [3] | 2.03 | 5.76 [4] | 4.26 [3] |
| **North Africa** | | | | | | |
| Egypt | 6,743 | 0.049 | 1.96 [5] | 1.48 [4] | 1.69 [5] | 1.54 [4] |
| Morocco | 4,973 | 0.028 | 2.04 [5] | 1.50 [3] | 1.82 [4] | 1.67 [4] |
| Tunisia | 3,511 | 0.036 | 1.44 [2] | 1.36 | 1.23 | 1.42 |
| **Asia** | | | | | | |
| Sri Lanka | 2,775 | 0.016 | 1.26 | 1.31 | 1.08 | 1.16 |
| Thailand | 2,257 | 0.040 | 1.81 [3] | 1.53 [2] | 1.67 [2] | 1.56 |
| **Latin America and Caribbean** | | | | | | |
| Bolivia | 4,615 | 0.025 | 1.98 [5] | 1.24 | 1.76 [3] | 1.33 |
| Brazil | 2,559 | 0.107 | 1.12 | 1.03 | 1.10 | 1.07 |
| Colombia | 1,896 | 0.049 | 1.30 | 1.56 [2] | 1.36 | 1.68 [2] |
| Dominican Rep. | 3,426 | 0.073 | 1.20 | 1.11 | 1.12 | 1.15 |
| Guatemala | 3,728 | 0.033 | 1.95 [5] | 1.22 | 1.72 [3] | 1.40 |
| Trimean | | | 1.71 | 1.35 | 1.39 | 1.42 |

1. Controlled for age, twin, sex, maternal age, birth order, mother's education, residence, economic status, and fate of previous child.
Significance levels refer to relative odds: 2. p < .10;  3. p < .05;  4. p < .01;  5. p < .001.
Note: P(ref) is the prevalence of the outcome in the reference group.

livia, the Dominican Republic, and Guatemala (not shown). The relationship between birth interval length and use of preventive child health services is weak: No consistent differences in the risk of not being vaccinated by length of birth interval were observed.

## Breastfeeding initiation
The chances of never being breastfed vary by the length of the birth interval (see Table 7). In most surveys, short birth-interval length is strongly associated with the child never being breastfed. Since this could be due to a higher proportion of very ill babies, neonatal survival was controlled in an attempt to ascertain and control for the effects of the poor child-health status at birth. However, although the control indeed reduces the relative risks, a higher risk of never having been breastfed remains for children in most countries who are born after short intervals. In several countries, long birth intervals are

also associated with an increased risk of the child never being breastfed, making the interpretation of these results difficult.

## Discussion

The findings presented here suggest that prenatal factors are more important than postnatal factors in the causal pathway between rapid childbearing and heightened risk of early childhood mortality. First, the evaluation of age patterns of mortality indicates that the effects of birth intervals, although not limited to the neonatal period, do become weaker later in infancy and thereafter. This pattern is very similar to the pattern found in the WFS.

Second, the analysis of health status and health-service utilization outcomes does not lend much support to the hypothesis of sibling competition and disease transmission. The effects of short birth intervals on nutritional status are rather moderate,[20] especially in comparison with the effect of maternal education on child anthropometric indicators in this set of countries, reported by Bicego and Boerma (1991): That study found more than a doubling of relative risks of stunting and being underweight among children of mothers with no education, compared with children of mothers with at least a secondary education. Thus, it seems very unlikely that measurement errors of the anthropometric indicators have caused these surprisingly weak effects. A plausible interpretation of the weak birth interval-nutritional status relationship is that the postnatal factors of nutritional intake and infectious-disease load – both primary determinants of nutritional status – do not figure prominently in explaining the birth interval-mortality relationship. This interpretation is further supported by the existence of very small or no effects of short birth intervals on diarrhoea prevalence, on child immunization coverage, and on medical service utilization problems during diarrhoea. However, it appears that none of these three dependent variables has been measured that well in DHS, and biases (toward no effect) may be the consequence. Yet, the uniform absence of strong effects in all countries does strongly suggest that sibling competition is, at best, of secondary importance in explaining the relationship between interval length and early childhood mortality.

Does the analysis of DHS data provide more direct evidence of the prenatal mechanisms? First, women with short birth intervals have shorter recuperative intervals between the end of lactation and the start of a new pregnancy than do women with longer intervals. The overlap of gestation and lactation is particularly stressful to the mother and the child. In the DHS surveys, the overlap of gestation and lactation was found in about 6 percent of pregnancies, but was almost two times more common if the birth interval was shorter than 24 months. Therefore, the joint effects of pregnancy and lactation on a mother's physiology and nutritional status may be a mechanism through which short preceding intervals affect child-health status. This may result in low birthweight children, prematurity, or impaired lactational abilities.

Second, short birth intervals are associated with a somewhat higher risk of not attending prenatal care at all, which is most pronounced in five of the seven DHS countries in Sub-Saharan Africa. This higher risk may be due to the lack of opportunities to attend prenatal clinics, since there is a young child to care for, although controlling for the survival status of the previous child did not have an effect. There may also be sociocultural or personal reasons for not attending prenatal care, since a rapid return to pregnancy is often considered undesirable and perhaps embarrassing. Another explanation is that a higher proportion of premature deliveries among women having short birth intervals contributes to the lower proportion attending prenatal care among short birth intervals, particularly if women tend to make the first visit to prenatal clinics late in pregnancy.

Women with long birth intervals (of three years or more) have moderately higher levels of attendance at prenatal care and are slightly more likely to deliver in institutions than women with shorter intervals. Both more opportunities and better motivation to have another child may contribute to these differences. On the other hand, in our analyses, controlling for use of maternity services, which has been suggested to be the cause of longer birth intervals and lower child mortality (Potter, 1988), did not have any effect on the birth spacing-child survival association.

Third, controlling for the survival status of the previous child in the mortality analysis does not lead to an increase of the effects of short intervals on mortality when the previous child is still alive. This finding does not suggest that sibling competition is not operating at all, but shows that the effects of increased intrafamilial mortality risks are stronger than are the effects of sibling competition.

Why is the effect of short birth intervals on mortality somewhat more pronounced at ages 1–6 months than during the neonatal period? If prenatal factors were the only mechanisms linking the length of preceding birth intervals and child survival, then one would expect the excess risk to be highest during the neonatal period. First, the absence of this pattern may be due to data quality problems in retrospective surveys. The observed pattern may have been caused by selective under-reporting of neonatal deaths; in longitudinal surveys, where under-reporting of neonatal deaths is much less of a problem, the effects of short birth intervals are most pronounced in the neonatal period. Second, it may suggest that breastfeeding practices play a mediating role, at least in some settings. The survival chances of children during the first half of infancy are strongly associated with breastfeeding. If impaired lactation is a consequence of short intervals, then this could explain some of the excess mortality risks for children with short preceding birth intervals during the first half of infancy. Children born after short birth intervals also had somewhat higher chances of not being breastfed, even after controlling for neonatal mortality, which may in part indicate that women who do not breastfeed have shorter birth intervals. Poor maternal health or low motivation to breastfeed (for example, if the child is not wanted) are possible explanations. The control for breastfeeding practices, however, did only slightly attenuate the association between short birth intervals and child mortality. An important caveat concerns the quality of retrospective reports on the duration of breastfeeding, which are required to estimate the effect of breastfeeding on mortality using DHS data. There are multiple problems including missing values, severe heaping, and inaccurate recall, which may, for example, vary by the mother's level of education, as was observed in Brazil (Huttly et al., 1990).

Furthermore, no information on the pattern of breastfeeding and supplementation is available, and these factors may be more important than duration per se in determining child health and survival.

Where do these findings lead? Clearly, research in several interrelated areas would foster a more complete understanding of the disadvantages associated with short birth intervals. The relationship between short intervals and maternal health and nutrition, weight gain during pregnancy, in-utero growth retardation, and prematurity must be better understood and described within the developing country context. A second area that needs to be further elucidated is the relationship between short preceding birth intervals and lactational performance. In addition, the sociocultural aspects of rapid new pregnancies need to be studied. For example, what are the consequences for care during pregnancy and during the first months of life? Further, theory and application need to be expanded to encompass consideration of social and biomedical interventions and opportunities for program intervention.

## Appendix

**Table 1A** Proportion of missing (or inconsistent) breastfeeding data among living children and deceased children (1–6 months and 7–23 months), and numbers of children never breastfed, breastfed but stopped before death, and breastfed until death, by age at death (1–6 months and 7–23 months)[a]

| Survey | Missing data among (%) | | | Breastfeeding among deceased children (N) | | | | | |
|---|---|---|---|---|---|---|---|---|---|
| | | | | Died at 1–6 months | | | Died at 7–23 months | | |
| | Sur- vivors[b] | Deaths 1–6 months | Deaths 7–23 months | Never | Stopped | Until death | Never | Stopped | Until death |
| **Sub-Saharan Africa** | | | | | | | | | |
| Burundi | 2.5 | 10.4 | 9.9 | 3 | 3 | 54 | 2 | 11 | 20 |
| Ghana | 2.5 | 4.8 | 12.1 | 3 | 10 | 47 | 1 | 26 | 60 |
| Mali | 9.9 | 4.2 | 8.9 | 0 | 4 | 65 | 0 | 13 | 76 |
| Senegal | 3.6 | 1.2 | 2.2 | 0 | 6 | 79 | 8 | 27 | 99 |
| Togo | 2.0 | 17.5 | 12.5 | 1 | 0 | 45 | 4 | 3 | 56 |
| Uganda | 1.2 | 8.5 | 5.8 | 2 | 10 | 95 | 5 | 34 | 105 |
| Zimbabwe | 0.8 | 7.9 | 10.8 | 0 | 7 | 28 | 0 | 15 | 18 |
| **North Africa** | | | | | | | | | |
| Egypt | 0.4 | 2.1 | 2.2 | 26 | 15 | 98 | 22 | 24 | 88 |
| Morocco | 4.3 | 8.1 | 16.5 | 15 | 30 | 57 | 4 | 26 | 36 |
| Tunisia | 0.0 | 0.0 | 0.0 | 8 | 23 | 17 | 1 | 16 | 10 |
| **Asia** | | | | | | | | | |
| Sri Lanka | 0.9 | 0.0 | 0.0 | 0 | 2 | 11 | 1 | 1 | 11 |
| Thailand | 0.7 | 0.0 | 18.2 | 4 | 2 | 16 | 0 | 2 | 7 |
| **Latin America and Caribbean** | | | | | | | | | |
| Bolivia | 0.5 | 6.3 | 3.5 | 11 | 33 | 90 | 10 | 72 | 56 |
| Brazil | 0.6 | 4.7 | 5.1 | 24 | 30 | 27 | 12 | 20 | 5 |
| Colombia | 1.4 | 0.0 | 0.0 | 6 | 4 | 9 | 3 | 7 | 3 |
| Dominican Republic | 0.1 | 7.1 | 6.3 | 17 | 25 | 23 | 7 | 39 | 14 |
| Guatemala | 0.4 | 1.1 | 1.0 | 18 | 12 | 56 | 7 | 32 | 57 |

[a] Among children of birth order two and higher.  [b] Excludes children still breastfed.

# Acknowledgments

The authors wish to thank James Trussell for giving his comments on the paper as a discussant at the DHS World Conference, 5–7 August 1991 in Washington DC, and gratefully acknowledge the support and advice of colleagues at the DHS during various stages of the study.

# Notes

1  As described by Jelliffe and Maddocks (1964), the maternal depletion syndrome results from the increasing and cumulative stress of successive pregnancies and lactation. This stress may result in specific nutrient deficiencies, such as vitamin D deficiency (osteomalacia) and iodine deficiency (goiter), or in general protein and calorie deficiency. Jelliffe and Maddocks described the syndrome among New Guinea highlanders, where women were responsible for most of the heavy work, had a very poor diet (almost exclusively sweet potato), and had repeated pregnancies and periods of prolonged lactation. Interestingly, maternal depletion in this context had probably nothing to do with close spacing of births, since postpartum sexual abstinence routinely lasted for 2–3 years in this population.

2  If short birth intervals are not a cause of premature delivery, then controlling for the length of gestation becomes very important, since over-representation of premature births in the very short birth-interval groups causes a spurious relationship between short intervals and mortality (Miller, 1989), especially for neonatal mortality. The effects on neonatal mortality risk of controlling for gestation are large for very short birth intervals, but smaller if the focus is on intervals lasting fewer than 18 or 24 months.

3  The effects of breastfeeding can also be counteractive; for example, curtailment of lactation in the previous pregnancy may lead to a short birth interval but may also lessen the nutritional depletion associated with prolonged lactation for the poorly nourished mother.

4  It has been argued that much of the birth-interval effect on child mortality in retrospective surveys was due to poor data quality (Potter, 1988). Recent analyses of WFS (Lantz et al., 1992) and DHS data (Hobcraft et al., 1991) have shown that data quality problems cannot account for the child spacing-child survival relationship in most surveys.

5  Such an effect may be due to specific medical or socioeconomic conditions. For example, in the case of neonatal mortality (for which intrafamilial mortality risks are probably most correlated), biological conditions such as hereditary diseases, birth trauma due to small pelvis, and propensity to deliver prematurely, are important. Behaviour may be important as well; for example, neonatal tetanus deaths may occur repeatedly, because all newborns in a family are given a special treatment whereby animal excreta is applied to the umbilical stump. It cannot, however, be excluded that the death of both the child who preceeds and the child who follows an interval is a consequence of a rapid succession of pregnancies. In other words, increased intrafamilial mortality risks can also be a consequence of rapid childbearing.

6  Anthropometric data were collected in 19 surveys in the period 1986–89. Trinidad and Tobago was not included in this study, because the overall sample size and, particularly, the numbers of deaths

were too small; further, the only regional survey in Ondo State, Nigeria, was also excluded. Brazil was included, although the anthropometric data were only collected in the northeast.

7   The analysis originally focused on short birth intervals lasting fewer than 18 months, but numbers in this category were too small in several countries for the analyses of morbidity and anthropometry.

8   The model is:

$$\ln (q_i/(1-q_i)) = b_0 + b_i X_i,$$

where $q_i$ is the probability of the outcome given the array of independent measures, $X_i$; and where $b_0$ is a constant and $b_i$ represents a series of unknown coefficients to be estimated via maximum-likelihood (Hosmer and Lemeshow, 1989).

9   The form of the model is:

$$\ln (h(t)_i / h_0(t)) = b_i X_i,$$

where $h(t)_i$ is the predicted hazard or mortality risk at age (month) t for an individual with the array of covariate values, $X_i$, $h_0(t)$ is the underlying and arbitrary hazard at age t, and $b_i$ represents the regression coefficients estimated by the partial-likelihood method of Cox (1972). All covariates, except breastfeeding, are fixed across the age intervals 1–6 months and 7–23 months.

10   Children born within two years of the survey are censored before reaching their second birthday (that is, before completing the 1–23 month period of observation). Hazards regression includes the survival experience of censored cases up to their age at censoring.

11   The maximum-likelihood estimate of $b_i$ is interpreted as the difference in the predicted log odds (or log hazard) of the outcome between those with the higher-risk characteristic and those with the reference characteristic. Exponentiation of $b_i$, thus, provides an estimate of the relative odds (or relative hazard) associated with that characteristic. In the case of postneonatal mortality, the estimated relative hazard can be viewed as a scalar which raises or lowers (depending on the sign of $b_i$) the underlying hazard uniformly (or proportionately) throughout the age ranges 1–6 months and 7–23 months.

12   It is not advisable to control for the duration of breastfeeding in the analysis of the effects of short intervals on neonatal mortality, since many children may not have been breastfed because of poor health (for a discussion of alternatives, see Elo and Miller, 1991).

13   In the hazards regression, two down-weighted observations are created that represent one child's experience before and after weaning. For instance, if a child stopped breastfeeding at exactly nine months of age and died (or was censored alive) at 18 months, two half-weighted nine months exposure cells are created that indicate breastfeeding and survival to nine months and nonbreastfeeding and survival through the next eight months and then death (or censoring) in the last month of observation.

14   According to the recalled data on breastfeeding status of the previous child and birth dates of the index child, more than 5 percent of the women continued to breastfeed during pregnancy in 12 of the 17 countries, and more than 10 percent continued in seven countries. According to the current status data, this does not appear to be genuine, and misdating of births or overestimation of breastfeeding duration is likely. This will be discussed in greater detail in a DHS Methodological Report on the evaluation of the quality of health data in DHS surveys, which is in preparation.

15   $RR = RO/\{(1-P_{ref}) + (RO \times P_{ref})\}$; where RR is the relative risk, RO the relative odds, and $P_{ref}$ the prevalence of the outcome in the reference group (that is, children with preceding birth intervals of 24–35 months).

16  In the presentation of results, the statistical significance of the estimate of the relative odds (derived from the estimated coefficient and its standard error) will be shown along side the converted relative risks as an approximation of the statistical significance of the relative risks.

17  The trimean is calculated as: $(Q_1 + 2Q_2 + Q_3) / 4$, where $Q_1$ equals the first quartile value, $Q_2$ equals the median value, and $Q_3$ equals the third quartile value.

18  More insight into the association between birth intervals and child survival can be gained by including data on birth weight. Such data were not collected in the DHS surveys during 1986–89, with the exception of the Bolivia DHS survey. The latter included data on the infant's subjective size at birth, as perceived by the mother. The effect of preceding birth intervals on neonatal mortality was reduced by about 10 percent after controlling for size at birth.

19  In some countries, the estimated relative risks are not the same as the risks shown in Table 3, due to exclusion of the missing values for breastfeeding in the analyses used to prepare Table 4.

20  The analysis of anthropometric data is based on living children, and therefore the results are subject to a survivor bias. If, for instance, birth interval length is associated with growth retardation, and (as has been shown) growth retardation leads to greater mortality risk, then the exclusion of dead children will bias estimates of the birth interval-nutritional status relationship towards zero. However, it has been shown that such a bias is small in the case of underweight and very small for stunting, and only becomes a problem when mortality levels are very high (Boerma et al., 1992).

## References

Aaby, P. 1988. *Malnourished or Overinfected: An Analysis of the Determinants of Acute Measles Mortality.* Copenhagen: Laegeforeningens Forlag.

Bicego, G.T. and J.T. Boerma. 1991. 'Maternal education and child survival: A comparative analysis of DHS data.' Paper presented at DHS World Conference, August 5–7, Washington DC.

Boerma J.T. and H.A.W. Van Vianen. 1984. 'Birth interval, mortality and growth in a rural area in Kenya.' *Journal of Biosocial Science* 16: 475–486.

Boerma, J.T., A.E. Sommerfelt, and G.T. Bicego. 1992. 'Child anthropometry in cross-sectional surveys in developing countries: An assessment of the survivor bias.' *American Journal of Epidemiology* 135: 438–449.

Brody D.J. and M.B. Bracken. 1987. 'Short interpregnancy interval: A risk factor for low birth weight.' *American Journal of Perinatology* 4: 50–54.

Cox, D. 1972. 'Regression models and life tables.' *Journal of the Royal Statistical Society*, Series B, 34: 187.

De Sweemer, C. 1984. 'The influence of child spacing on child survival.' *Population Studies* 38: 47–72.

Doyle, P., D. Morley, M. Woodland, and J. Cole. 1978. 'Birth intervals, survival and growth in a Nigerian village.' *Journal of Biosocial Science* 10: 81–94.

Elo, I.T. and J.E. Miller. 1991. 'Ever-breastfed status and health at birth.' Paper presented at the IUSSP Seminar on Measurement of Maternal and Child Mortality, Morbidity, and Health Care: Interdisciplinary Approaches.

Fedrick, J. and P. Adelstein. 1973. 'Influence of pregnancy spacing on outcome of pregnancy.' *British Medical Journal* 4: 753–756.

Ferraz, E.M., R.H. Gray, P.L. Fleming, and T.M. Maia. 1988. "Interpregnancy interval and low birth weight: Findings from a case control study." *American Journal Epidemiology* 128: 1,111–1,116.

Goldberg, H.I. and F.G. M'Bodji. 1985. "Birth intervals and undernutrition in rural Senegal.' In *Proceedings of the IUSSP International Conference in Florence* Vol. 2, Ordina Editions. Pp. 67–78.

Gray, R.H. 1990. '"Epidemiologic methods and case control studies of mortality and morbidity.' In *Measurement and Analysis of Mortality: New Approaches*. Eds. J. Vallin, S. D'Souza, and A. Pallon. Oxford: Carendon Press.

Gubhaju, B.B. 1985. 'The effect of previous child death on infant and child mortality in rural Nepal.' *Journal of Biosocial Science* 16: 231–236.

Hobcraft, J. 1991. 'Family formation patterns and child survival: A comparative analysis.' Paper presented at the annual meeting of the Population Association of America, March 21–23, Washington, DC.

Hobcraft, J., J.W. McDonald, and S.O. Rutstein. 1985. 'Demographic determinants of infant and early child mortality: A comparative analysis.' *Population Studies* 39: 363–385.

Hosmer, S. and S. Lemeshow. 1989. *Applied Logistic Regression*. New York: John Wiley and Sons.

Huttly, S.R.A., F.C. Barros, C.G. Victora, J.U. Beria, and J.P. Vaughan. 1990. 'Do mothers overestimate breast feeding duration? An example of recall bias from a study in southern Brazil.' *American Journal of Epidemiology* 132: 572–575.

Jansen, A.A.J., W. Gemert, B. Thiuri, and S.A. Lakhani. 1984. 'Growth of infants of low and normal birth weight.' In *Maternal and Child Health in Rural Kenya*. Eds. J.K. Van Ginneken and A.S. Muller. Beckenham: Croom Helm. Pp. 197–206.

Jelliffe, D.B. and I. Maddocks. 1964. 'Ecologic malnutrition in the New Guinea Highlands.' *Clinical Pediatrics* 3: 432–438.

Koenig, M.A., J.F. Phillips, O.M. Campbell, and S. D'Souza. 1990. 'Birth intervals and childhood mortality in Bangladesh.' *Demography* 27: 251–266.

Lang, J.M., E. Lieberman, K.J. Ryan, and R.R. Monson. 1990. 'Interpregnancy interval and risk of preterm labor.' *American Journal of Epidemiology* 132: 304–309.

Lantz, P., M. Parten, and A. Palloni. 1992. 'Using retrospective surveys for estimating the effects of breastfeeding and childspacing on infant and child mortality.' *Population Studies* 46: 121–140.

Lieberman, E., J.M. Lang, K.J. Ryan, R.R. Monson, and S.C. Schoenbaum. 1989. 'The association of inter-pregnancy interval with small for gestational age births.' *Obstetrics and Gynecology* 74: 1–5.

Majumder, A.K. 1990. 'Child survival and its effects on mortality of siblings in Bangladesh.' *Journal of Biosocial Science* 22: 333–347.

Mavalankar, D. and R.H. Gray. 1991. 'Interpregnancy interval and risk of preterm labor' (letter). *American Journal of Epidemiology* 133: 958–959.

Merchant, K., R. Martorell, and J.D. Haas. 1990. 'Maternal and fetal responses to the stresses of lactation concurrent with pregnancy and of short recuperative intervals.' *American Journal of Clinical Nutrition* 52: 280–288.

Miller, J.E. 1989. 'Is the relationship between birth intervals and perinatal mortality spurious? Evidence from Hungary and Sweden.' *Population Studies* 43: 479–495.

Miller, J.E., J. Trussell, A.R. Pebley, and B. Vaughan. 1992. 'Birth spacing and child mortality in Bangladesh and the Philippines.' *Demography* 29: 305–318.

Millman, S.R. and E.C. Cooksey. 1987. 'Birth weight and the effects of birth spacing and breastfeeding on infant mortality.' *Studies in Family Planning* 18: 202–212.

Palloni, A. 1989. 'Effects of inter-birth intervals on infant and early childhood mortality.' In *Differential Mortality: Methodological Issues and Biosocial Factors*. Eds. L. Ruzicka, G. Wunsch, P. Kane. Oxford: Clarendon Press. Pp. 163–188.

Palloni, A. and S. Millman. 1986. 'Effects of birth intervals and breastfeeding on infant and early child mortality.' *Population Studies* 40: 215–236.

Pebley, A.R. and S. Millman. 1986. 'Birthspacing and child survival.' *International Family Planning Perspectives* 12: 71–79.

Potter, J.E. 1988. 'Birth spacing and child survival: A cautionary note regarding the evidence from the WFS.' *Population Studies* 42: 443–450.

Retherford, R.D., M.K Choe, S. Thapa, and B.B. Gubhaju. 1989. 'To what extent does breastfeeding explain birth-interval effects on early childhood mortality?' *Demography* 26: 439–450.

Sullivan, J.M., G.T. Bicego, and S.O. Rutstein. 1990. 'Assessment of the quality of data used for the direct estimation of infant and child mortality in the Demographic and Health surveys.' *DHS Methodological Reports* No.1. Columbia: MD. Institute for Resource Development.

Van Steenbergen, W.M., J.A. Kusin, S. Kardjati, and C. De With. 1989. 'Energy supplementation in the last trimester of pregnancy in East Java, Indonesia: Effect on breast-milk output.' *American Journal of Clinical Nutrition* 50: 274–279.

Winikoff, B. 1983. 'The effects of birth spacing on child and maternal health.' *Studies in Family Planning* 14: 231–245.

12

# Maternal education and child survival: a comparative study of survey data from 17 countries

*George T. Bicego and J. Ties Boerma*

Social Science & Medicine, *vol. 36, no. 9, 1993, pp. 1207–1227.*

## Abstract

A uniform analytical methodology was applied to survey data from 17 developing countries with the aim of addressing a series of questions regarding the positive statistical association between maternal education and the health and survival of children under age two. As has been observed previously, the education advantage in survival was less pronounced during than after the neonatal period. Strong but varying education effects on postneonatal risk, undernutrition during the 3–23 month period, and non-use of health services were shown – although a large part of these associations are the result of education's strong link to household economics. Differential use of basic health services, though closely tied to a mother's educational level, does little to explain the education advantage in child health and survival. However, the issue of the actual quality of services measured in the DHS is raised. Other issues concerning the roles of the pattern of family formation and differential physical access to health services are explored and discussed.

childhood mortality; education; comparative

## Introduction

A considerable body of research has demonstrated the statistical association between education of mothers and childhood mortality in developing countries. Cleland and van Ginneken (1) have reviewed the works of Cochrane et al. (2) using data from 33 countries, and the United Nations (3) using data from 15 countries – to find that each one year increment in maternal education corresponds on average to a 7–9% decline in indirectly calculated measures of childhood mortality. Rutstein (4), using WFS data of 41 countries, showed that the education advantage, with few exceptions, is more pronounced after as opposed to during infancy.

While one of the most common findings in the child survival literature, the education-mortality relationship remains one of the least understood. Several lines of inquiry are relevant. First, to what extent is the observed relationship merely a function of education's link to economic status? Previous studies have been encumbered by the unavailability of data that captures variation in household wealth or disposable income. Two large comparative studies have examined the effect of maternal education, net of economic controls that range in character from paternal occupation and education to household latrine and water facilities (3, 5). The broad conclusion drawn from these studies is that a large part – approximately one half – of the education-mortality relationship is accounted for by the various adopted indices of household economic condition. The Hobcraft et al. study (5) using direct estimation procedures that allow age-specific analysis, found the net education effect to be much stronger during the 1–5 age segment than during infancy; in only 9 of 24 countries did the education effect remain statistically significant for neonatal and postneonatal mortality after inclusion of economic controls.

Second, if the education-mortality association (or a part of the association) is indeed causal, what behaviors serve to mediate the education advantage in child health and survival? Of the many theories that attempt to explain the relationship[1], perhaps the most relevant and intuitive from the standpoint of child health policy relate to education-conditioned use of health services (modern and traditional) and pattern of family formation (age at initiation, pace and size). The evidence for such causal connections however, is inconclusive. While participation in mass immunization programs may not be education-related (8, 9), there exists considerable evidence to support the thesis that, in many societies, better educated mothers more commonly use maternal and child health services than less educated mothers (10–14). Results of a follow-up study of Filipino children show that each one-year increment in maternal education increases the probability of preventive health service use by about 4% during any month during the first year of life (15). Data from a small-scale study in Indonesia indicate that educated women have greater awareness of correct immunization schedules; the authors conclude that it is possession of this specific knowledge rather than formal education per se that leads a mother to ensure that her children receive available vaccines (16).

Barbieri (17), applying multivariate methods to the Senegal DHS data, concluded that the effect of maternal education on child survival does not operate through differential health service utilization or family formation pattern. Cleland and van Ginneken (1) linked results from two previous studies that use WFS data (5,18) to show convincingly that differences in the distribution of births by birth order, maternal age at birth, and birth interval length do essentially nothing to explain the education advantage.

A third important line of inquiry involves possible modification of the education effect on survival depending on the level of access to modern health services. Does greater physical access to health services widen or narrow the differences between children of more educated and those of less educated mothers in the use of child-health related services and ultimately in the child survival chances? A review of previous studies leads to mixed conclusions. Results of Orubuloye and Caldwell (19) indicate that access to medical services in rural Nigeria amplifies the maternal education effect on childhood mortality. The authors reason that only in settings with access to services can the increased autonomy and abilities conferred by education be fully employed by mothers towards the improvement of child health. On the other hand, the results of Rozenzweig and Schultz (20), using census data for urban Colombia, and Bicego (21), using survey data of rural Haiti, suggest that greater physical access to health services improves survival to a greater extent among the children of less educated than for children of more educated women, thereby narrowing education differentials. The latter findings are consistent with results from ecological studies of China (22) and Costa Rica (23), where education differentials in childhood mortality have narrowed over a period of increasing access to health services. Similarly, Palloni (24) in an aggregate level study of Latin American countries, argued that individual assets and characteristics (e.g. maternal education) are less important as determinants of mortality risk in settings of greater access to basic resources and services.

Lastly, above it was described how the education-mortality relationship, even after control for economic status, tends to be more pronounced at older as opposed to younger ages of childhood. This age-pattern to the education effect may reflect a consequence of poor nutrition and repeated episodes of infectious (but non-fatal) disease that, while related to behavioral inputs at younger ages, are manifest in terms of mortality risk only at later ages. Mosley and Becker (25) have shown that such cumulative deterioration in health, termed frailty, should be an important consideration when evaluating models of childhood mortality risk in developing countries. While cross-sectional data are severely limited in the extent to which previous morbidity, nutritional inputs, and changes in nutritional status can be measured, it is argued in this paper that analysis of the determinants of cross-sectional nutritional status can provide useful information regarding causal pathways through which household socioeconomics impact survival chances.

There seems no inherent reason to assume, *a priori*, that the answers to the questions raised above are the same in all contexts. On the other hand, it would be of considerable utility for social researchers and policy-makers alike to identify some underlying pattern of results common to a group of culturally-diverse countries that would provide clues concerning pathways of influence. This is where comparative analysis can prove useful. In the present study, we address these issues using a uniform conceptual framework and analytical method, applied to DHS survey data from 17 countries representing a wide range of socio-demographic and epidemiologic conditions.

## Conceptual and analytical framework of the study

A conceptual framework is shown in Figure 1 that represents the posited relationship among maternal education, key confounders and intermediate variables, and measures of health outcome. The framework builds on the earlier conceptual models of Mosley and Chen (26) and Van Norren and Van Vianen (27), with modifications based on the limitations and structure of the DHS data. Explicit here, as in the original Mosley-Chen framework, is that there exists a finite number of variables, called proximate or interme-

**Figure 1** Conceptual framework for the analysis of the effects of maternal education on child survival

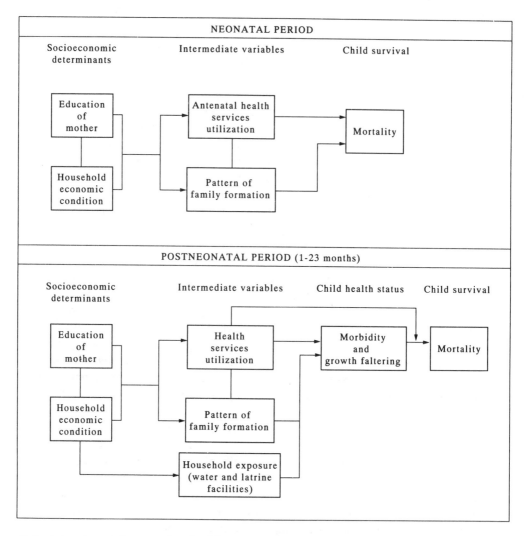

diate determinants (e.g. modern health services), through which background socioeconomic factors (e.g. maternal education) must operate to influence survival chances.

Household economic status and sanitary conditions (exposure to disease), are important determinants of childhood mortality and may, at the same time, be associated with a mother's level of education and use of health services. The DHS data contain information that allows a measure of control over the perturbing influence of these variables on estimation and inference[2], more information than was available for previous studies using WFS data. The first phase of analysis focuses on maternal education as a determinant of early childhood mortality, controlled for economic status, and the particular role of health services use and family formation pattern in mediating the relationship. Physical sanitary conditions (as opposed to exposure-related behaviors) are conditioned by economic status (either measured or unmeasured in this study) and are not considered a potential mediating variable in the education-health outcome relationship. Rural-urban residence is regarded as a crude proxy for physical access to modern health services, so that the potential for variation in the effect of education on mortality risk across 'access' strata is examined through use of education/urban-rural interaction terms. Separate conceptual models are posited for neonatal mortality, and mortality after the first month, the rationale for which is elaborated in later sections.

Ideally, we would wish to have age-specific measures of past illnesses, nutritional inputs and growth that would allow controls for health heterogeneity in our study populations (26). The DHS morbidity and nutritional status data are cross-sectional, of course, and thus restricted to living children, making use of a single statistical model (including both morbidity and mortality measures on all children born during a period in time, living and dead at survey) unfeasible. Furthermore, previous studies have suggested that under-reporting of recent morbidity, diarrhoeal illness in particular, in survey data tends to be greater among less educated women (29, 30), attenuating estimates of the education-morbidity relationship. More objective assessment of past illnesses and poor nutrition, on the other hand, may be obtained through use of anthropometric measures collected in most of the DHS surveys. In this study, maternal education's effect on the risk of stunting or long-term growth faltering (low height for-age) and underweight status (low weight-for-age) at survey is estimated using the same analytical framework as was used for mortality analysis, in order to determine whether growth retardation may be an important precursor in the pathway from low educational status to heightened mortality risk after the first month of life. An assumption underlying such cross-analysis interpretation is that the large majority of early childhood deaths (after the neonatal period) in our study populations are due to repeated bouts of infection and deteriorating nutritional status This assumption appears quite reasonable under conditions of moderate to high child mortality (26, 27).

Lastly, does lacking formal education increase the probability that a mother will not utilize the modern health system? Essentially, this isolates for closer examination a piece of the conceptual framework outlined above. Here, measures of non-use of health services are posited as dependent measures or outcomes. All other antecedent variables remain in the model and variation between 'access' (urban-rural) strata in the effect of education on non-use is examined under the proposition that greater access to basic health services leads to greater homogeneity in the actual use of services.

## Data and analytical methods

### The data
The data of 17 DHS surveys conducted over the period 1987–90 were used in these analyses: four of Latin America and the Caribbean (Bolivia, Colombia, Dominican Republic and Guatemala), eight of Sub-Saharan Africa (Burundi, Ghana, Kenya, Mali, Senegal, Togo, Uganda and Zimbabwe), three of North Africa (Egypt, Morocco, Tunisia) and two of Asia (Thailand and Sri Lanka). All births since the cutoff date for col-

lection of health information (5–6 years before the survey) were included in the analysis of childhood mortality and in the analysis of health service utilization. For analysis of anthropometric outcome, all surviving children, aged 3–23 months at survey were included. Variable definitions and constructions are provided below.

- *Mortality.* Information on survival status at the time of the survey and the age at death (in single months) is drawn from the (complete) birth histories. Two age segments are investigated; the neonatal period (zero completed months or less than thirty-one days), and the period between 1 and 23 completed months of age. Heaping of age at death at 12 months is common in survey data of this type (31). Collapsing the conventional post-neonatal (1–11 months) and toddler (12–23 months) periods serves to avoid biases introduced by any relationships between age at death misreporting and the explanatory variables. Further, the increasingly small number of deaths at older ages and the heavy right-censoring precludes statistically relevant results for a separate toddler model, especially in the low mortality countries (e.g. Thailand, Colombia, and Sri Lanka).[3] This age segment (1–23 months) will henceforth be referred to, unconventionally, as the postneonatal period.

  Under-reporting of child deaths is a problem common to birth history data. Although impossible to access with any precision, it is probable that some child deaths have been omitted in the survey data under study and that such under-reporting is more likely among uneducated mothers.[4] If so, the result would be a downward bias in the estimate of the education-mortality relationship. Thus, the reader may choose to consider the results of the study lower-bound estimates.

- *Stunting and underweight status.* Height and weight were measured for children aged 3–36 or 3–60 months at the time of the survey, depending on the survey.[5] In this study we examine stunting (low height-for-age) and underweight status (low weight-for-age) among children aged 3–23 months.[6] A child is considered stunted if the recumbent length for age is more than two standard deviations below the NCHS/WHO reference median. A child is considered underweight if her weight-for-age is more than two standard deviations below the NCHS/WHO reference median. Wasting was originally considered for study, but the number of wasted children was determined to be prohibitively small in nearly all of the countries.

  Cross-sectional data on child anthropometry is biased in that only survivors to the survey date are measured. For purposes of this study, if growth faltering is related to both education on one hand and survivorship on the other (both very likely), then estimates of the education-growth faltering relationship will be attenuated by selection bias. Previous work has shown, however, that the extent of bias is small for the case of low weight-for-age and negligible for low height-for-age (32).

- *Non-use of health services.*
  - *Non-use of tetanus toxoid during the 'index' pregnancy (NoTT):* All children were assigned to either use or non-use categories based on their mothers' responses to a question whether she received any injection to prevent tetanus in her child during that pregnancy.

- *Non-use of antenatal services (NoANC):* All children were assigned to either use or non-use categories based on whether their mother responded that, during that pregnancy, she received prenatal care from a doctor, nurse, or trained midwife. NoANC and NoTT are used as independent (explanatory) variables in the neonatal mortality analysis, and as dependent (outcome) measures in later analyses.
- *Index of non-use of health services (NoHSU):* For analysis of postneonatal mortality (1–23 months) and anthropometric outcome (3–23 months), an index that intends to capture variation in a mother's propensity to use modern health system was constructed. The index is based on the joint distribution of NoANC (described above) and NoDS, non-use of delivery services, which is a dichotomous variable that indicates whether or not the mother went to the hospital or clinic for delivery, or otherwise had a medically supervised delivery. One point is assigned for each of the behaviors NoANC and NoDS, so that the index (NoHSU) runs from a best score of 0 (medical supervision during both pregnancy and delivery) to a worst score of 2 (lacking any medical super vision during pregnancy and delivery). In lieu of any information concerning use of health services expected to impact health and survival during the 1–23 month age period[7], this index, while lacking the specific interpretation carried by variables used for the neonatal period, does serve to identify mother/child units at high risk of non-use. If a mother fails to contact the modern health system throughout pregnancy and delivery, it follows that the mother is considerably less likely (than women with a better NoHSU score) to have sought out and received other child health services after delivery.

- *Family formation pattern (bio-demographic profile).* Information on preceding birth interval length, birth order and maternal age at birth are derived from the birth histories. Birth interval length is classified as short (<24 months) or not, birth order as first, 2–5, or 6+, and maternal age at birth as at less than 20 years, 20–34 years or 35+ years. First order births are placed in the reference birth interval category (i.e. 24+ months). Each of these variables has been shown to be important correlates of early childhood mortality in developing countries.

- *Indicators of water-borne exposure to disease.* Heightened exposure to water-borne entero-pathogens is expected to increase the risk of potentially fatal diarrhoeal diseases. The level of household exposure will, in part, be related to the pathogenicity of household drinking water, and whether or not the household has adequate excreta disposal facilities. Two variables are constructed from the household data that intend to capture such variation. For one variable (WATER), children are classified into a high-risk exposure group if the child lives in a household using non-piped drinking water. For the second variable (LATRINE), the child is considered at higher risk if living in a household without some sort of latrine. In the more developed countries (e.g. Colombia, Dominican Republic) where the distribution of these data warranted, an additional category was broken out for children living in households with a flush toilet. It should be reiterated that these physical exposure variables are not viewed as mediating factors in the education-health outcome relationship[8], but merely as variables which through their connection to (unmeasured) economic factors on one hand and health outcome on the other, may help to provide a better control for economic condition of households beyond what is captured in the economic index *per se*.

- *Socioeconomic factors. Maternal education:* Mothers were asked what level of education they ever attended and, within that level, how many years. Three educational levels are considered here: no education, some primary but no secondary, and some secondary education. The number of completed years required to finish primary school varied among countries: 5 years in Colombia, Morocco, and Sri Lanka; 6 years in Guatemala, Egypt, Tunisia, Burundi, and Togo; 7 years in Thailand, Kenya, Uganda, Zimbabwe, and Senegal; 8 years in Bolivia, Dominican Republic, and Ghana; and 9 years in Mali. Where the percentage of births whose mothers had some secondary school was less than 10% (400–500 births, in practice), the primary and secondary categories were collapsed. Thus, in Morocco, Tunisia, Burundi, Mali, Senegal and Togo referred to here as 'B' countries, only two categories (no education and any education) are analyzed. In the remaining 11 'A' countries, all three levels are maintained in the analyses.

- *Index of household economic status:* No data was collected in the DHS surveys on household income *per se*. However, three types of data intended to capture variations in household wealth and disposable income were collected. These data are used to construct an index that serves as a control variable in all analyses. The first type of data is on possession of a radio and a television; two points are assigned for television, one for a radio if no television is owned. The second type considers the type of materials used in floor construction, a non-dirt floor is assigned two points. The third type relates to ownership of a motorized means of transportation: two points are assigned for either a car, truck or tractor, one point for a motorcycle if no car, truck, or tractor is owned. This results in an index with a minimum score of 0 points and a maximum score of 6 points.[9]

Table 1 gives a summary of mortality rates, stunting and underweight prevalences, and distributions of the study population of births by mother's educational level and level of health services utilization for the 17 countries considered here. It is worth here remarking at the wide variation in both health outcome and explanatory factors encompassed by these countries. These variations will come into play later in the interpretation of findings.

## Basic statistical models

Six dependent variables are examined in this study: neonatal mortality, postneonatal mortality, stunting and underweight at the time of survey, non-use of tetanus toxoid during pregnancy and non-use of antenatal services. All of these, except postneonatal mortality, were analyzed as dichotomous outcomes using the logistic regression model:

$$\ln \frac{(q_1)}{(1-q_1)} = b_0 + b_i X_i \text{, or}$$

$$\text{logit } q_i = b_0 + b_i X_i,$$

where $q_i$, is the probability of the outcome given the array of independent measures, $X_i$; and where $b_o$ is a constant and $b_i$, represents a series of unknown coefficients to be estimated via maximum-likelihood (33). In the case of postneonatal mortality, we use a Cox hazards regression model, obviating the exclusion of a large number of children born within 2 years of survey.[10]

$$\text{In } \frac{h(t)_i}{h_0(t)} = b_i X_i,$$

where $h(t)_i$ is the predicted hazard or mortality risk at age (month) $t$ for an individual with the array of covariate values, $X_i$, $h_0(t)$ is the underlying and arbitrary hazard at age $t$, and $b_i$ represents the regression coefficients estimated by the partial-likelihood method of Cox (34). All covariates are fixed across ages 1–23 months.

Independent measures are reference parameterized, with the theoretically low-risk category serving as reference. The maximum-likelihood estimate of $b_i$ is interpreted as the difference in the predicted log odds (or log hazard) of the outcome between those with the higher-risk characteristic (i.e. no education or primary education) and those with the reference characteristic (i.e. secondary education in 'A' countries, any education in 'B' countries). Exponentiation of $b_i$, thus, provides an estimate of the relative odds (or relative hazard) associated with that characteristic. In the case of postneonatal mortality, the estimated relative hazard can be viewed as a scalar which raises or lowers (depending on the sign of $b_i$) the underlying hazard uniformly (or proportionately) throughout the age range 1–23 months.[11]

The relative odds will overstate the relative risk to very different degrees when the prevalence of the outcome is high and varies widely across comparison groups (35), as it does in these analyses regarding anthropometric status and non-use of health services (see Table 1). This of course would result in a misleading base for comparison amongst countries. Therefore, in the analyses of anthropometric status and non-use of health services use (as outcome measures), relative odds were converted to relative risks.[12] For analysis of neonatal mortality, which in no country exceeds five percent, the conversion to relative risks was deemed unnecessary and relative odds were interpreted directly as relative risks.

## Model estimation and inference

Since our primary interest is to estimate effects of introducing the intermediate variables and confounders on the relationship between mother's education and child health endpoints, we do not attempt to identify the most parsimonious model that fits the data. Rather, we follow the change in the coefficients for education, related to the addition of key confounders and intermediate variables, to draw inference on intervening mechanisms. The process of model estimation is thus related to the causal/temporal ordering of factors shown in the conceptual framework in Figure 1 and represented in the generalized sequence of equations:

**Table 1** Number of births, mortality ratios, prevalences of stunting and underweight status, and percentage distributions of births by maternal education and various indices of health services utilization. 17 DHS countries

| Country | Births | Neonatal mortality rate | Postneonatal mortality ratio | % No education | % Primary education | % No tetanus toxoid | % No ANC | Index of health service use (%) | | Children 3–23 months at survey | % Stunted | % Under weight |
|---|---|---|---|---|---|---|---|---|---|---|---|---|
| | | | | | | | | Low | Moderate | | | |
| Bolivia | 5757 | 0.032 | 0.061 | 18.9 | 59.5 | 76.0 | 50.7 | 42.3 | 20.1 | 1726 | 29.7 | 12.8 |
| Colombia | 2684 | 0.018 | 0.014 | 8.0 | 58.9 | 61.6 | 26.9 | 16.4 | 22.7 | 840 | 21.1 | 11.0 |
| Dom. Rep. | 4718 | 0.032 | 0.040 | 10.9 | 66.9 | 11.9 | 5.6 | 2.6 | 13.9 | 1193 | 20.5 | 12.7 |
| Guatemala | 4581 | 0.033 | 0.050 | 49.5 | 40.5 | 86.2 | 65.8 | 58.3 | 19.8 | 1440 | 52.4 | 30.4 |
| Egypt | 8548 | 0.036 | 0.042 | 51.5 | 31.7 | 87.6 | 45.6 | 36.8 | 35.6 | 1223 | 29.4 | 14.4 |
| Morocco[a] | 6050 | 0.041 | 0.039 | 85.0 | 8.9 | ND | 75.2 | 62.8 | 22.7 | 1930 | 22.6 | 14.9 |
| Tunisia[a] | 4439 | 0.026 | 0.023 | 55.4 | 34.8 | 66.8 | 42.4 | 23.0 | 27.4 | 1275 | 15.6 | 10.1 |
| Sri Lanka | 3990 | 0.016 | 0.010 | 11.6 | 30.5 | 13.2 | 3.8 | 1.6 | 14.0 | 1260 | 25.3 | 38.3 |
| Thailand | 3660 | 0.020 | 0.013 | 7.9 | 73.8 | 34.5 | 19.0 | 13.3 | 17.6 | 1164 | 16.7 | 18.6 |
| Ghana | 4089 | 0.043 | 0.050 | 44.9 | 26.1 | 29.1 | 16.4 | 15.7 | 43.5 | 1206 | 23.1 | 28.3 |
| Kenya | 6913 | 0.030 | 0.046 | 25.5 | 51.4 | 9.7 | 22.3 | 13.2 | 43.2 | ND | ND | ND |
| Uganda | 4915 | 0.042 | 0.078 | 37.5 | 51.8 | 43.6 | 12.5 | 11.7 | 48.0 | 1592 | 36.9 | 23.2 |
| Zimbabwe | 3334 | 0.027 | 0.029 | 18.5 | 62.4 | 20.1 | 7.5 | 6.7 | 23.3 | 940 | 25.9 | 10.3 |
| Burundi[a] | 3769 | 0.034 | 0.053 | 75.3 | 19.6 | 36.2 | 17.7 | 17.2 | 55.8 | 1164 | 38.4 | 32.6 |
| Mali[a] | 3311 | 0.044 | 0.073 | 81.9 | 16.4 | 71.6 | 57.7 | 49.7 | 13.6 | 712 | 20.5 | 29.4 |
| Senegal[b] | 4253 | 0.045 | 0.067 | 83.2 | 12.8 | 68.9 | 37.3 | 34.3 | 26.6 | 424[b] | 20.5 | 20.0 |
| Togo[a] | 3098 | 0.039 | 0.048 | 66.9 | 25.1 | 28.4 | 33.8 | 25.5 | 25.8 | 1379 | 29.7 | 24.7 |

[a] 'B' countries, those with less with 10% of births in secondary education category.
[b] Children 6–23 months at survey studied.
ND–no data collected.

**Table 2** Relative risks of neonatal mortality associated with maternal education. Gross effects, effects controlled for economic status (equation 2), effects with addition of family formation variables (equation 3) and health service use variables (equation 4) and interaction effects (rural vs urban)

*'A' Countries*

| Country | Neonatal mortality rate (/00) | No education vs secondary education | | | | | Primary vs secondary education | | | | |
|---|---|---|---|---|---|---|---|---|---|---|---|
| | | Equation (1) (gross) | Equation (2) | Equation (3) | Equation (4) | Interaction | Equation (1) (gross) | Equation (2) | Equation (3) | Equation (4) | Interaction |
| Bolivia | 32 | 2.59*** | 2.34*** | 2.33** | 1.64 | 1.92 | 1.94** | 1.79** | 1.69** | 1.41 | 1.82 |
| Colombia | 18 | 4.60*** | 3.77** | 4.56** | 4.46** | 0.23 | 2.74** | 2.53** | 2.80** | 2.80** | 0.93 |
| Dominican R. | 32 | 1.75 | 1.53 | 1.66 | 1.50 | 2.13 | 1.20 | 1.12 | 1.15 | 1.09 | 1.23 |
| Guatemala | 33 | 1.07 | 0.78 | 0.82 | 0.72 | 1.96 | 1.10 | 0.82 | 0.90 | 0.81 | 1.25 |
| Egypt | 36 | 1.82*** | 1.62** | 1.53** | 1.48* | 2.12* | 1.69** | 1.62** | 1.59*** | 1.57** | 1.21 |
| Thailand | 20 | 4.52** | 2.93* | 2.20 | 2.20 | UD | 3.67** | 2.60* | 2.27 | 2.40 | UD |
| Sri Lanka | 16 | 1.30 | 1.10 | 1.09 | 1.74 | UD | 0.85 | 0.75 | 0.75 | 0.71 | UD |
| Ghana | 43 | 1.07 | 0.96 | 0.84 | 0.80 | 1.27 | 1.47* | 1.45* | 1.32 | 1.30 | 1.03 |
| Kenya | 30 | 1.71** | 1.39 | 1.66** | 1.57* | 0.64 | 1.16 | 1.00 | 1.09 | 1.07 | 1.71 |
| Uganda | 42 | 1.13 | 0.88 | 0.92 | 0.85 | 0.15** | 0.95 | 0.76 | 0.79 | 0.75 | 0.34** |
| Zimbabwe | 27 | 1.28 | 1.22 | 1.11 | 1.11 | 0.68 | 1.14 | 1.12 | 1.09 | 1.11 | 0.79 |
| trimean | 32 | 1.65 | 1.40 | 1.45 | 1.31 | 1.19 | 1.30 | 1.18 | 1.21 | 1.14 | 1.14 |

*'B' Countries*

None vs any education

| Country | Neonatal mortality rate | Equation (1) (gross) | Equation (2) | Equation (3) | Equation (4) | Interaction |
|---|---|---|---|---|---|---|
| Morocco | 41 | 1.28 | 1.05 | 1.05 | 1.00 | 1.47 |
| Tunisia | 26 | 1.39 | 1.31 | 1.34 | 1.27 | 1.24 |
| Burundi | 34 | 1.25 | 1.14 | 1.26 | 1.17 | 0.56 |
| Mali | 44 | 2.32*** | 1.78* | 1.73* | 1.62 | 1.00 |
| Senegal | 45 | 1.09 | 0.95 | 1.04 | 0.88 | 0.91 |
| Togo | 39 | 0.75 | 0.74 | 0.76 | 0.73 | 5.59*** |
| trimean | 40 | 1.25 | 1.10 | 1.16 | 1.07 | 1.13 |

*Estimated effect significant at $P < 0.10$; ** at $P < 0.05$; *** at $P < 0.01$.
UD—Undefined; no deaths in reference category (i.e. children of urban mothers with secondary education).

$$\text{logit } q_1 = b_0 + b_1 X_1, \qquad\qquad (1)$$

$$\text{logit } q_{1,2} = b_0 + b_1 X_1 + b_2 X_2, \qquad\qquad (2)$$

$$\text{logit } q_{1,2,3} = b_0 + b_1 X_1 + b_2 X_2 + b_3 X_3, \qquad (3)$$

$$\text{logit } q_{1,2,3,k} = b_0 + b_1 X_1 + b_2 X_2 + b_3 X_3 + \dots b_k X_k \quad (4)$$

where equation (1) includes only the maternal education parameters; equation (2) adds the index of household economic status (and the exposure variables), and equations (3) (or 3 and 4) add the proximate determinants in sequence. When evaluating the hypothesis regarding interaction of physical access to health services (proxied by urban-rural residence) with education, an interaction term is added to the equation, along with the urban-rural (main effect) dummy variable. A test of the hypothesis that the estimated education and interaction effects (i.e. on mortality, stunting, etc.) are not different from 1.0 (the null hypothesis) due merely to chance probability was accomplished using the Wald statistic,[13] the square of the ratio of the estimated coefficient to its standard error, compared against a $X^2$ distribution with one degree freedom:

$$(b_i / \text{SE}(b_i))^2 \sim X^2 \text{ ( 1 df )}.$$

Sex of child and the multiplicity of the birth are included in the mortality and anthropometric status models, so as to adjust for potential imbalance in these risk related variables across key study variables.


## Results

The concern and challenge of comparative analysis is in seeking to identify common patterns across countries, while maintaining an objective eye to the possibility of real variation among countries. The results of this study are presented in a way that hopefully facilitates comparisons amongst countries. While countries are grouped regionally for purpose of easy location of results for specific countries, regional generalizations were not the intent of the analysis and indeed were avoided because of the obvious lack of regional representativeness. At the risk of tempting the reader to 'average-away' interesting exceptions to otherwise common patterns, trimeans[14] are provided to assist the reader in summarizing results.

### Maternal education and neonatal mortality
The probability of dying in the first month of life varies from a low of 16 per thousand in Sri Lanka to a high of 43 per thousand in Ghana. Table 2 shows the estimated effects of mother's education on neonatal mortality. While the clear pattern is for low or no education to be associated with higher mortality risk, in 10 of 17 countries studied, the gross education effects are small and not statistically different from the null value of

1.00. Of the 6 countries showing significant gross effects, two low mortality countries, Colombia and Thailand have the greatest education differentials. As expected, children of women lacking any education fare worst, and (with few exceptions) children of secondary educated women experience the lowest probability of neonatal mortality. But in the cases of Togo, Ghana and Senegal, children of uneducated women (after controlling for economic status in the case of Ghana and Senegal) are at lowest risk of neonatal death. It is plausible that at least part of this unusual finding could be explained by (1) differential omission of births not surviving the neonatal period or (2) a tendency to report neonatal deaths to have occurred in the first completed month, related to educational level. It may on the other hand be true that to a certain extent, the tendency for such differential omission and age at death misreporting occurs in all settings, but that only in settings with genuinely weak education effects on neonatal survival do these effects become apparent.

The extent to which economic status of the household confounds the education-neonatal mortality also varies widely; inclusion of the economic index (equation 2) erases on average about 35% (not shown) of the excess risk associated with no education and 16% of excess risk associated with primary education in 'A' countries (with statistically significant estimates), and 40% of the excess risk in Mali, the only 'B' country with significantly elevated neonatal risk associated with education. Interestingly, the effect of inclusion of variables that capture variation in the pattern of family formation (equation 3), is either insubstantial or works to amplify the education advantage. Kenya is the most notable in this regard, here suggesting that less education is associated with family formation patterns that reduce rather than increase neonatal mortality risk, ceteris paribus. Addition of the health service use variables in equation (4) (non-use of tetanus toxoid and non-use of antenatal care during the index pregnancy) generally tends to move the education coefficients towards the null value (suggesting that these variables operate to mediate in part the education advantage), but the effects are small. Only in Bolivia, is the drop in the education effect substantial – about 50% of the none/secondary effect and about 40% of the primary/secondary effect. More typical is the case of Egypt, where the health service use variables play a smaller role in explaining the education advantage (about 10% of the none/secondary contrast and less than 5% of the primary/secondary contrast).

Interaction effects vary considerably across countries. Rural areas (with assumed lower access to modern health services) show a stronger education effect than urban areas in 8 of 17 countries, but only in Egypt and especially in Togo is the effect statistically significant. For example, in Togo the relative risk of neonatal mortality associated with education is more than five times greater among rural children ($RR_{none/sec.} = 1.45$) than among urban children ($RR_{none/sec.} = 0.26$). Thus, the unusual national-level effect mentioned above for Togo is explained by the unusually high neonatal mortality among children of secondary educated women in towns. Only in Uganda is the education effect significantly greater among urban ($RR_{none/sec.} = 3.42$) than among rural children ($RR_{none/sec.} = 0.51$); thus, the national-level estimates effectively mask an underlying urban-rural difference.

In sum, the association between maternal education and neonatal survival varies from virtually no effect to moderately strong effects. A substantial part of the education advantage is explained by education's link to economic status of the household, and is about as likely to be more pronounced in higher-access urban areas as in lower-access rural areas. The intermediate (behavioral) variables, with few exceptions, do relatively little to explain how the education advantage may be effected.

## Maternal education and postneonatal mortality (1–23 months)

The approach to analysis of postneonatal risk differs from neonatal risk analysis in three ways: first, a hazards regression is used to estimate effects; second, equation (2) includes not only the economic index but also variables related to household water supply and sanitary conditions, reportedly important precursors to mortality during this age segment conditioned by measured and unmeasured economic actors; and lastly, an index of health service utilization is used in equation (4) that intends to capture variation in a mothers propensity to use modern health services important to health and survival during the 1–23 month period. Notice that the range of mortality probabilities is much wider during these ages (an 8-fold difference between lowest and highest levels) than during the neonatal period (less than 3-fold difference). Consequently, for the countries with relatively low mortality (Sri Lanka, Thailand and Colombia), estimates of education effects on postneonatal mortality are subject to substantial statistical imprecision. In these cases, reference cells for study of interaction (i.e. urban children of mothers with secondary education) contain no deaths, resulting in undefined parameter estimates.

Table 3 shows that, with the exceptions of Bolivia, Colombia, Mali and Burundi, the effect of maternal education on mortality risk is more pronounced during ages 1–23 months than during the neonatal period. Apart from the case of Thailand, where estimates are relatively unstable, the education advantage is most pronounced in Guatemala ($RR_{none/sec.} = 4.10$; $RR_{prim./sec.} = 4.43$) and Egypt ($RR_{none/sec.} = 3.08$; $RR_{prim./sec.} = 2.21$), although none/secondary gross effects for Bolivia, Dominican Republic, and Zimbabwe are also above $RR = 2.0$ even after controlling for economic status.

The education-postneonatal mortality relationship is confounded by economic status of the household to roughly the same extent as was observed in analysis of the neonatal period; among 'A' countries with significant gross effects, 40% of the excess risk related to lacking any maternal education and 30% related to primary education may be explained by economic condition; among 'B' countries, 50% of excess risk is accounted for by economic condition. As was observed in the neonatal analysis, addition of the family formation variables tends to push the estimated education effect away rather than towards the null value, again suggesting that in some countries (see Kenya, in particular), lacking any education is correlated with safer categories of the family formation variables. This observation does not, however, hold universally; in Guatemala, Dominican Republic, and Thailand, a substantial drop in the education effect is observed in equation (3).

Addition of the index of health service use moves the education effect towards the null value in most countries, but this pattern is pronounced only in the cases of Zim-

**Table 3** Relative risks of postneonatal mortality (1–23 months) associated with maternal education. Gross effects, effects controlled for economic status (equation 2), effects with addition of family formation variables (equation 3) and health service use index (equation 4), and interaction effects (rural vs urban)

| 'A' Countries | Postneonatal mortality ratio(/00) | No education vs secondary education | | | | | Primary vs secondary education | | | | |
|---|---|---|---|---|---|---|---|---|---|---|---|
| Country | | Equation (1) (gross) | Equation (2) | Equation (3) | Equation (4) | Interaction | Equation (1) (gross) | Equation (2) | Equation (3) | Equation (4) | Interaction |
| Bolivia | 61 | 2.46*** | 2.01** | 2.01** | 1.78** | 0.76 | 2.28*** | 2.01*** | 1.93** | 1.78** | 0.51 |
| Colombia | 14 | 1.15 | 0.47 | 0.47 | 0.46 | UD | 1.19 | 0.76 | 0.91 | 0.91 | UD |
| Dominican R. | 40 | 2.56*** | 2.11*** | 1.84* | 1.69 | 0.26** | 1.86*** | 1.59* | 1.44 | 1.39 | 0.27 |
| Guatemala | 50 | 5.58*** | 4.10** | 3.56** | 3.52** | 0.22 | 5.70*** | 4.43** | 4.14** | 4.06** | 0.16 |
| Egypt | 42 | 4.10*** | 3.08*** | 3.17*** | 2.83*** | 0.28*** | 2.49*** | 2.21*** | 2.23*** | 2.14*** | 0.31** |
| Thailand | 12 | 11.70** | 7.17** | 5.20 | 4.57 | UD | 9.49** | 6.11** | 5.52 | 5.31 | UD |
| Sri Lanka | 10 | 2.64** | 1.45 | 1.52 | 1.44 | UD | 0.90 | 0.63 | 0.67 | 0.65 | UD |
| Ghana | 50 | 1.65** | 1.31 | 1.30 | 1.30 | 2.08* | 1.42 | 1.26 | 1.24 | 1.26 | 1.53 |
| Kenya | 46 | 2.20*** | 1.51** | 1.73** | 1.73** | 0.56* | 1.77*** | 1.47*** | 1.47*** | 1.46** | 0.57* |
| Uganda | 78 | 1.54* | 1.36 | 1.44 | 1.44 | 0.71 | 1.35 | 1.15 | 1.26 | 1.33 | 0.84 |
| Zimbabwe | 28 | 2.26** | 2.39** | 2.77*** | 2.27** | 0.47 | 1.29 | 1.40 | 1.48 | 1.11 | 0.47 |
| trimean | 39 | 2.48 | 1.98 | 1.92 | 1.82 | 0.47 | 1.77 | 1.52 | 1.54 | 1.45 | 0.46 |

| 'B' Countries | Postneonatal mortality ratio | None vs any education | | | | |
|---|---|---|---|---|---|---|
| Country | | Equation (1) (gross) | Equation (2) | Equation (3) | Equation (4) | Interaction |
| Morocco | 39 | 2.55*** | 1.57 | 1.60 | 1.33 | 0.98 |
| Tunisia | 23 | 1.45* | 1.20 | 1.23 | 1.19 | 0.49* |
| Burundi | 53 | 1.00 | 1.19 | 1.22 | 1.27 | 0.91 |
| Mali | 73 | 1.73** | 1.45* | 1.54* | 1.59* | 1.26 |
| Senegal | 67 | 1.67** | 1.41 | 1.45 | 1.44 | 0.58* |
| Togo | 48 | 1.40* | 1.19 | 1.25 | 1.14 | 1.09 |
| trimean | 53 | 1.56 | 1.31 | 1.35 | 1.22 | 0.88 |

*Estimated effect significant at $P < 0.10$; ** at $P < 0.05$; *** at $P < 0.01$.
UD—undefined; no deaths in reference category (i.e. children of urban women with secondary education) or no observations in one of contrasted subgroups.

Table 4 Relative risks of stunting among children aged 3–23 months at survey associated with maternal education. Gross effects, effects controlled for economic status (equation 2), effects with addition of family formation variables (equation 3) and health service use index (equation 4), and interaction effects (rural vs urban). Stunted if $< -2$ SD below NCHS/WHO reference median height-forage

'A' Countries

| Country | % Stunted | No education vs secondary education | | | | | Primary vs secondary education | | | | |
|---|---|---|---|---|---|---|---|---|---|---|---|
| | | Equation (1) (gross) | Equation (2) | Equation (3) | Equation (4) | Interaction | Equation (1) (gross) | Equation (2) | Equation (3) | Equation (4) | Interaction |
| Bolivia | 29.7 | 2.34*** | 1.81*** | 1.78*** | 1.55** | 1.69 | 1.72*** | 1.46** | 1.43** | 1.28 | 1.30 |
| Colombia | 21.1 | 3.74*** | 2.89*** | 2.36** | 1.98** | 2.77** | 1.93*** | 1.65*** | 1.51** | 1.34 | 0.61 |
| Domin. Rep. | 20.5 | 4.30*** | 2.78*** | 2.58*** | 2.54*** | 1.41 | 2.92*** | 2.09*** | 1.98** | 1.96** | 1.00 |
| Guatemala | 52.4 | 2.34*** | 1.70** | 1.62** | 1.48* | 0.24** | 1.70*** | 1.29* | 1.22 | 1.17 | 0.38 |
| Egypt | 29.4 | 1.68*** | 1.28** | 1.16 | 1.15 | 0.98 | 1.31* | 1.08 | 1.02 | 1.00 | 1.02 |
| Thailand | 16.7 | 2.93*** | 2.02** | 2.03** | 1.95*** | 0.41 | 2.81*** | 2.09*** | 2.16*** | 2.15** | 0.61 |
| Sri Lanka | 25.3 | 2.30*** | 1.56*** | 1.56*** | 1.43** | 2.30 | 1.83*** | 1.39*** | 1.39*** | 1.36** | 0.68 |
| Ghana | 23.1 | 1.35** | 1.23* | 1.21 | 1.17 | 0.81 | 1.31** | 1.19 | 1.21 | 1.13 | 0.88 |
| Uganda | 36.9 | 1.82*** | 1.36** | 1.44** | 1.33* | 0.90 | 1.59** | 1.27 | 1.31* | 1.27 | 1.18 |
| Zimbabwe | 25.9 | 2.26*** | 1.69** | 1.62** | 1.46 | 1.11 | 1.76*** | 1.35** | 1.32* | 1.25 | 1.50 |
| trimean | 25.6 | 2.32 | 1.65 | 1.64 | 1.52 | 1.10 | 1.74 | 1.39 | 1.36 | 1.27 | 0.89 |

'B' Countries

| Country | % Stunted | None vs any education | | | | |
|---|---|---|---|---|---|---|
| | | (Equation 1) (gross) | Equation (2) | Equation (3) | Equation (4) | Interaction |
| Morocco | 22.6 | 2.07*** | 1.43** | 1.43** | 1.24 | 1.14 |
| Tunisia | 15.6 | 1.60*** | 1.27 | 1.27 | 1.18 | 1.89** |
| Burundi | 38.4 | 1.36** | 1.16 | 1.17 | 1.16 | 0.57* |
| Mali | 20.5 | 1.13 | 0.92 | 0.95 | 0.93 | 0.87 |
| Senegal | 20.5 | 2.05** | 1.72* | 1.68 | 1.68 | 0.67 |
| Togo | 29.7 | 1.22* | 1.09 | 1.15 | 1.15 | 1.45 |
| trimean | 22.9 | 1.51 | 1.23 | 1.24 | 1.18 | 1.00 |

Note: In Senegal, the age range of children is 6–23 months.
*Estimated effect significant at $P < 0.10$; ** at $P < 0.05$; *** at $P < 0.01$.

babwe, Bolivia, and Dominican Republic, where 30, 22 and 19% of the education effect is explained by differential use of services, and Morocco, where 45%, of the (non-significant) effect is explained.

In contrast to the neonatal period, the education effect tends to be more pronounced in the urban than the rural setting. Among 'A' countries, the relative risk of postneonatal mortality related to maternal education is about twice as large among urban children than among rural children. In Egypt, Dominican Republic, Kenya, Tunisia and Senegal, this pattern is particularly remarkable. For example, in urban Egypt, postneonatal mortality is 4.81 times greater among children of uneducated women and 3.39 times greater among children of women with primary education than among those with secondary education, ceteris paribus. In rural Egypt, the corresponding relative risks are 1.32 and 1.03.

In sum, postneonatal mortality risk is roughly twice as sensitive to the effects of maternal education as neonatal risk, after controlling for economic condition of the household. Both risk-elevating behaviors (high-risk biodemographic profile of births) and risk-diminishing behaviors (greater use of health services) appear to be associated with higher maternal education. Measures of these behaviors, however, do relatively little on the whole to explain how the education effect is mediated. It does appear clear that there exists a tendency among the countries studied here for the education advantage in postneonatal survival to be more pronounced in urban settings as compared to the rural areas, which is in contrast to observations on the neonatal period when risk is equally sensitive to maternal education in the lower-access rural setting. These observations are further discussed in the last section.

### Maternal education and growth faltering (children aged 3–23 months)

Stunting and low weight-for-age are not independent phenomena. Since a child's weight is in part a function of her height, many children who are stunted will also be underweight and visa versa. It is thus expected that some risk factors for stunting would also predispose towards being underweight. However, short-term seasonal fluctuations in food availability and disease prevalence will disproportionately effect a child's cross-sectional weight (and weight for-age), while a child's linear growth (and height-for age) is less sensitive to such fluctuations and thus better indicates long-term patterns of undernutrition and recurrent infection. It is probably also the case that stunting (deceleration in linear growth) reflects physiologic adaptation to routine and chronic nutritional deficits, and does not necessarily indicate increased susceptibility to disease and death. This is reflected in previous studies showing that stunting is much less closely associated with mortality risk than low weight-for-age (36, 37). Among the 17 countries studied here, the prevalence of stunting ranges from a high in Guatemala (52%) to a low in Tunisia (16%); the percentage of children underweight is highest in Sri Lanka (38%) and lowest in Tunisia (10%). While stunting tends to be more common (trimean of 24.7%) than underweight status (19.9%), in four countries (Sri Lanka, Mali, Ghana and Thailand), children are more likely to be underweight than stunted.

*Stunting (low height-for-age).* Table 4 shows that stunting of children early in life is strongly related to maternal education, with the notable exceptions of Mali and Togo where the estimated gross effects of education are on the small side. On average, the education advantage is less pronounced for stunting than for postneonatal mortality, especially after including the control for economic status of the household. Among 'A' countries, the introduction of the economic index (equation 2), reduces the excess risk associated with no education by 47%, excess risk associated with primary education by 50% and among 'B' countries excess risk drops by 52%. However, even after controlling for economic status, children of women with no education are at least twice as likely to be stunted in Colombia, Dominican Republic and Thailand as children of secondary educated women.

Introduction of the family formation variables (equation 3) does little to change the education coefficients. Only in the case of Colombia and Egypt is the education-stunting relationship appreciably explained through differentials in the biodemographic profiles of births. In the remaining countries, either there is observed no mediating effect of these variables or the effect is to move the education effect away from the null value as was observed in the mortality analyses. Among 'A' countries showing significant education effects in equation, addition of the health services use index results in a drop in the no education effect of 20%, and in the primary education effect of 16%. Among 'B' countries, only Morocco has a significant equation (3) effect, 44% of which is explained through use of health services.

Regarding differences in the education effect between urban-rural strata, no general pattern is observed across countries. The education advantage is more pronounced in the rural areas of Colombia and Tunisia, but greater in the urban areas of Guatemala and Burundi. In the remaining countries, no significant interaction effects were observed.

*Underweight status (low weight-for-age).* The gross relationship between maternal education and underweight status is more pronounced than the education-stunting relationship (Table 5), and is roughly of the same magnitude as was estimated in the postneonatal mortality analysis. This is, however, largely due to greater confounding with economic status; 56% of the excess risk associated with no education is related to economic status, and 61% of excess risk associated with primary education among 'A' countries. Among 'B' countries, 56%, excess risk associated with education is due to confounding with economic condition. Thus, larger education effects on low weight-for-age (compared to the stunting model) are largely erased in equation (2), and reversed (when compared to the postneonatal mortality model). A discussion of this pattern is taken up later.

As already observed in the analyses of mortality and stunting, the relationship between education and low weight-for-age is, in most countries, little affected by inclusion of family formation variables (equation 3). Yet, in the exceptional case of Egypt, the education coefficient drops 30% (equation 3), suggesting that the education effect is in part related to education's link to the distribution of births by birth order, birth interval, and maternal age (i.e. less educated women tend to exhibit higher risk reproductive patterns). The remaining countries show similar, but more modest effects, no effects, or effects that operate in the opposite direction. Use of health services appears even less important in mediating the education-underweight relationship (average change in excess risk in equation (4) among countries with significant no education effects = 10%) than in mediating the education-stunting relationship (20%).

No general pattern was observed regarding interaction effects; the only significant interaction occurred in Guatemala, where the relative risk associated with no education in the urban setting was 3.5, compared to 1.1 in the rural setting.

## Maternal education and health service use

The effects of maternal education on two measures of health service utilization: (1) non-use of tetanus toxoid during pregnancy (NoTT) and (2) non-use of modern health system during pregnancy (NoANC), are examined in Table 6 and Table 7. Notice that the percentage non-use varies in the extreme, especially regarding anti-tetanus injection.[15]

*Non-use of tetanus toxoid during pregnancy (NoTT).* The strength of the education-NoTT varies widely from virtually no gross effect observed at the national level in Colombia and Guatemala to strong effects in the Dominican Republic, Sri Lanka, Ghana, Kenya, Uganda, Burundi and Togo (Table 6). Even after control for economic condition of the household, NoTT is about twice as likely among children of non-educated women as those with secondary education in the Dominican Republic, Sri Lanka, Ghana, and Kenya and as those with any education in Togo. The extent to which the gross education effect is confounded by economic status also varies considerably; for example, in Uganda 46% of the gross education effect (none/secondary) is explained by variation in economic status, whereas in Bolivia, only three percent is so explained.

Differences in the pattern of family formation are apparently not a major factor in explaining the education-NoTT relationship. Only in the case of Thailand does the introduction of these variables substantially diminish the size of the education effect (39%). On average among 'A' countries, only nine percent of the excess risk associated with no education is erased in equation (3), and only 13% of the excess risk associated with primary education; among 'B' countries, the excess risk explained is 7%.

In 14 of the 17 countries studied here, NoTT is more closely tied to maternal education in the rural areas than in urban areas. Kenya is a particularly notable case; in the rural milieu, NoTT is 2.64 times more likely among children of uneducated women and 1.76 times more likely among children of primary educated women as among children of women with secondary education. In urban Kenya, non-use is more prevalent among the educated ($RR_{none/sec.} = 0.69$; $RR_{prim./sec.} = 0.83$). This pattern of greater NoTT among the educated is observed clearly in Guatemala, Colombia, Zimbabwe, and to lesser extent in Egypt, and while not evident in other countries may still be an underlying phenomenon that tends to attenuate the education effect generally. This finding is discussed in a later section.

*Non-use of antenatal services (NoANC).* Of the dependent variables studied here, NoANC is most closely linked to levels of maternal education. Among the 'A' countries, the level of excess risk of NoANC associated with no education ranges from 70% in Kenya to 2100% in the Dominican Republic; excess risk associated with primary education ranges from 31% in Kenya to over 700% in Thailand (Table 7). These enormous differentials in NoANC are, on average, reduced by only 26% for both the none/secondary and primary/secondary contrasts with the introduction of the economic index

**Table 5** Relative risks of underweight among children aged 3–23 months at survey associated with maternal education. Gross effects, effects controlled for economic status (equation 2), effects with addition of family formation variables (equation 3) and health service use index (equation 4), and interaction effects (rural vs urban). Underweight if $< -2$ SD below NCHS/WHO reference median weight-forage

'A' Countries

| Country | % Underweight | No education vs secondary education | | | | | Primary vs secondary education | | | | |
|---|---|---|---|---|---|---|---|---|---|---|---|
| | | Equation (1) (gross) | Equation (2) | Equation (3) | Equation (4) | Interaction | Equation (1) (gross) | Equation (2) | Equation (3) | Equation (4) | Interaction |
| Bolivia | 12.8 | 1.96** | 1.35 | 1.23 | 1.04 | 2.76 | 1.43* | 1.12 | 1.06 | 0.91 | 2.66 |
| Columbia | 11.0 | 2.10** | 1.63 | 1.40 | 1.30 | 1.35 | 1.74* | 1.43 | 1.31 | 1.27 | 0.98 |
| Domin. Rep. | 12.7 | 4.01*** | 2.39** | 2.07** | 1.88** | 1.57 | 2.69*** | 1.85** | 1.62* | 1.57* | 0.52 |
| Guatemala | 30.4 | 3.64*** | 2.33** | 2.29** | 2.14** | 0.31* | 2.48*** | 1.71* | 1.70* | 1.65 | 0.33* |
| Egypt | 14.4 | 4.19*** | 2.48** | 2.03** | 2.06** | 2.00 | 3.42*** | 2.40*** | 2.10*** | 2.10** | 1.10 |
| Thailand | 18.6 | 3.53*** | 2.23** | 2.22** | 2.12** | 0.43 | 2.91*** | 2.08*** | 2.15*** | 2.11** | 1.07 |
| Sri Lanka | 38.1 | 1.58*** | 1.15 | 1.14 | 1.01 | 1.14 | 1.32*** | 1.04 | 1.04 | 1.00 | 0.60 |
| Ghana | 28.3 | 1.16 | 1.10 | 1.07 | 1.05 | 1.22 | 1.11 | 1.00 | 0.96 | 0.93 | 1.28 |
| Uganda | 23.2 | 1.79** | 1.44* | 1.49* | 1.39 | 1.37 | 1.28 | 1.10 | 1.15 | 1.11 | 1.10 |
| Zimbabwe | 10.3 | 3.35*** | 1.78 | 1.92* | 2.05* | UD | 1.78* | 1.04 | 1.23 | 1.19 | UD |
| trimean | 18.2 | 2.61 | 1.74 | 1.65 | 1.56 | 1.34 | 1.82 | 1.32 | 1.32 | 1.26 | 0.94 |

'B' Countries

| Country | % Underweight | None vs any education | | | | |
|---|---|---|---|---|---|---|
| | | Equation (1) (gross) | Equation (2) | Equation (3) | Equation (4) | Interaction |
| Morocco | 14.9 | 3.36*** | 1.85** | 1.75*** | 1.51 | 0.43 |
| Tunisia | 10.1 | 1.36* | 1.01 | 1.06 | 0.97 | 1.15 |
| Burundi | 32.6 | 1.31** | 1.10 | 1.10 | 1.10 | 1.36 |
| Mali | 29.4 | 1.12 | 0.99 | 1.00 | 0.96 | 0.72 |
| Senegal | 20.0 | 3.15*** | 3.02** | 3.12** | 2.99** | 0.67 |
| Togo | 24.7 | 1.66*** | 1.43** | 1.52*** | 1.52*** | 1.44 |
| trimean | 22.3 | 1.72 | 1.29 | 1.31 | 1.25 | 0.93 |

Note: For Senegal, the age range for children is 6–23 months
*Estimated effect significant at $P < 0.10$; ** at $P < 0.05$; *** at $P < 0.01$.
UD—undefined; no children underweight in reference group (i.e. urban mothers with secondary education).

**Table 6** Relative risks of non-use of tetanus toxoid associated with maternal education. Gross effects, effects controlled for economic status (equation 2), effects controlled for family formation (equation 3) and interaction effect (rural vs urban)

### 'A' Countries

| Country | % Non-use | No education vs secondary education | | | | Primary vs secondary | | | |
|---|---|---|---|---|---|---|---|---|---|
| | | Equation (1) (gross) | Equation (2) | Equation (3) | Interaction | Equation (1) (gross) | Equation (2) | Equation (3) | Interaction |
| Bolivia | 76.0 | 1.33*** | 1.32*** | 1.32*** | 1.19 | 1.14 | 1.13 | 1.13 | 0.99 |
| Colombia | 61.6 | 1.01 | 0.99 | 0.96 | 1.89*** | 1.08** | 1.08** | 1.06 | 1.42** |
| Dom. Rep. | 12.0 | 2.92*** | 2.60*** | 2.45*** | 1.66 | 1.63*** | 1.51*** | 1.43** | 1.18 |
| Guatemala | 86.2 | 1.02 | 1.01 | 1.01 | 1.23 | 0.93 | 0.93 | 0.93 | 0.84 |
| Egypt | 87.6 | 1.07** | 1.07** | 1.06** | 1.57*** | 1.03* | 1.03* | 1.02 | 1.52*** |
| Thailand | 34.5 | 1.69*** | 1.56*** | 1.34*** | 2.47*** | 1.09 | 1.01 | 0.95 | 2.30*** |
| Sri Lanka | 13.2 | 2.05*** | 1.91*** | 1.93*** | 1.63 | 1.48*** | 1.41*** | 1.31*** | 1.05 |
| Ghana | 29.1 | 2.35*** | 1.90*** | 1.87*** | 1.07 | 1.63*** | 1.47*** | 1.42*** | 0.80 |
| Kenya | 9.7 | 2.01*** | 1.96*** | 1.90*** | 3.75*** | 1.33*** | 1.33** | 1.33** | 2.12*** |
| Uganda | 43.6 | 2.10*** | 1.59*** | 1.59*** | 0.96 | 1.69*** | 1.33*** | 1.32** | 1.10 |
| Zimbabwe | 20.1 | 1.33** | 1.24** | 1.21 | 1.50* | 1.13 | 1.00 | 1.05 | 2.75*** |
| trimean | 38.6 | 1.63 | 1.52 | 1.40 | 1.54 | 1.34 | 1.27 | 1.25 | 1.27 |

### 'B' Countries

| Country | % Non-use | None vs any education | | | |
|---|---|---|---|---|---|
| | | Equation (1) (gross) | Equation (2) | Equation (3) | Interaction |
| Tunisia | 66.8 | 1.19*** | 1.18*** | 1.14*** | 1.31*** |
| Morocco | ND | ND | ND | ND | ND |
| Burundi | 36.2 | 1.85*** | 1.66*** | 1.64*** | 0.87 |
| Mali | 71.6 | 1.75*** | 1.47*** | 1.48*** | 1.07 |
| Senegal | 68.9 | 1.51*** | 1.35*** | 1.33*** | 1.57*** |
| Toto | 28.4 | 2.18*** | 1.93*** | 1.91*** | 1.64** |
| trimean | 59.7 | 1.71 | 1.48 | 1.48 | 1.30 |

*Estimated effect significant at $P < 0.10$; ** at $P < 0.05$; *** at $P < 0.001$; ^ at $P < 0.01$.
ND—no data available on use of tetanus toxoid.

**Table 7** Relative risks of non-use of antenatal care associated with maternal education. Gross effects, effects controlled for economic status (equation 2), effects controlled for family formation (equation 3) and interaction effect (rural vs urban). 17 DHS counties

### 'A' Countries

| Country | % Non-use | No education vs secondary education | | | | Primary vs secondary | | | |
|---|---|---|---|---|---|---|---|---|---|
| | | Equation (1) (gross) | Equation (2) | Equation (3) | Interaction | Equation (1) (gross) | Equation (2) | Equation (3) | Interaction |
| Bolivia | 50.7 | 6.28*** | 6.11*** | 6.01*** | 0.88 | 4.21*** | 3.99*** | 3.82*** | 0.89 |
| Columbia | 26.9 | 6.34*** | 5.10*** | 4.53*** | 0.86 | 3.93*** | 3.35*** | 3.13*** | 1.28 |
| Dom. Rep. | 5.6 | 22.29*** | 14.29*** | 12.94*** | UD | 6.84*** | 5.01*** | 4.53*** | UD |
| Guatemala | 65.8 | 5.83*** | 4.42*** | 4.23*** | 0.75 | 3.95*** | 2.73*** | 2.59*** | 0.81 |
| Egypt | 45.6 | 3.07*** | 2.61*** | 2.39*** | 0.63*** | 2.25*** | 2.03*** | 1.83*** | 0.77* |
| Thailand | 19.0 | 18.70*** | 11.96*** | 9.27*** | 1.26 | 8.36*** | 5.16*** | 4.44*** | 0.73 |
| Sri Lanka | 3.8 | 6.95*** | 6.17*** | 5.84*** | 1.95 | 2.07*** | 1.89*** | 1.76** | 1.38 |
| Ghana | 16.4 | 5.34*** | 3.55** | 3.39*** | 0.55 | 2.61*** | 2.12*** | 2.04*** | 0.40* |
| Kenya | 22.3 | 1.72*** | 1.61*** | 1.55*** | 1.14 | 1.31*** | 1.25*** | 1.24*** | 1.03 |
| Uganda | 12.5 | 5.90*** | 3.26*** | 3.37*** | 0.44 | 2.87*** | 1.76** | 1.84*** | 0.54 |
| Zimbabwe | 7.5 | 5.29*** | 4.94*** | 5.06*** | 0.47 | 3.30*** | 3.26*** | 3.42*** | 0.98 |
| trimean | 21.1 | 5.95 | 4.75 | 4.50 | 0.76 | 3.21 | 2.71 | 2.58 | 0.81 |

### 'B' Countries

| Country | % Non-use | None vs any education | | | |
|---|---|---|---|---|---|
| | | Equation (1) (gross) | Equation (2) | Equation (3) | Interaction |
| Morocco | 75.2 | 2.12*** | 1.81*** | 1.80*** | 1.13 |
| Tunisia | 42.4 | 2.19*** | 1.90*** | 1.69*** | 0.84 |
| Burundi | 17.7 | 3.00*** | 2.59*** | 2.54*** | 0.63 |
| Mali | 57.7 | 2.30*** | 1.80*** | 1.79*** | 0.93 |
| Senegal | 37.3 | 5.34*** | 3.72*** | 3.65*** | 1.05 |
| Togo | 33.8 | 2.66*** | 2.46*** | 2.35*** | 1.59** |
| trimean | 42.1 | 2.50 | 2.17 | 2.14 | 0.99 |

*Estimated effect significant at $P < 0.10$; ** at $P < 0.05$; *** at $P < 0.01$.
UD—undefined; no non-users with secondary education in rural area.

in equation (2). Among 'B' countries non-use is from 2 to 5 times more likely among uneducated women as women with any education, and 27% of this effect is explained by education's link to economic status of the household.

As in the analysis of NoTT, the pattern of family formation by and large does little to explain how the education effect is mediated (on average, 9% of the education effect is so explained among 'A' countries, and 7% among 'B' countries). In Thailand and Tunisia, however, the change in the education effect from equations (2) to (3) is 25% and 24%, respectively, suggesting that in these cases, the biodemographic profile of children (birth interval length, birth order, and maternal age at birth) may play a role in the education-NoANC relationship.

The interaction effect observed in several countries regarding NoTT (i.e. greater education advantage in the rural areas) is not seen in the analysis of NoANC, with the exception of Togo. Indeed, among 'A' countries, it is more common to find that the education effect on NoANC is more pronounced in the urban than in the rural setting. However, only in the case of Egypt was this pattern found statistically significant.

## Summary and discussion

This study examined the DHS data of 17 developing countries with the aim of addressing a set of questions regarding the statistical association of maternal education with child health and survival. Multivariate logistic and hazards regressions were used to estimate the education effect on neonatal mortality, postneonatal mortality (1–23 months), stunting (3–23 months), underweight status (3–23 months), and non-use of selected health services. Several points emerged from the analysis.

1 While this study has found significantly elevated risks of dying throughout the first 2 years of life associated with low levels of mother's education, mortality risk during the 1–23 month period is more than twice as sensitive to the education effect than during the neonatal period. In only 5 of 17 countries did the education effect remain statistically relevant after controlling for economic condition of the household. These findings are consistent with similar results of Hobcraft et al. (5) and with the hypothesis that personal assets (including maternal education) condition key risk-modifying behaviors to a greater extent as the child ages and thus as household-based decisions regarding susceptibility and exposure to disease become increasingly important in delineating mortality risk. That there exists important exceptions to this pattern (Bolivia, Colombia, Mali and Burundi), however, makes this generalization less compelling as a model on which to base interpretations for individual countries outside this particular analysis.

2 In this study, variations in the strength of the education effect between urban and rural settings were examined. It has been suggested that physical access (i.e. proximity in terms of distance and travel time) is an important (co)factor in determining use of modern health services, and that education may confer skills and attitudes that help women overcome these hurdles. If this is true, education differentials should be larger, ceteris paribus, in areas where health services are more difficult to reach. Yet, in general, the results for postneonatal mortality indicate the opposite; to wit, the education advantage

in survival is more pronounced in urban areas. An alternative hypothesis is that an urban environment imposes unique and difficult challenges on mothers regarding social and economic integration. An urban mother may need to engage more actively in the public domain, having less reliance on familial mechanisms of support to maintain and improve the health of her children. These results may indicate that, rather than physical access to modern health services, it is access to broader social and economic support systems that is limiting in the urban context. Lacking education is plainly maladaptive in towns, in the rural areas, less so. Furthermore, educated women in the rural areas, may still be under considerable social pressure to maintain traditional (but harmful) practices concerning patterns of nutrition, and the recognition and treatment of illnesses. Such constraints are probably less compelling within the urban socio-cultural landscape. Yet, in light of significant exceptions to this observed 'pattern' (e.g. Ghana, Mali, Togo), it seems imprudent to generalize broadly from these results without more detailed anthropological investigation. Still, these findings do corroborate broadly one view of Caldwell, that education enhances a woman's ability to manipulate critical aspects of the modern world, particularly regarding bureaucratic institutions that often dominate many aspects of urban life in developing countries (6).

Why is the pattern described above not observed as widely during the neonatal period? One explanation is that neonatal risk is more closely linked than is postneonatal risk to adverse pregnancy outcomes (e.g. intra-uterine growth retardation, prematurity, obstetrical trauma, etc.), as well as exposure and susceptibility to the tetanus pathogen in some of these countries – outcomes that are more easily modified by medical technology. Thus, immediate physical access to modern health technologies, both curative to reduce case-fatality from poor pregnancy outcome, and preventive in terms of hygienic delivery and tetanus toxoid use, may indeed be more relevant in the case of neonatal survival than for the postneonatal period. Personal assets (i.e. education) that help overcome impediments to physical access to these medical technologies are likely to be important in the rural setting.

3 The magnitude of the education advantage in growth faltering (during the 3–23 month period) roughly parallels that observed regarding effects observed on mortality during the 1–23 month period, a finding tending to support the hypothesis outlined in equation (1). It should however be considered that these estimates are likely to be biased slightly downwards by selection out of the sample of dead children (32). Interestingly, the economic condition of the child's household appears more closely tied to growth faltering than mortality, and thus operates to confound the education-stunting/underweight relationship to a greater degree than in the education-mortality relationship. This is summarized by way of trimeans in Figure 2, which shows clearly that the strength of the education-underweight relationship in particular is attenuated markedly from a level above to a level below that of education-postneonatal mortality in all 3 analytical subgroup contrasts. A plausible reading of this pattern is that: (A) while the economic status strongly constrains decisions on well-child care (especially, nutritional inputs), it figures less importantly once a child becomes ill, and (B) maternal education is important in conditioning decisions on both preventive and curative care, including timely recognition of and response to serious disease symptoms. In any case, these results

**Figure 2** Trimean of education effect on neonatal mortality, postneonatal mortality (1–23 months), stunting (3–23 months), underweight status (3–23 months). Gross effects, effects controlled for economic status (equation 2), and effects after inclusion of family formation variables (equation 3) and health services use variables (equation 4). Graphs A and B are based on trimeans of 11 'A' countries; graph C is based on trimeans of 6 'B' countries.

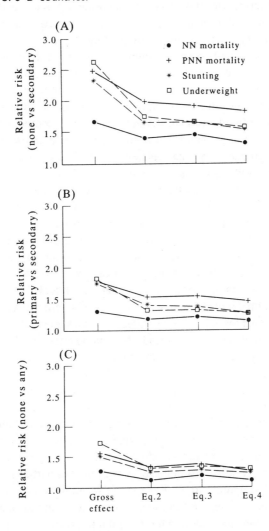

point clearly to increased acute and chronic undernutrition as likely biological stepping stones on the path between low maternal education and poor survival chances.

The distinction between education's impact on preventive versus curative action could be best addressed in longitudinal study of well versus sick children, to determine whether knowledge and perceptions of illness, a woman's autonomy in the household and other characteristics presumably related to education, impact on the path from health to sickness (including serious growth faltering) or from sickness to death to different degrees. The answer to these questions has obvious relevance for the allocation of resources to basic preventive child health programs as well as programs of food supplementation. It seems unlikely that cross-sectional and retrospective survey data of the type available from the DHS will ever provide adequate information that would serve to link treatment behaviors with mortality risk modification. Such analysis requires large numbers of children who died very close to the survey date, and for whom morbidity and treatment could be considered somewhat reliable. We already know that the quality of morbidity data diminishes very rapidly with time since survey and that reported treatment patterns may well be biased by mortality outcome.

4  There was observed a difference between urban and rural strata in the strength of the relationship between maternal education and reported non-use of tetanus toxoid; to wit, the education advantage, with a few exceptions, being more pronounced in the rural setting. In many countries, this pattern is the result of high reported non-use among the (secondary) educated in towns and may relate to greater use of private doctors, who, recognizing the considerably diminished risk of neonatal tetanus among their clients (i.e. urban elite), will often be less diligent in administering tetanus toxoid. In the rural setting (where the education-NoTT relationship is moderate to strong and in the expected direction in all countries), the hypothesis of Rozenzweig and Schultz may be invoked; namely, that where severe obstacles of access exist, education is key in placing a woman at a relative advantage in terms of securing these particular services (20). If so, then reducing such obstacles (improving physical access) could well improve use by uneducated rural mothers. In areas where neonatal tetanus still figures prominently as a cause of early infant death, such improved access could prove a important step towards better survival prospects.

5  Reported non-use of antenatal care (NoANC) was found enormously sensitive to the effects of maternal education. Even after controlling for economic status of the household and the biodemographic profile of the pregnancy, NoANC was 55 to 1300% higher among the uneducated than women with secondary education. Naturally, many more births are characterized by 'no antenatal care' than eventually will go on to die, and it was shown in the mortality analysis that only a small part of the education effect operates through differential non-use of health services. The most parsimonious explanation for these findings is that the education-NoANC relationship is genuine but that the types of services typically delivered in these settings (and in part captured in the DHS questionnaire) do relatively little to modify mortality risk. Few would argue that a single antenatal visit (of unknown character and quality), for instance, will substantially enhance child survival prospects during the neonatal or postneonatal period. In any case, this study can not (and did not intend to) evaluate ANC efficacy. Especially for the analysis of postneonatal risk, information related to use of services that could be expected to specifically enhance survival were unavailable from the DHS-I data for both living and dead children (e.g. immunizations, treatment of illness, details on the specific type of antenatal services received, etc.). Even if such data were available, the cross-sectional nature of the data would make causal interpretation of the relationship between use and survival tenuous at best. It is, on the other hand, significant that in

both high and low access settings, more educated women will use health services to a much greater extent than the uneducated.

6  With few exceptions, birth order, birth interval of a child, and the age of the mother do little to explain education-related differentials in mortality and growth faltering. Unexpectedly, in some countries studied here – most notably the case of neonatal and post-neonatal risk in Kenya – less education appears to be associated with a safer rather than riskier biodemographic profile of births. That the pattern of family formation can not appreciably explain the education advantage in child survival was previously observed in a re-analysis of Hobcraft et al. (5, 18) results by Cleland and Van Ginneken (1) and by Barbieri (17) in an analysis of the Senegal DHS data.

## Acknowledgements

The authors wish to thank Meredith John, Wamucii Njogu and Elisabeth Sommerfelt for their helpful comments on an earlier version of this paper, presented at the DHS World Conference, August 1991, Washington, DC.

## Notes

1  See Caldwell (6) and Schultz (7) for a review of the behavioral mechanisms that have been advanced to explain the education-mortality relationship.

2  See Trussell and Menken (28) for a review of problems related to unobserved heterogeneity in observational studies of child survival.

3  Indeed, this is why mortality after the second birthday is not examined at all. In all but the high mortality countries of West Africa, the number of deaths from the second to the fifth birthday is too small for meaningful analysis.

4  See Sullivan et al (13) for an assessment of the quality of DHS mortality data. In general, this study of 22 countries (including those used here) indicate no gross under-reporting of early childhood deaths. Age at death reporting was on the other hand a serious problem, especially heaping at 12 months, in countries of Sub-Saharan Africa.

5  In Senegal, a 1 in 3 sub-sample of households was selected for collection of anthropometric data. All surviving children 6–36 months old in the selected household were measured.

6  This age range was chosen so as to correspond as closely as possible with that used in the analysis of postneonatal mortality (i.e. 1–23 months).

7  Information (from the DHS-I) concerning use of health services among children deceased before the survey date were restricted to those variables considered here.

8  Unfortunately, most of the DHS surveys did not collect any data on exposure-related behaviors, that could be potentially conditioned by a mother's level of education.

9  In Bolivia, only the third type of household economic information was collected, so that the range of possible score was 0 to 2.

10  Children born within 2 years of the survey are censored before reaching their second birthday (i.e. before completing the 1–23 month period of observation). Hazards regression includes the survival of censored cases up to their age at censoring.

11  While the proportionality assumption is never fully satisfied with real data, sharp departures or changes in the direction of covariate effects with increasing age will tend to mask or attenuate true effects. Checks on proportionality of hazards across the age range 1–23 months were accomplished by inspecting educational level-specific survival curves. Also, when the numbers of deaths allowed, separate 1–6 months and 7–23 months regressions were run and examined for substantial age-varying effects. In no case were such effects large enough to alter the substantive conclusions drawn from the estimated effects of education on postneonatal mortality (1–23 months) presented in this paper.

12  Using the formula, $RR = RO / \{ 1 - p_{ref}) + (RO \quad p_{ref})\}$; where $RR$ is the relative risk, $RO$ the relative odds, and $p_{ref}$ the prevalence of the outcome in the reference group (i.e. children of women with secondary education).

13  The Wald statistic has the property that when the estimated coefficient is very large, the tests of statistical significance is conservative (i.e. leading one to fail to reject more frequently than most other tests the null hypothesis that, for instance, there is no relationship between education level and mortality) (33).

14  The trimean is calculated as $(Q_1 + 2Q_2 + Q_3)/4$; where $Q_1$ equals the first quartile value, $Q_2$ equals the median value, and $Q_3$ equals the third quartile value.

15  This was the principal rationale for transforming the estimates of relative odds to relative risks, thereby facilitating comparisons across countries with divergent non-use levels. However as a result, the distinction between statistically significance and practical relevance becomes a bit blurred. For example, small differences between education categories in absolute risk of non-use in high non-use countries (and thus small relative risks) may be found statistically significant, while in lower non-use settings, the same absolute difference in risk of non-use between education groups results in larger relative risks that are statistically non-significant. In other words, the sample size and prevalence of the outcome (non-use), in addition to the strength of the education-non use relationship, have bearing on statistical significance. Also, it is important to remember that any risk factor so prevalent as to make these considerations relevant (say, above 30%) is unlikely to be a key proximate determinant of any very rare outcome, like mortality. In any case, the practical importance of relative differences should be borne in mind in drawing conclusions from these results.

# References

1  Cleland J. and Van Ginneken J.K. Maternal education and child survival in developing countries: the search for pathways of influence. *Soc. Sci. Med.* 27, 1357–1368, 1988.

2  Cochrane S., O'Hare D. and Leslie J. The effects of education on health. *World Bank Working Papers*, No 405. World Bank, Washington, DC, 1980.

3  United Nations *Socio-Economic Differentials in Child Mortality in Developing Countries*. Department of International Economic and Social Affairs, New York, 1985.

4 Rutstein S.O. Socio-economic differentials in infant and child mortality: Preliminary Tables. *WFS Comparative Studies, Cross-national Summaries* International Statistical Institute, the Hague, Netherlands, 1984.

5   Hobcraft J., McDonald J. and Rutstein S.O. Socioeconomic Factors in Infant and Child Mortality: A Cross-National Comparison. *Pop Stud.* 38, 193–223, 1984.

6   Caldwell J.C. Education as a factor in mortality decline: an examination of Nigeria data. *Pop. Stud.* 33, 395–413, 1979.

7   Schultz T. Studying the impact of household, economic and community variables on child mortality. In *Child Survival: Strategies for Research* (Edited by Mosley W.H. and Chen L.C.) pp. 215–236, Population and Development Review 10, Suppl. Population Council, New York, 1984.

8   Friede A., Waternaux C., Guyer B., de Jesus A. and Filip L. An Epidemiological Assessment of Immunization Programme Participation in the Philippines. *Int. J. Epidemiol.* 14, 135–141, 1985.

9   Belcher D., Nicholas D., Ofusu-Amaah S. and Wurapa F.A. Mass immunization campaign in rural Ghana. *Publ. Hlth Rep.* 93, 170–176, 1978.

10  Boerma J.T., Sommerfelt A.E., Rutstein S.O. and Rojas G. *Immunization: Levels, Trends, and Differentials.* DHS Comparative Studies, No. 1. Institute for Resource Development, Columbia, MD, 1990.

11  Tekce B. and Shorter F. Determinants of child mortality: a study of squatter settlements in Jordan. In *Child Survival: Strategies for Research* (Edited by Mosley W.H. and Chen L.C.) pp. 257–280, Population and Development Review 10, Suppl. Population Council, New York, 1984.

12  Benyoussef A. and Wessen A. Utilization of health services in developing countries –Tunisia. *Soc. Sci. Med.* 8, 287–304, 1974.

13  Caldwell J.C., Reddy P. and Caldwell P. The social component of mortality decline: an investigation in south India employing alternative methodologies. *Pop. Stud. 37,* 185–205, 1983.

14  Mbacke C. and van de Walle E. *Socio-economic Factors and Access to Health Services as Determinants of Child Mortality.* IUSSP Seminar on Mortality and Society in Sub-Saharan Africa, Yaoundé, Cameroon, 1987.

15  Cebu Study Team. Underlying and proximate determinants of child health: the Cebu longitudinal health and nutrition study. *Am. J. Epidemiol. 133,* 185–201.

16  Streatfield K., Singarimbun M. and Diamond I. Maternal education and child immunization. *Demography* 27, 447–455, 1990.

17  Barbieri M. New evidence on the impact of maternal education on infant and child mortality in Senegal. Paper presented at the 1990 Annual Meeting of the Population Association of America, Toronto, Canada, May 3–5, 1990.

18  Hobcraft J., McDonald J. and Rutstein S.O. Demographic determinants of infant and early childhood mortality. *Pop. Stud. 39,* 363–385, 1985.

19  Orubuloye I.O. and Caldwell J.C. The impact of public health services on mortality: a study of mortality differentials in a rural area of Nigeria. *Pop. Stud. 29,* 259, 1975.

20  Rozenzweig M.R. and Schultz T.P. Child mortality and fertility in Colombia: individual and community effects. *Hlth Policy Educ.* 2, 305, 1982.

21  Bicego G. Trends, age-patterns, and determinants of childhood mortality in Haiti. Ph.D. dissertation, The Johns Hopkins University, Baltimore, MD, 1990.

22  Yang S. and Dowdle N.B. Trends and levels of mortality in China. *Int. Symp. on China s One-per Thousand Population Sample Survey,* Beijing, 1985.

23  Rosero-Bixby L. The case of Costa Rica. In *Health Policy Social Policy and Mortality Prospects* (Edited by Vallin J. and Lopez A.). IUSSP, Ordina, Liege, 1985.

24  Palloni A. Health conditions in Latin America and policies for mortality change. In *Health Policy, Social Policy and Mortality Prospects* (Edited by Vallin J. and Lopez A.). IUSSP, Ordina, Liege, 1985.

25  Mosley W.H. and Becker S. Demographic models for child survival: implications for program strategy. In *Child Survival Programs: Issues for the 1990s*. The Johns Hopkins University Institute for International Programs, Baltimore, Maryland, 1990.

26  Mosley W.H. and Chen L.C. An analytical framework for the study of child survival in developing countries. In *Child Survival: Strategies for Research* (Edited by Mosley W.H. and Chen L.C.), pp. 22–45, Population and Development Review 10, Suppl. Population Council, New York, 1984.

27  Van Norren B. and Van Vianen H.A.W. *The Malnutrition-Infections Syndrome and Its Demographic Outcome in Developing Countries: A New Model and Its Application.* Programming Committee for Demographic Research, Publication No. 4. The Hague, Netherlands, 1986.

28  Trussell J. and Menken J. Estimating levels, trends and determinants of child mortality in countries with poor statistics. In *Child Survival: Strategies for Research* (Edited by Mosley W.H. and Chen L.C.) pp. 325–346, Population and Development Review 10, Suppl. Population Council, New York.

29  Tsui A.O., DeClerque J. and Mangani N. Maternal and sociodemographic correlates of child morbidity in Bas Ziere: the effects of maternal reporting. *Soc. Sci. Med. 26*, 701–713, 1988.

30  Boerma J.T., Black R.E., Sommerfelt A.E., Rutstein S.O. and Bicego G.T. Accuracy and completeness of mother's recall of diarrhoea occurrence in pre-school children in the demographic and health surveys. *Int. J. Epidemiol. 20* 1073–1080.

31  Sullivan J., Rutstein S.O. and Bicego G. Assessment of the quality of DHS data used in the direct estimation of infant and child mortality. In *Assessment of the Quality of DHS-I Data.* Institute for Resource Development, DHS Methodological Reports, No. 1, Columbia, MD, 1990.

32  Boerma J T., Sommerfelt A.E. and Bicego G.T. Child anthropometry in cross-sectional surveys in developing countries: an assessment of survivor bias. *Am. J. Epidemiol.* 135, 438 449, 1992.

33  Hosmer D. and Lemeshow S. *Applied Logistic Regression.* Wiley, New York, 1989.

34  Cox D. Regression models and life tables. *J. R. Stat. Soc. Series B* 34, 187, 1972.

35  Gray R. Epidemiologic methods and case-control studies of mortality and morbidity. Paper presented at the IUSSP Seminar on Comparative Studies of Mortality and Morbidity: Old and New Approaches to Measurement and Analysis, Siena, Italy, 1986.

36  Serdula M. Diet, malnutrition, and mortality in sub-Saharan Africa. Paper presented at the IUSSP semimar on Mortality and Society in Sub-Saharan Africa, Yaounde, Cameroon, 1987.

37  Garenne M., Maire B., Fontaine O., Dieng P. and Briend A. *Risques de Deces associés a Différents Etats Nutrittionnels chez l'Enfant d'Age Prescolaire.* O.R.S.T.O.M., O.R.A.N.A., Dakar, Senegal, 1987.

13

# The contribution of demographic and health surveys to explanatory studies of child survival in developing countries

## Introduction

Large-scale collection of health data in cross-sectional demographic surveys is a relatively new area. DHS surveys have collected information on indicators of various levels of the Mosley-Chen conceptual framework. These include the demographic outcome (child mortality, causes of death), health status indicators (birth weight, anthropometry and child morbidity), indicators of the proximate determinants (utilization of preventive and curative health services, feeding practices, fertility patterns) and underlying or 'remote' determinants such as education of the mother and father, residence, religious denomination and ethnicity. Mortality information is normally collected using a complete birth history of the mother; child health data are collected for all children born during the five years preceding the survey.

First, the quality of health data in DHS surveys is reviewed. This includes data on proximate determinants, child morbidity, anthropometry and causes of death. Subsequently, the contribution of DHS surveys to enhancing our understanding of the determinants of child survival is assessed. Finally, a re-consideration of the goals of health data collection in DHS surveys is proposed. By reducing the length of the core questionnaire to a few key health indicators, more space would be available for in-depth research conducted in conjunction with demographic and health surveys.

## Data quality

### Proximate determinants
While acknowledging the limited possibilities of assessing the validity of health data, the quality of data on proximate determinants collected in DHS surveys appears fairly satisfactory, particularly when viewed at the descriptive level. Generally, the data are

internally consistent, and comparison with other data sources did not reveal important differences (Chapter 3). This implies that DHS surveys can provide basic statistics on preventive and curative health services utilization and basic features of feeding patterns at the international, national and subnational levels for health planning and monitoring and evaluation. The main problems identified were missing values on utilization of maternity care and past feeding patterns for deceased children and inaccurate recall and reporting of duration of breastfeeding (and other recalled duration variables). At the individual level, however, it appears some variables suffer from a considerable level of misclassification, which affects individual level analyses of the determinants of child survival (e.g. recalled duration of breastfeeding).

Demographic surveys can provide very reliable data on immunization coverage by collecting data from the child's health card and supplementing this information with mother's recall of immunizations. The quality of the immunization coverage estimates and differentials depends upon the proportion of mothers able to show their children's cards to the interviewer.

The collection of curative health care data is dependent on the reporting of morbidity events for the two weeks preceding the survey. Since morbidity data are considered biased (see next section), this may affect the quality of data on health-seeking behaviour during illnesses. In addition, data on type of treatment (e.g kind of drugs given, amount of fluids used) are not reliable.

Surveys also do not appear to be useful instruments to gather data on utilization of non-modern health facilities. There may be fairly complete reporting of the presence of traditional birth attendants assisting during delivery, but visits by traditional healers are greatly underreported.

## Child morbidity

Decades of experience with the collection of child mortality data have shown the strengths of demographic surveys through indirect and direct techniques. The collection of data on health status and causes of death is, on the other hand, relatively new to demographic surveys (Gray, 1989).

The analysis of morbidity data (diarrhoea, acute respiratory illness and fever) reveals that respondents' bias and misreporting are common, even within a short recall period of two weeks (Chapter 4). This problem is not unique to demographic surveys; also in epidemiological surveys there is considerable diversity in definitions of disease and study designs, and therefore results are difficult to compare (Chapter 5). Increased efforts are required in the especially difficult area of morbidity to develop better measurement methods, although recall and reporting problems are likely to persist, especially in comparing cross-sectional surveys undertaken in different cultural settings. Intercountry studies with a standardized methodology, such as the BOSTID study on acute respiratory infections in ten countries (Selwyn, 1990), could help solve some of them.

Validation studies by epidemiologists are also needed (Kalter, 1991). For instance, data from Machakos, Kenya, showed a 4–7 fold increase in reported incidence of diarrhoea if the respondents were prompted (asked directly about the occurrence of diarrhoea), compared with the incidence derived from mothers who were first asked whether the child had been ill since the last visit and, only if the answer was affirmative, were then prompted about the occurrence of diarrhoea (Leeuwenburg et al., 1984). A recent study in Ghana showed that overreporting of symptoms or conditions is likely if the respondent is prompted (Ross et al., 1994). Spontaneously reported health problems were considered more useful. Hitherto, DHS surveys have prompted respondents about the presence of diarrhoea, symptoms of acute respiratory infections and fever. This may also have affected data on treatment patterns, one of the proximate determinants in the conceptual framework. Epidemiological studies may help further surveys to improve basic questions on morbidity or other issues.

Questionnaires have also been improved based on quality assessments of cross-sectional surveys. During the first 19 DHS surveys, respondents were first asked whether their child had suffered diarrhoea in the last 24 hours, and, if not, whether the child had suffered diarrhoea in the last two weeks. On average 11.0% of children had had diarrhoea in the last 24 hours and 10.3% within the last two weeks but not in the last 24 hours prior to the survey (unweighted average of 19 countries). Since most diarrhoea episodes are acute and end within one week, this is an unexpectedly high proportion of children with diarrhoea in the last 24 hours compared with the remainder of the last two weeks (see Chapter 4 for details). The order of the questions was reversed in 20 subsequent DHS surveys. The respondents were first asked about diarrhoea in the last two weeks, followed by a questions on diarrhoea in the last 24 hours. On average, 7.0% of children had diarrhoea in the last 24 hours, and 9.5% had diarrhoea in the remainder of the last two weeks (unweighted average of 20 surveys), a more plausible finding. It seems very likely that reversal of the order of the questions had a significant impact on the results.

Generally, we need to be very cautious when using reported illness prevalence data in surveys to assess the disease burden in children. Minor improvements in data collection are still possible and also much needed, if only to improve our assessment of treatment patterns for common illnesses in childhood.

## Anthropometry

Anthropometric data are considered good indicators of the nutritional and health status of children, and are perhaps the best indicator of frailty, in spite of shortcomings pointed out in Chapter 2. Birth weight is a key indicator of the health and nutritional status of newborn and mother. The main source of birth weight data in developing countries is health facilities, with associated problems of limited coverage and selection bias. In the cross-sectional demographic surveys data on birth weight can be collected to obtain national estimates of the incidence of low birth weight (Chapter 9). Data from 15 DHS surveys showed that the mother's recall of numerical birth weight and the mother's estimates of the relative size of the baby at birth can be used to obtain a national estimate of the incidence of low birth weight. The level of misclassification, however, was too large to use reported data on subjective size as an indicator of low birth weight at the individual level. Survey data on subjective size at birth are therefore of limited value for explanatory studies.

In cross-sectional surveys, the sample of children for whom anthropometric measurements are available is not representative of all children in a birth cohort, since only children surviving to the survey date are measured. This survivor bias may have implications for studies of trends and differentials in anthropometric indicators. The effect of the survivor bias was assessed by reviewing evidence from longitudinal studies on the prevalence of malnutrition among deceased children and among surviving children and by analyzing data from 17 DHS surveys (Chapter 10). It was concluded that comparisons of anthropometric data across geographic units, population subgroups, and calendar time are marginally affected by the survivor bias, unless mortality differences between the birth cohorts are very large (more than 50 per 1000 births).

Generally, it is possible to collect good quality data on child anthropometry, with minor problems of digit heaping and missing values. Since data on the ages of children are perhaps more accurate in demographic surveys than in other surveys (data on birth date and completed years are collected in the context of a complete birth history) and a standardized methodology is followed (Sommerfelt and Boerma, 1994), it can be concluded that the inclusion of anthropometry in demographic surveys is apt to make a major contribution to our knowledge of child health status in developing countries.

## Causes of death

The verbal autopsy method is a method of collecting data on causes of death from the relatives of the deceased. Only a few validation studies of the verbal autopsy method have been carried out, and more are needed in different cultural contexts (Gray, 1992). In Namibia, a validation study was carried out in conjunction with a national DHS survey, focusing on malnutrition, diarrhoea, pneumonia, malaria and measles. The study results suggested that verbal autopsy data can be useful to ascertain the leading cause of death in childhood, but are probably not adequate for health impact evaluation. Exceptions are well-defined, locally recognized conditions, such as measles and perhaps neonatal tetanus. For most illnesses misclassification is quite common, and the usefulness for assessment of trends or health impact evaluation rather limited (see also WHO, 1992). The main purpose of including cause of death questions in demographic surveys should therefore be limited to establishing the leading causes of infant and child mortality. The inclusion of verbal autopsy modules in seven DHS surveys did produce unsatisfactory results, in part due to poor questionnaire design in the initial surveys (Chapter 6). A fairly short, well-structured questionnaire included in demographic surveys may, however, provide useful results for health planning purposes, as was shown in Cameroon and Namibia (Balépa et al., 1992, Katjiuanjo et al., 1993).

One strength of demographic surveys is the collection of age-specific mortality data. Since several biomedical causes of death have distinct age patterns, age-specific mortality may be used to obtain an idea about the relative importance of certain causes of death. Neonatal tetanus is perhaps the disease with the most pronounced age pattern of mortality. As many as 90% of neonatal tetanus deaths occur between 4 and 14 days of age, when mortality due to perinatal causes (prematurity, birth trauma, congenital anomalies, etc.) has dropped considerably. Birth history data from 37 national DHS surveys were analyzed to assess the quality of neonatal mortality data and to estimate levels and trends in mortality occurring at 4–14 days (Chapter 8). It was shown that mortality at 4–14 days has declined considerably during the last decade in most developing countries, concomitant with the development and expansion of programmes to reduce neonatal tetanus. Demographic surveys can thus provide indirect information about neonatal tetanus mortality.

The data also point to a major problem of the population-based neonatal tetanus mortality surveys which were popular in the 1980s. Even though it has been common knowledge among demographers for a while that the use of a recall period of 12 months to obtain mortality data leads to considerable underestimation of mortality, this method has been used in at least 40 national surveys on neonatal tetanus mortality during the 1980s. Most surveys missed as many as half of the neonatal deaths. Such problems could be avoided in the future by increased involvement of demographers in epidemiological and health management-oriented surveys (e.g. immunization coverage surveys, household surveys on diarrhoea case management).

## Understanding the determinants of child survival: contribution of surveys

Two of the most important determinants of child survival in developing countries are birth spacing and maternal education. Have surveys made an important contribution to our understanding of how they affect child survival?

### Preceding birth intervals
Many studies have demonstrated the importance of the length of preceding birth intervals for the survival chances of young children (United Nations, 1994). Little is known about the actual biological and behavioural mechanisms responsible for this relationship. Data from 17 DHS surveys were used to investigate the relative importance of prenatal mechanisms (e.g. maternal depletion) and postnatal factors (e.g. sibling competition) (Chapter 11). It was shown that the effects of short birth intervals on nutritional status are rather moderate, and there is only a weak relationship between interval length and lower attendance at antenatal care services. No consistent association exists with morbidity or other health services utilization variables. These findings, in the light of the strong persistent effect of short interval length on early infant mortality, indicate that prenatal mechanisms are more important than postnatal factors.

It appears better data on the child's health status at birth are required to firmly establish the specific prenatal causal mechanisms involved. Such data may be derived from retrospective surveys, but recalled data on birth weight or size at birth are not good enough for explanatory individual level analysis, while reliable data on duration of gestation or prematurity are even more difficult to collect (Chapter 9, Elo and Miller, 1992). More detailed data on the course of pregnancy, maternal health and previous births may also be required. To evaluate postnatal mechanisms further, the unit of data collection and analysis may have to be the family rather than the individual child to obtain new insights. Such approaches are beyond the possibilities of a standard demographic survey.

## Maternal education

Maternal education has a strong and positive impact on the survival of the children and has been postulated to affect it through a wide range of proximate determinants (Cleland and Van Ginneken, 1988, Caldwell, 1979). Recently, a forum in the *Health Transition Review* was organized to encourage exploration of the mechanisms whereby increases in maternal education are converted into low child mortality (Caldwell, 1994). Authors of contributions to this forum appear to agree that, as Caldwell puts it: "...the full exploration of the mechanisms with obtaining of clinching proof has hardly begun" (Caldwell, 1994, p. 224).

DHS and other surveys were considered useful in further examinations of the parental education-child mortality relationship, in spite of some data quality and measurement problems (Brockerhoff and de Rose, 1994). The need was acknowledged for statistical approaches documenting the associations between demographic, social, and economic characteristics on the one hand and health practices and child mortality on the other (Ewbank, 1994).

An example of a comparative study using data from 17 DHS countries was presented in Chapter 12. Maternal education has a strong association with child survival, with the greatest influence occurring after the neonatal period. Maternal education also has a strong effect on child anthropometry and on non-utilization of health services, although some of these associations are the result of education's strong link to household economics. Differential use of health services, although closely tied to a mother's educational level, did little to explain the educational advantage for child survival. This comparative study adds to the growing body of evidence in this area, but a detailed assessment of behaviours modified by more and better education and measurement of its effects on health and mortality are clearly outside the realm of cross-sectional surveys. Anthropological investigations and longitudinal studies are more suited to explore these factors.

## Obstacles

During the past decade much progress has been made in understanding the determinants of child survival. The main contributions of demographic surveys concern the provision of a wealth of data on levels, differentials and trends in infant and child mortality and the establishment of the relative magnitudes of the effect of certain characteristics on infant and child mortality after controlling for other underlying determinants of child survival. One particular strength is the collection of age-specific mortality data (e.g. within infancy). Demographic surveys are also useful to explore pathways of influence and to identify the role of proximate determinants, using individual level data.

A number of factors inherent in cross-sectional surveys, however, limit their usefulness. Quality assessment of DHS data shows that such surveys provide useful information at the descriptive level, but do not seem to extend further at the explanatory level. For virtually all variables, there is considerable misclassification: individuals with A are classified as B and vica versa. As long as there is no overall trend in the misclassification towards A or B, the descriptive statistics will be useful and valid. For explanatory analyses, however, the misclassification poses a severe problem and undermines the search for causal pathways.

In addition to the problem of data quality, a large number of variables cannot be measured adequately in a cross-sectional survey. DHS surveys collect data on a limited number of key indicators guided by the Mosley-Chen framework, which are generally accepted as important indicators of the coverage of essential services to promote child survival. However, a simple comparison of aggregate data from DHS surveys already challenges the usefulness of this exercise. A comparison between Namibia and Nigeria shows us that Namibia scores better on virtually all health indicators, and child mortality is less than half that of Nigeria, which supports the importance of measuring these indicators. If we, however, compare Namibia and Zambia, no major differences can be discerned on most indicators of maternal and child health collected by DHS: immunization coverage, antenatal and delivery care, feeding patterns, family planning use, anthropometry, etc. The level of mother's education was only slightly higher in Namibia. Infant and child mortality levels in Zambia are, however, more than twice as high as in Namibia. The differences are presumably not due to data quality problems, since data collection procedures are well-standardized, and there are no indications of more serious data quality problems with either survey. Thus, the only explanation is that mortality differences between the countries are caused by characteristics not included in DHS questionnaires.

In particular, the quality of care dimension is lacking in DHS and other cross-sectional surveys. Behavioural responses to prevent or treat child illness are difficult to measure in pre-coded questions. The quality of health services received after taking a child to a health facility and treatment compliance are equally difficult to measure in cross-sectional surveys.

Causal pathways can only be partially explored in retrospective cross-sectional surveys. For instance, we can separately examine the effect of mother's education on selected proximate determinants, on morbidity and child anthropometry, and on mortality. It is, however, not possible to assess the mechanisms through which education affects infant and child mortality at the individual level since anthropometric data, morbidity data and data on health services utilization or other proximate determinants are not available for dead children. Furthermore, when certain proximate determinants are available for this type of analysis (e.g. use of delivery care, duration of breastfeeding), data quality problems are more commonly pronounced for deceased children, introducing potential biases in estimating model effects.

The lack of time specificity of retrospective data calls into question the reliability of results. Mortality data refer to a prolonged period preceding the survey, while several of the underlying, proximate determinants and health status indicators are measured at the time of the survey.

## Where to go from here?

It appears that we have almost exhausted the number of 'unexpected' explanatory findings in surveys. More attention needs to be paid to study designs prior to the survey. To move past the current impasse in our understanding of key behavioural and biological influences of disease and death, we need to craft more innovative investigative methods from the outset. These new approaches should aim to link the conventional large-scale sample surveys with more in-depth targeted studies in the areas of biological health assessment and qualitative evaluation of behavioural response by caretakers to current episodes of illness.

The primary aim of the collection of health data in demographic surveys should be to collect data on a very limited number of key health indicators, which are important for health planning and implementation. Such data can be easily and reliably collected. A short questionnaire section will suffice to collect basic child health information. Secondly, the survey may be used to obtain more insight into the determinants of child survival and the effects of health and social interventions. This could be done for a subsample of the main survey respondent, using both qualitative and quantitative methods.

### Focusing on key indicators

A sharp reduction in the length of the standard health section used in demographic surveys is needed. The information collected on child health should focus on a small number of key indicators of the operation of the proximate determinants and health status of children, which would still fulfill the need for national indicators such as those used for monitoring the health goals of the World Summit for Children. These include:

- Maternity: proportion of women using antenatal care and delivering in health facilities during past year. These are reliable indicators of the utilization of health services during a very critical period for mother and child. No attempt should be made to collect data on the quality of services.

- Family planning: proportion of women currently using and ever used family planning methods. Knowledge of specific family planning methods can also be included. More detailed questions on family planning and fertility can be asked, depending on the survey objectives with regard to fertility and family planning.

- Water and sanitation: proportion of households using latrine or other sanitary facilities and proportion of households having piped treated water supply (or from protected safe source). Both are indicators of exposure to water-borne infections, which have relevance beyond the child survival perspective.

- Immunization: coverage of measles and other vaccines among one-year-old children. Immunization is our most important child survival intervention, and vaccination coverage is still the best indicator of utilization of preventive health services. For most one-year olds a written record of immunizations received is available. If a country or region regularly conducts national immunization coverage surveys, it is not necessary to collect such information in the context of a DHS (even though DHS may provide additional information on differentials).

- Feeding: breastfeeding status by age. From current status data the proportion of children still breastfed at 0, 1, 6, 12 and 24 months can be derived. Information on supplementary feeding may be useful for the whole population, but it is probably more cost-effective to collect such information on a smaller sample.

- Curative health services: whether the mother knows when to seek health services. Ideally, we would like to know what the mother actually does when the child is ill. Generally, this information is collected by asking whether the child is ill or has been ill in the last two weeks, and, if so, what was the treatment-seeking behaviour. In the large surveys, however, it may be more useful to focus on whether the mother knows what she is supposed to do, irrespective of a reported illness. This avoids the bias introduced by subjective morbidity reporting by the mother. In an in-depth interview with a smaller sample, more detailed information can be collected on actual behaviour.

- Child anthropometry: the collection of weight and height of children. While costly, anthropometric data collection can readily be incorporated into cross-sectional surveys and provides an excellent opportunity for a biological assessment of the nutritional status of children in a population. In particular, the study of trends in anthropometric status may provide essential information for health planners and enhance our understanding of the determinants of child survival. A simple alternative would be the mid-upper arm circumference, although this measure is not very useful for children under 1 year of age and provides less detailed data on, for example, chronic malnutrition.

The focus of the child health questionnaires is generally on children under five years old. This is presumably associated with the concept of the under-five clinic in developing countries. In practice, such clinics are, however, seldom visited by children aged 3 and 4 years. Furthermore, children aged 3 and 4 are rather different from younger children. Anthropometric indicators do not change much after the third birthday, mortality levels have fallen to relatively low levels, breastfeeding has been ended, immunization has been completed (or not), etc. It is therefore not cost-effective to include three- and four-year-olds routinely in surveys. The sample size can be reduced considerably by excluding those children. The focus should be on children under 3, as was done in the third phase of DHS.

### In-depth studies in conjunction with surveys

By limiting the main survey questionnaire to the basic descriptive information required for the whole population, opportunities are created for in-depth studies. Employing current status data as selection criteria, special questionnaires, physical examination or even biological assessment methods can be used to obtain in-depth data. For example, we may ask to see the medicines given to a child with diarrhoea on the day of the survey, we can attempt to obtain a dietary history for the day of interview for undernourished children, we can obtain serum or stools for laboratory analysis. The information obtained may be of good quality and very detailed. When a respondent reports a recent death of her child, a fairly detailed verbal autopsy questionnaire study can be administered, including questions on health services utilization prior to death. If a woman does not use antenatal care services, a detailed inquiry can be made. A similar approach can be used for the collection of family planning-related data. A detailed questionnaire could be used to compare child care practices in a sub-sample of educated and non-educated mothers.

Thus, with more creative design, large-scale cross-sectional surveys may throw more light on the determinants of child survival. For instance, a case-control design (as first suggested by Gray, 1986) can be employed to study the proximate determinants of child death, morbidity or poor nutrition. For every child with a selected health outcome or characteristic, one to four appropriate controls can easily be selected from the survey sample. Alternatively, a follow-up study of a sub-sample can be planned to collect in-depth information, e.g. among women who have just delivered of are about to deliver.

Perhaps most importantly, an integrated design provides an opportunity for the use of qualitative methods and techniques. Hitherto, qualitative research has mainly been used prior to the quantitative survey to obtain, for instance, locally appropriate terms for the survey questions, but could just as well follow such a survey. The integration of quantitative and qualitative data, often a painstaking exercise, becomes easier. Macro-surveys would retain their large-scale character, but simultaneously provide a basis for the merger of anthropological data and quantitatively oriented studies. Indeed, much of the information collected in surveys could be replaced by in-depth interviews. For instance, a set of 40 recorded interviews with mothers whose children have not been vaccinated may be more revealing than asking 5000 mothers a pre-coded question on the reason for non-utilization of health services amidst another 100 other structured questions on a wide range of topics. Linking the qualitative data to survey data on, for example, the mother's level of education or immunization coverage in the region could make such information even more relevant, both from research and programmatic perspectives.

The design of a short-core survey questionnaire also allows more flexibility in large-scale surveys, like DHS. Such flexibility is needed to be able to incorporate other topics such as adult health or economic aspects of health. It also paves the way for including a more biological assessment of illnesses in nationally representative surveys, e.g. through collecting blood samples on filter paper. Finally, it gives countries a better chance to focus their DHS survey on the topics that are considered a priority problem by the countries themselves.

Is it feasible to change the methodology of demographic and health surveys, limit the main questionnaire, and include integrated in-depth studies? Reducing the DHS questionnaire to less than half of its current length (by reducing the family planning and health sections) will give the interviewer a chance to add special questionnaires on morbidity, cause of death, use of health services, etc. if necessary (affirmative answer on screening question in main questionnaire). In other cases, for a subsample, a special interviewer or team may be required, for instance, if blood is to be taken or a qualitative interview needs to be conducted. Logistically, this may be possible with only limited additional costs. No major problems are expected during data processing and analysis, although more time may be required for analysis of some in-depth studies. This, however, should not delay the publication of the basic descriptive report of the survey.

Capacity building has been a weakness of both DHS and WFS. Surveys are conducted at maximum speed, and while the local institutions often turn out to be effective organizations in terms of field work, they are only a temporary part of the process. The proposed design with integrated in-depth and especially follow-up studies will certainly take more time, but should lead to a greater involvement of local institutions, notably universities. Collaboration with institutions in developed countries may further enhance the quality of the study and the aspects of training and capacity building. In that case survey programmes like DHS may contribute to both multidisciplinary research and capacity building in developing countries.

In conclusion, cross-sectional surveys have made an important contribution to our present knowledge of the determinants of child survival in developing countries. Surveys need to continue to provide information on levels, trends and differentials in child mortality, nutritional status and health practices. The collection of health data in demographic surveys is useful and has provided us with important information on the determinants of child survival in developing countries. On the other hand, it must be acknowledged that much of the information collected on aspects of child health in demographic surveys is not very useful, particularly when trying to explain child survival levels, trends and differentials. To move past the current impasse in our understanding of key behavioural and biological influences of disease and death, we need to re-consider health data collection in surveys. New approaches are needed. These should aim to link the conventional large-scale sample surveys with more in-depth targeted studies in the areas of biological health assessment and qualitative studies of health behaviour.

## References

Balépa M, Fotso M and Barrere B (1992). Enquete Demographique et de sante, Cameroun 1991. Direction Nationale du Récensement, Yaounde and Macro International Inc., Columbia, Md.

Brockerhoff M and de Rose L (1994). Parental education and child survival: can the DHS tell us anything new? *Health Transition Review* 4: 192–196.

Caldwell JC (1994). How is greater maternal education translated into lower child mortality? *Health Transition Review* 4: 224–229.

Caldwell JC (1979). Education as a factor in mortality decline: an examination of Nigerian data. *Population Studies* 33:395–413.

Cleland JC and Van Ginneken JK (1988). Maternal education and child survival in developing countries: searching for pathways of influence. *Social Science and Medicine* 27: 1357–1368.

Elo and Muller (1992). Ever-breastfed status and health at birth. In Boerma JT (ed.). *Measurement of maternal and child mortality, morbidity and health care: interdisciplinary approaches*. Liege: Derouaux-Ordina, pp.309–331.

Ewbank DC (1994). Maternal education and theories of health behaviour: a cautionary note. *Health Transition Review* 4: 214–223.

Gray RH (1989). The integration of demographic and epidemiologic approaches to studies of health in developing countries. In: Ruzicka L, Wunsch G and Kane P (eds.). *Differential mortality: methodological issues and biosocial factors*. Oxford: Clarendon Press, pp. 36–63.

Gray RH (1986). Epidemiologic methods and case-control studies of mortality and morbidity. Paper presented at IUSSP seminar on Comparative studies of mortality and morbidity: old and new approaches to measurement and analysis, Siena, Italy 7–12 July 1992.

Kalter H, Gray RH, Black RE et al. (1991). Validation of the diagnosis of childhood morbidity using maternal health interviews. *International Journal of Epidemiology* 20:193–198.

Katjiuanjo P, Titus S, Zauana M et al. (1993). Namibia Demographic and Health Survey 1992. Ministry of Health and Social Services and Columbia, Maryland: Macro International Inc.

Leeuwenburg J, Gemert W, Muller AS et al. (1984). The incidence of diarrhoeal disease. In: Van Ginneken JK and Muller AS (eds.). *Maternal and child health in rural Kenya: an epidemiological study*. London: Croom Helm, pp.109–118.

Ross DA, Huttly SRA, Dollimore N et al. (1994). Measurement of the frequency and severity of childhood acute respiratory infections through household surveys in Northern Ghana. *International Journal of Epidemiology* 23: 608–616.

Selwyn BJ (1990). The epidemiology of acute respiratory tract infection in young children: comparison of findings from several developing countries. *Reviews of Infectious Diseases* 12 (Supplement 8): S 870–S888.

Sommerfelt AE and Boerma JT (1994). Anthropometric status of young children in DHS-I surveys: an assessment of data quality. In: An assessment of the quality of health data in DHS-I surveys. *DHS Methodological Reports* No. 2, Calverton, Maryland: Macro International Inc., pp. 125–142.

United Nations (1994). The health rational for family planning: timing of births and child survival. Department of Economic and Social Information and Policy Analysis. Population Division. STA/ESA/SER.A/ 141. New York.

WHO (1992). The measurement of overall and cause-specific mortality in infants and children. Report of a joint WHO/UNICEF consultation, 15–17 December 1992, WHO/ESM/UNICEF/CONS/92.5, Geneva.

# Summary

# Child survival in developing countries:

# can demographic and health surveys help to understand

# the determinants?

Since its inception in 1985, the global Demographic and Health Surveys programme (DHS) has included the collection of data on maternal and child health in its surveys. To the present, more than 50 nationally representative DHS surveys have been completed, making DHS the leading source of population-based data on maternal and child health in the developing world. This thesis is an attempt to assess the contribution of health data collection in demographic cross-sectional surveys, notably DHS, to our understanding of the determinants of child survival in developing countries.

To this end, we need to have a framework conceptualizing how determinants affect child survival. The Mosley-Chen framework for the study of child survival in developing countries was published in 1984 and has dominated child survival research since then. The framework is particularly suitable for cross-sectional surveys and has had a major influence on DHS. In *Chapter 2* the Mosley-Chen framework is presented, and its advantages and limitations discussed. Even though there are a number of important limitations, it is concluded that the framework should continue to guide child health data collection and analysis and in surveys, as it is instrumental for interdisciplinary communication in child survival research.

The ten chapters are based on analyses of DHS data and address two questions. The first one, dealt with in Chapters 3 to 10, relates to data quality and concerns the measurement of health indicators in demographic surveys. The second is whether these health data collected in demographic surveys can actually enhance our understanding of the determinants of child survival in developing countries and is the focus of Chapters 11 and 12.

*Chapter 3* synthesizes the results of an extensive evaluation of health data quality in the first 27 DHS surveys. It is shown that health data quality is satisfactory for most variables and suitable for estimates of national or regional health indicators. At the individual level, however, it appears there is considerable misclassification. Morbidity reporting is one of the most problematic areas of health interview surveys. *Chapter 4* illustrates some of the problems associated with the collection of data on childhood diarrhoea in DHS surveys, showing how an ostensibly minor issue such as the order of questions may affect the ultimate prevalence value.

An external validation of survey data on child health can be carried out through a substantive comparison between the results of demographic surveys and longitudinal epidemiological studies. In *Chapter 5* results are compared for child morbidity (diarrhoea and respiratory infections), vaccination, and neonatal tetanus mortality. There is good consistency between both sources for most indicators.

Knowledge of the biomedical causes of death may also improve our understanding of the determinants of child survival. Chapters 6, 7, and 8 are concerned with collection of data on causes of death in surveys. A validation study of the verbal autopsy method was carried out in Namibia prior to the DHS survey (*Chapter 6*) to improve the questionnaire and to facilitate the interpretation of the child mortality data generated. It was concluded that the verbal autopsy technique is adequate for some causes of death (such as measles and tetanus), but less useful for others (such as malaria and pneumonia).

*Chapter 7* analyzes the results obtained in seven DHS surveys through a verbal autopsy module and indicates that the best possible outcome to be expected is a general picture of the leading causes of child death in a population.

*Chapter 8* shows how age-specific mortality data from DHS surveys can be used to assess the magnitude of neonatal tetanus mortality. In most DHS surveys, these data are considered fairly accurate, and if tetanus is an important cause of neonatal death, 4-14 days mortality can be used to obtain an estimate of the magnitude.

*Chapter 9* examines the usefulness of recalled data on the size of the child at birth to obtain better estimates of the incidence of low birthweight. It appears that for most countries surveys can provide an estimate of the incidence by including two specific questions to questions (recalled birthweight and subjective size at birth). Such an estimate would be superior to estimates based on only health facility data. At the individual level, however, recalled data on size at birth do not appear to be sufficiently accurate.

Child anthropometric data have been collected from surviving children in most DHS surveys. *Chapter 10* utilizes the availability of both child mortality and anthropometric data in the same anthropometric survey to assess the potential impact of a survivor bias on estimates of undernutrition. Only if child mortality is very high does the survivor bias influence estimates of undernutrition from anthropometric data.

Child spacing and maternal education are two of the most important determinants of child survival in developing countries. *Chapter 11* presents a comparative analysis of

17 DHS countries using the Mosley-Chen conceptual framework in an attempt to assess why the preceding birth interval has such a strong effect on child survival. It is shown that the influence of short intervals on nutritional status is rather low, and there is only a weak relationship between interval length and reduced attendance at antenatal care services. No consistent association exists with morbidity or other health services utilization variables. These findings indicate that prenatal mechanisms are more important than postnatal ones in the association short birth intervals – high child mortality.

The same approach was used to study the link between mother's education and child survival (*Chapter 12*). Maternal education has a strong association with child survival, with its most significant influence occurring after the neonatal period. It also has a clear effect on child anthropometry and on non-utilization of health services, although some of these associations are the result of education's powerful link to household economic status. Differential use of health services, although closely tied to a mother's educational level, did little to explain the educational advantage in child survival.

Finally, the contribution of DHS and other surveys to our understanding of the determinants of child survival in developing countries is reviewed (*Chapter 13*). There is no doubt that they have generated a wealth of information on a limited number of indicators of maternal and child health in developing countries. With regard to the determinants of child survival, it appears that we have almost exhausted the number of 'unexpected' explanatory findings in surveys. More attention needs to be paid to study designs prior to the survey. To move past the current impasse in our understanding of key behavioural and biological influences of disease and death, we need to develop more innovative investigative methods. These new approaches should aim to link the conventional large-scale sample surveys with more in-depth targeted studies in the areas of biological health assessment and qualitative evaluation of a caretaker's behavioural response to a current episode of child illness. The primary aim in demographic surveys should be to collect data on a very limited number of key health indicators, which are important for health planning and implementation. Such data can be easily and reliably collected and a short questionnaire section will suffice. Secondly, the survey may be used to obtain more insight into the determinants of child survival and the effects of health and social interventions. This could be done for a subsample of the main survey respondent, using both qualitative and quantitative methods. This approach would also strengthen the training and capacity building component of DHS, as institutions in developing countries should be involved in the survey for a prolonged period.

# Samenvatting

## Kindersterfte in ontwikkelingslanden

## Kunnen demografische en gezondheidsenquêtes helpen de onderliggende factoren te begrijpen?

In 1985 werd het Demographic and Health Surveys programma (DHS) opgezet, gericht op het ondersteunen van enquêtes in ontwikkelingslanden. In de DHS enquêtes worden gegevens verzameld over de gezondheid van moeders en kinderen. Tot op heden heb-ben meer dan vijftig landen een nationale DHS enquête gehouden en DHS enquêtes zijn momenteel een van de belangrijkste bronnen van nationale en regionale gegevens over de gezondheid van kinderen. Dit proefschrift is een evaluatie van de bijdrage van demografische enquêtes, met name DHS, aan de studie van de factoren die de kinder-sterfte in ontwikkelingslanden beïnvloeden.

Om te kunnen begrijpen welke rol die onderliggende factoren spelen in de overleving-skansen voor kinderen, moeten we ze onderbrengen in een conceptueel model. Het Mosley-Chen model dat is ontwikkeld voor de studie van kindersterfte in ontwikkeling-slanden, werd voor het eerst gepubliceerd in 1984 en heeft vanaf dat moment het onder-zoek naar kindersterfte gedomineerd. Dit model is met name geschikt voor dwarsdoorsnede-onderzoek en heeft grote invloed gehad op DHS. In *Hoofdstuk 2* wordt het Mosley-Chen model beschreven en wordt ingegaan op de voor- en nadelen die eraan verbonden zijn. Hoewel er een aantal belangrijke beperkingen worden gecon-stateerd, is de voornaamste conclusie dat dit model een nuttig instrument blijft voor de verzameling en analyse van gegevens over gezondheid van en sterfte onder kinderen, vooral omdat het de interdisciplinaire communicatie bevordert.

De tien hoofdstukken die volgen zijn gebaseerd op analyse van DHS gegevens en er lig-gen twee vragen aan ten grondslag. De eerste vraag, behandeld in *Hoofdstuk 3 tot en met 10*, betreft de kwaliteit van de gegevens en het meten van gezondheidsvariabelen in demografische enquêtes. De tweede vraag is of de verzameling van deze gegevens in demografische enquêtes ook ons begrip verhoogt van de factoren die kindersterfte in ontwikkelingslanden bepalen. Deze vraag wordt besproken aan de hand van twee voor-beelden in Hoofdstuk 11 en 12.

*Hoofdstuk 3* geeft een synthese van de uitgebreide evaluatie van de resultaten inzake de kwaliteit van gezondheidsgegevens in de eerste 27 DHS enquêtes. Het blijkt dat de kwaliteit van de meeste gegevens dusdanig is dat betrouwbare schattingen van nationale en regionale gezondheidsindicatoren mogelijk zijn. Op individueel niveau is er echter sprake van aanzienlijke misclassificatie, wat de analyse van de onderliggende factoren verzwakt. De ziekterapportages behoren tot de meest problematische onderdelen van de enquêtes waarmee gezondheid wordt gemeten. *Hoofdstuk 4* illustreert enkele van de problemen die zich voordoen bij het verzamelen van gegevens over diarree bij kinderen in DHS enquêtes. Het laat zien hoe een ogenschijnlijk irrelevant detail zoals de volgorde van de gestelde vragen de uiteindelijke prevalentiewaarde van diarree kan beïnvloeden.

Een externe validatie van enquêtegegevens over de gezondheidstoestand van kinderen kan worden uitgevoerd door het vergelijken van resultaten tussen demografische enquêtes en epidemiologische studies met een longitudinaal karakter. In *Hoofdstuk 5* worden de resultaten vergeleken voor ziekten bij kinderen (diarree en luchtweginfecties), vaccinaties, en sterfte bij pasgeborenen als gevolg van tetanus. Voor de meeste indicatoren stemmen de gegevens van beide bronnen goed met elkaar overeen.

Kennis over de biomedische doodsoorzaken zou eveneens ons begrip van de onderliggende factoren van kindersterfte kunnen verbeteren. De hoofdstukken 6, 7 en 8 gaan over het verzamelen van gegevens over doodsoorzaken middels enquêtes. Een validatiestudie van de zogenaamde `verbale autopsiemethode' voor het vaststellen van mogelijke doodsoorzaken bij kinderen werd uitgevoerd in Namibië, voorafgaand aan een nationale DHS enquête (*Hoofdstuk 6*). De doelstelling was om te komen tot een betere vragenlijst en om de interpretatie van gegevens over kindersterfte in de nationale enquête te vergemakkelijken. Uit de conclusie kwam naar voren dat de verbale autopsiemethode zeer bruikbaar is voor bepaalde doodsoorzaken (zoals mazelen en tetanus), maar minder accuraat voor andere oorzaken (zoals malaria en longontsteking).

*Hoofdstuk 7* geeft een analyse van de resultaten van zeven DHS enquêtes waarin een verbale autopsiemodule was opgenomen. Het beste resultaat dat met dergelijke modules verkregen kan worden, is een algemeen beeld van de meest voorkomende doodsoorzaken onder kinderen.

*Hoofdstuk 8* laat zien hoe leeftijdsspecifieke sterftegegevens in DHS enquêtes kunnen worden gebruikt om de omvang van het probleem van neonatale sterfte door tetanus vast te stellen. De kwaliteit van deze gegevens was in de meeste DHS enquêtes behoorlijk goed en als tetanus een belangrijk gezondheidsprobleem is, kan de sterfte tussen 4 en 14 dagen worden gebruikt om een schatting te maken van de omvang van het tetanusprobleem.

*Hoofdstuk 9* onderzoekt het nut van subjectieve gegevens over de grootte van een kind bij de geboorte, namelijk zoals de moeders zich die herinneren en daarover rapporteren.

Dergelijke schattingen verdienen de voorkeur bover schattingen die uitsluitend zijn gebaseerd op geboorten in gezondheidsinstellingen. Het blijkt dat enquêtes voor de meeste landen acceptabele schattingen opleveren als er twee vragen met betrekking tot geboortegewicht worden opgenomen: het numerieke gewicht (indien bekend) en de subjectieve grootte van het kind bij de geboorte (heel klein, klein, gemiddeld etc.). Dergelijke schattingen blijken structureel beter dan wanneer ze uitsluitend op gezondheidsgegevens zijn gebaseerd. Op individueel niveau echter zijn deze gegevens niet accuraat genoeg.

In de meeste DHS enquêtes worden gegevens verzameld over de anthropometrie van kinderen (lengte en gewicht). Dergelijke gegevens kunnen alleen worden verzameld over levende kinderen. *Hoofdstuk 10* maakt gebruik van de unieke beschikbaarheid van zowel gegevens over kindersterfte als anthropometrische gegevens in één enquête om de potentiële invloed van een 'survivor bias' op schattingen van het voorkomen van ondervoeding vast te stellen. Alleen als de kindersterfte erg hoog is, beïnvloedt de 'survivor bias' de schattingen van het niveau van ondervoeding.

Twee van de belangrijkste factoren die de overlevingskansen van kinderen in ontwikkelingslanden beïnvloeden, zijn geboorte- intervallen en het opleidingsniveau van de moeder. *Hoofdstuk 11* bevat een vergelijkende analyse van 17 DHS enquêtes die gebruik maken van het Mosley-Chen model. Met de analyse wordt geprobeerd te bepalen waarom de lengte van het voorafgaande geboorte-interval zo'n sterke invloed heeft op de overlevingskansen van een kind. De studie laat zien dat het effect van korte intervallen op de voedingstoestand van kinderen tamelijk gering is. Er is slechts een beperkte relatie tussen geboorte-interval en verminderd gebruik van zwangerschapsklinieken, en er is geen direct verband vast te stellen met ziekteprevalentie of gebruik van andere preventieve en curatieve gezondheidsdiensten. Korte geboorte-intervallen hebben een sterkere invloed op vroege zuigelingensterfte en kindersterfte. Deze bevindingen laten zien dat factoren gedurende de zwangerschap belangrijker zijn voor de relatie tussen geboorte-interval en kindersterfte dan factoren na de geboorte.

Dezelfde benadering wordt gebruikt om het verband tussen het opleidingsniveau van moeders en kindersterfte te bestuderen (*Hoofdstuk 12*). Een hoger opleidingsniveau van de moeder is in sterke mate gekoppeld aan betere overlevingskansen van haar kinderen, met de grootste invloed na de eerste levensmaand. Er is eveneens een aantoonbaar effect op de anthropometrie van kinderen en op het gebruik van gezondheidsdiensten, hoewel een deel van deze verbanden kan worden teruggevoerd op het krachtige verband tussen opleidingsniveau en het economische niveau van het huishouden. Maar ofschoon verschillen in het gebruik van gezondheidsdiensten sterk gerelateerd zijn aan het opleidingsniveau van de moeder, kan het verband tussen het voordeel van een betere opleiding en kindersterfte vanuit deze verschillen niet verklaard worden.

Tot slot wordt geëvalueerd wat de bijdrage is van DHS en andere enquêtes aan de studie van de factoren die de kindersterfte in ontwikkelingslanden beïnvloeden (*Hoofdstuk*

*13*). Er bestaat geen twijfel over dat DHS en andere enquêtes een schat aan informatie hebben opgeleverd over een beperkt aantal indicatoren ten aanzien van de gezondheid van moeders en vooral kinderen in ontwikkelingslanden. Wat betreft de factoren die kindersterfte beïnvloeden lijkt het er op dat we niet meer mogen rekenen op nieuwe `on-verwachte' verklarende bevindingen in enquêtes. Het is nu tijd om meer aandacht te besteden aan het opzetten van de studie die aan een enquête voorafgaat. Om uit de huidige impasse te raken van wat de bepalend gedragsfactoren en biologische factoren zijn die ziekte en sterfte beïnvloeden, moeten we ons meer richten op het ontwikkelen van innovatieve methoden. In dergelijke nieuwe benaderingen zouden conventionele enquêtes met grote steekproeven direct verbonden moeten worden met diepte-onder-zoek, gericht op enkele geselecteerde onderwerpen. Voorbeelden daarvan zijn het me-ten van de biologische gezondheid of de kwalitatieve evaluatie van het gedrag van verzorgers bij ziekte van een kind. Aanbevolen wordt dat het verzamelen van gegevens van een zeer beperkt aantal indicatoren, van belang voor het plannen en uitvoeren van gezondheidsprogramma's, het primaire doel zou moeten zijn van demografische en-quêtes. Dergelijke gegevens kunnen vrij eenvoudig worden en op een betrouwbare manier worden verzameld en het opstellen van een korte vragenlijst is daarvoor vol-doende. Ten tweede zou de enquête kunnen worden gebruikt om beter inzicht te krijgen in de factoren die de kindersterfte beïnvloeden en om de effecten van maatschappelijke en gezondheidsinterventies te meten. Dergelijk onderzoek kan worden uitgevoerd on-der een deel van de ondervraagden uit de hoofdenquête en gebruikmakend van kwanti-tatieve en kwalitatieve methoden (gericht op specifieke groepen, bijvoorbeeld kinderen met diarree op de dag van de enquête, ondervoede kinderen). Deze benadering zou de kwaliteit van de training kunnen verbeteren en een versterking zijn van de lokale en in-stitutionele capaciteit die beide onderdeel uitmaken van DHS. Daarvoor is het nodig dat de instituten voor een veel langere periode in de enquête betrokken kunnen worden dan nu het geval is.

CIP DATA KONINKLIJKE BIBLIOTHEEK, DEN HAAG

Boerma, Jan Ties

Child survival in developing countries : can demographic and health surveys help to understand the determinants? / Jan Ties Boerma. - Amsterdam : Royal Tropical Institute
Thesis Universiteit van Amsterdam. - With ref. -With summary in Dutch.
ISBN 90-6832-099-8
NUGI 742
Subject heading: child survival ; developing countries / demographic surveys / health surveys


© 1996 Royal Tropical Institute - Amsterdam
Cover design: Ad van Helmond - Amsterdam
Printer: Krips Repro - Meppel
ISBN 90 6832 099 8
NUGI 742